What others are saying about John Thorp

I have witnessed, first hand, the healing power of John Thorp's revolutionary energy technology. The results speak for themselves and open a new door in promoting health and wellness.

Denis Waitley, author "The Seeds of Greatness"

Microcurrent has been an important part of my practice for over ten years now. The addition of the Electro-Acuscope / Myopulse device introduced to me by John Thorp has made a very significant difference in how we approach treatment of patients using this technology. The outcomes we have witnessed continue to be amazing given the relative simplicity of the effort required to administer treatment. The specific core treatments developed by the Thorp Institute for use of the Acuscope / Myopulse unit are outstanding. The training provided is comprehensive and easily assimilated and their availability for support to practitioners serves as a guarantee for success using the equipment. John Thorp's expertise and enthusiasm are infectious in that positive way that guarantees successful outcomes. A book that can spread the information about such wonderful techniques leading to so many successful outcomes is an incredibly important step in maximizing awareness about the many benefits from the use of such therapies and my sincere hope is that John's efforts will make this wonderful treatment option available to everyone.

Catherine Willner, M.D.
Durango Neurological Associates, PC
Durango CO

As a doctor of Oriental medicine I used the Acuscope and Myopulse on patients that do not respond to traditional Chinese Medicine. After treating my patients using the protocols developed by John Thorp, I get about a 90% efficacy on patients that I have failed with using traditional Chinese medicine. I also want to say that John Thorp has gone above the call of duty when it comes to support in the use of these instruments. I have called John and he immediately gets back to me regarding questions I have in the use of his advanced treatment protocols. I have not found another company that has this kind of support in the United States.

Don Snow, D.O., M.D.

I first saw John for a chronic painful condition after I broke my leg skiing. The doctors told me I would be limping around forever. I found John and I do not limp anymore and I am pain free. A few years ago I got Carpal Tunnel Syndrome from signing about 400,000 books, saw John and the pain diminished dramatically. He also helped me with some detoxification issues that I had and I saw all this black stuff come out on these plates. I just feel blessed to know that John and this therapy exist and when I find something as good as this I want to share it with the world.

Jack Canfield, co-author "Chicken Soup for the Soul"

As head of the Bioenergetics department at Sanoviv Medical Institute, I have personally witnessed the results of the Acuscope and Myopulse for the past three years. The Thorp certified Acuscope and Myopulse and their training program are the best you can find anywhere in the world in the field of Bioenergetics. The instruments are only as good as the training you receive, and Thorp Institute has delivered a training program that is unlimited and supports our technicians 100%.

Luc Lemaire, D.C.

My Husband had a tooth extracted and was in excruciating pain. John Thorp happened to be at the hospital where my husband was and treated him for the pain. Within one hour, my husband reported that his pain was 90% gone. That made a believer out of me. I have added this technology to my medical practice and have been continually amazed with the results.

Sherri Tenpenny, D.O., Osteomed II, Cleveland, OH

I met John Thorp over five years ago and was impressed with the microcurrent technology he was representing. I contracted Rheumatoid Arthritis and was on a combination of medications, which prevented me from working. I purchased the instruments and attended the comprehensive Training Program. Soon I was able to stop taking 90% of my pain medications and return to my job as a physical therapist. I was so amazed with my results that I wanted to share this wonderful technology with others. Currently I am the lead trainer for Thorp Institute.

Linda Perry, R.P.T., M.P.T,

We had one patient here at Sanoviv that suffered with chronic headaches. He had this pain for over 7 years and in one treatment using the Acuscope that pain was gone and it has not returned. I have also seen tremendous results with patients that suffer from Fibromyalgia. After just a few sessions their pain begins to subside and they are amazed at the results. I have been often called the miracle man with the miracle machine.

Dr. Fernando Medina, M.D.

I was diagnosed with Multiple Sclerosis over twenty years ago. Due to my Multiple Sclerosis I suffered leg pain and spasms and had to use Botox injections to relieve the pain and the spasms. I was originally treated for my chronic pain in my low back and legs at Sanoviv Medical Institute. After a series of treatments using the Acuscope and Myopulse I no longer require the Botox injections in my legs that I used for the spasms and pain. It has relieved me of my chronic back pain and has even helped me with my balance. We immediately purchased the instruments from John Thorp and received their unlimited training. Not only has it helped me but it has also helped my husband who is a professional golfer and has some knee pain. I highly recommend the use of these instruments and the training given by the Thorp Institute.

Jan Mills

FROM STUNTMAN

to

ELECTRO MEDICINE MAN

A true story with forewords by

Mark Victor Hansen and Stephen Sinatra MD

by John Stuart Thorp

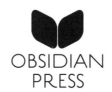

OBSIDIAN
PRESS

FROM STUNTMAN to ELECTRO MEDICINE MAN

Published by:
Obsidian Press
P.O. Box 2825
Peoria, Arizona 85380

ISBN 978-0-615-38609-6

FOREWORD

You want the healer's healer. You want the leading edge healer that electronically can turn disease back into effortless, healed ease.

Allow me to introduce you to an amazing man. A great, important friend of mine. A human treasure dedicated to keeping well people totally well; healing sick folks; teaching everyone the truth of high-level wellness using electronic technology; and he is busy training, educating, motivating and inspiring a ready army of well-qualified, competent healing professionals who facilitate the desperately needed wellness and health revolution. His name is John Thorp. You may not know him yet; however, I predict that he is destined to become intimately more famous over time. Why? Because he is doing what needs to be done to solve our healthcare crisis. John is a quietly effective master healer and teacher of healers. Word about him is spreading like a wild-fire on a windy day.

A decade ago, John regenerated my ailing hips. Medical doctors wanted to replace them with titanium hips that would need to be redone every decade. I thought that at fifty years old, healing might be okay, but at 70, 80, 90 it could be slow, ugly, and painful. I plan to live to be 127 with options for renewal; I didn't want to be cut out, zipped up, respectively.

John miraculously ran his electronic Acuscope and Myopulse over my hips and, voila, I could see the dials light up and radiate as my hips came bouncing back into life one light at a time. Best of all, the pain abated after the first session. I did the entire treatment protocol. I regularly revisit John and his practitioners for a tune-up. I want to be radiantly alive and physically healthy. John and I want the same for you.

You are about to read the story of a man who has overcome the odds to the betterment of everyone. Read, reap, share this breakthrough man, his thinking and technology with all whom you love and care about. They will thank you in their prayers. I thank John for healing me, keeping me healthy, and being my great friend and skiing colleague.

Happy Reading!

Mark Victor Hansen
Co-creator, #1 New York Times best selling series *Chicken Soup for the Soul*®; Co-author, *Cracking the Millionaire Code.*

FOREWORD

BY DR. STEPHEN SINATRA, MD

The first time I met John Thorp was in November, 2008, when our paths intersected at an anti-aging clinic in southern California. I was there as a patient looking for alternative solutions to avoid joint replacement surgery. John was summoned by the clinic's director to help ease the pain and suffering in my right hip.

Thorp utilized biophysical instruments known as Electro-Acuscope and Myopulse micro-current therapies. As a simple probe makes contact with the skin's surface, these devices actually deliver very minute quantities of electrical current to cells and tissues. This minute current, in turn, fosters the production of endogenous adenosine triphosphate (ATP) in the cellular mitochondria, where energy production takes place.

Immediately, I saw the potential value in Thorp's approach. After studying electrical medicine techniques for the past seven years or more, I resonated with this type of bioenergetic therapy because it goes directly to the heart of the matter: the cellular level.

After all, as a cardiologist and author of a book entitled *The Sinatra Solution: Metabolic Cardiology* —a term I coined to describe treating heart disease at the level of cellular energy—healing the body by nourishing and balancing cellular dynamics is a basic for me now. Call me a slow learner. I came to that seemingly simple realization after practicing traditional drug and cut medicine for almost 40 years! It never ceases to amaze me how remarkable the human body really is, and how competent it is to heal itself, if nurtured and supported properly. For example, when the heart is nourished with nutrients that support basic enzymatic cellular processes, more ATP will be generated, and cardiac function is significantly improved.

As physicians, our primary focus is to "rescue" patients by treating their symptoms in hopes of easing their suffering. Although modern technologies—like pharmaceutical and surgical interventions—frequently work, there remain many people who continue to suffer despite our best efforts. Maybe that's because we addressed the symptom, but missed the underlying cause of their "dis-ease".

Over the years I have observed that the body has an incredible "innate" intelligence for healing itself. Many times it's key that the physician figure out how to redirect the body's natural energies so that seemingly miraculous healing can occur. Supporting the body with natural healing organic foods, clean "energetic" waters with higher pH levels (alkaline), vitamins, minerals, phytonutrients, exercise, and mind/body interventions is key. And complimenting that multifaceted approach, it is a must to implement detoxification strategies to support the body to heal naturally. A healing relationship is also crucial to success.

It is imperative that both healer/physician and the recipient of their care (the patient) align in their positive intention to promote optimum health and wellness. A shared belief in the power to heal is fostered through such a mindful and reciprocal healing relationship, and the patient is empowered by the belief or faith of the healer.

Frequently, gifted healers can literally inculcate into their patients the belief that they can and will get well with such positive belief that patients do, indeed, get well.

But why do we become ill in the first place?

It is my firm belief that the reason we become sick, whether it be heart disease or any other illness, is because our bodies succumb to assaults from so many fronts: physical and emotional traumas as well as toxicity from outside sources like chemicals and heavy metals.

Our technological advances are also creating new challenges to our bodies. We are constantly bombarded by "bad vibes" in the form of abundant and relentless wireless microwaves that are now a part of our high tech environment. Look at the network of cell towers out there! These chaotic frequencies can disturb the body's balanced electrical state (yes, the body IS electric all by itself) and render it more vulnerable to breakdown.

These factors, coupled with nutrient depletion, create mitochondrial vulnerability, which often contributes to pathology and disease. Appreciating the importance of the integrity of the cellular membrane—as well as the receptor sites on that membrane—is basic to understanding the emerging science behind "metabolic medicine."

Simply stated, a healthy cell wall or membrane allows nutrients in and toxins out. It must BREATHE, so to speak. To be healthy, the cell's membrane must "inhale" as it ushers in the nutrients that support its metabolism, as well as "exhale" to safely expel the waste of those chemical reactions out to be excreted.

The integrity of a healthy membrane is threatened by external agents such as heavy metals like mercury, trans-fats from the diet, or excessive wireless smog, to mention a few. When one or more of these entities penetrates the cell membrane, defensive reactions occur.

With chronic exposure and insult, the normal functioning of the cellular machinery tends to wax and wane. The cells have more and more trouble "breathing," and mitochondrial dropout occurs. When this happens, the cell ages prematurely. The influx of vital of hormones, minerals, and nutrients is restricted while waste products accumulate.

Over time, microbial (bacterial, viral, parasitic) invasion occurs, setting the stage for acidic environments (low pH) and anaerobic metabolism (low oxygen). This cascade results in tremendous cellular vulnerability—and eventually disease of the cells and tissue.

As a cardiologist, I can attest to the importance of supporting energy production in individual heart cells to preserve the mitochondria in those cells. I project that this emphasis will become the focus of a new emerging field in cardiovascular medicine: "metabolic cardiology." I feel this term describes the favorable biochemical interventions we are starting to employ to directly improve energy metabolism in heart cells. When cellular metabolic functions are supported by ATP energy production, a rejuvenation and revitalization of cellular networks occur.

You see, ATP not only helps to create energy and pulsation, it also restores and repairs the cells. Yes, ATP will repair the cell! It took me 35 years of practicing cardiology to learn this one key concept: the heart is all about ATP! Another key to cardiac health: the restoration of the heart's energy substrate charge is accomplished by supporting its cells with coenzyme Q10 and L-carnitine. These naturally occurring compounds increase the turnover of ATP. Additionally, magnesium and D-ribose enhance the production of endogenous ATP in the body. Because your heart or any other tissue cannot naturally catch up with an ATP deficit quickly, targeted nutraceuticals are crucial to continue ATP production and maintain vital bodily functions. So much for the nutraceutical side of the story.

The electroceutical side of maintaining optimum health includes balancing the body's energy with low, harmonizing frequencies from other sources. For example, one can use an Ondamed machine, or a Rife technology. Other possible interventions to target the body's inherent electrical energy system include magnets, infrared saunas, Reiki, or even the laying on of hands. The simplest and easiest is grounding to the earth. Touching the bare feet to the ground (earth, grass, sand, concrete) discharges the body of toxic EMF (electromagnetic fields) while accumulating vital, enriched electrons that are abundant in the earth. All support the harmonious electrical energy charge in the body.

After all, our body is 70% water, and we carry a potent electrical charge. Ask any cardiologist who has performed an EKG or has shocked a heart out of ventricular fibrillation with a large amount of electric charge (watts) and he/she will tell you that the body is indeed electrical. Or, ask a neurologist who evaluates electrical brain waves detected by EEG's… you get the picture.

If we agree that we are electric, then assisting the body with harmonious, minute amounts of electrical energy will support healing.

For example, small amounts of electrical energy will heal non-displaced bone fractures in places where the blood supply is inefficient. Hospitals have been using TENS units for years to promote bone healing. So giving the body electroceutical support is another way to enhance endogenous ATP production, allowing the cells to heal themselves.

This is what John Thorp's Acuscope and Myopulse do. His electrical devices support the production of ATP in the cells, which eventually supports the healing process in the body local to where the current is being delivered. So what does a Hollywood stunt man bring to the energy medicine table?

John Thorp is a talented guy. When you read his book you will learn how this athlete, dare-devil, iron-man, and wild surfer developed the clinical protocols designed for this new technology. In essence, John's path included many unpredictable injuries resulting from his occupational and recreational interests. He relied on healing himself with his own technologies and he has become a messenger in the process.

When John was about to work on my right hip, I told him that the x-rays showed that there was "bone on bone" in that joint; no cartilage cushion at all. It ached! I limped. And my range of motion in that hip was severely restricted. He shrugged his shoulders and proceeded to "one up" me. John pulled up his pant legs and showed me a grossly deformed knee that still supports him in triathlons: stunningly swollen and twisted compared to his "normal" knee. I couldn't figure out HOW he even walked on it! (Still can't.)

Because John healed himself "against all odds," he knows that his technologies can heal others. This Hollywood stunt man has been employing electrostimulation therapies for healing for the last 24 years. What can we learn from him?

Simply stated, when you read this book, you will absolutely discover that John is a messenger for all of us. In my professional opinion, his recovery was nothing short of miraculous. After refusing surgery and maintaining his intention and belief that he could heal his own body, John is truly a living testimony to his own therapy.

I highly recommend this book to anyone who wishes to participate in their own healing. John's methods can help with detoxification, energy production, and ATP fortification in cells. His Myopulse and Acuscope units can offer an alternative healing methodology that really works. When you, the reader, fully comprehend John's passion, search, and struggle to live his own life to the fullest, you can understand why he felt it so important to bring this exciting "good vibe" technology forth to others.

This type of treatment is available to you, too. You can try to find a certified Electrotoxicologist therapist local to you, or order a unit to heal yourself.

Be well. I support you all in your belief that you can heal yourself.

DEDICATION

For my wife, Lisa, for her encouragement and love,

My father and mother, Al and Eva, who instilled a faith in me that is impenetrable,

My sister and brother-in-law, Betty Jo and Jim Nash, for their unceasing love,

And in memory of Duff King, a great pilot and my wingman flying hang gliders over the cliffs of Makapuu in Hawaii. And to all my fellow pilots who have departed this earth plane, no longer visible to us but soaring effortlessly above. "BLUE SKIES AND FOR THOSE WHO DARE!"

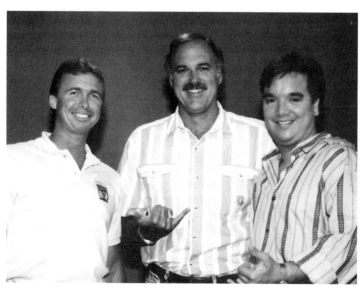

From L to R:
John Thorp, Duff King and John Noland
on the set of "Sports Rap"

ACKNOWLEDGMENTS

I would like to acknowledge my family and friends who have contributed to this book and this journey:

Thanks to Dennis McKenna, Randy Craft, Bernie Dohrmann, Mark Victor Hansen, Jack Canfield, David Backstrom, Kim Scott, Nick Nicholas, Tom Hauptman, Phil Carr, and Baron Hilton II, who have all unconditionally loved me.

A special thanks to Felipe Pomar with whom I have spent my days surfing and writing this book on a little Indonesian island called Rote.

Finally, sincere thanks to my editors: Eve Hogan, who helped edit this book and married me to my wife Lisa; Marcus Brutlag, who I shared a few waves with, whose writing skills surpass my own and who helped in bringing this book to its final stages; and Tony Maldi a true friend and great surfer that tried his best to direct me to the right people in support of my vision. Thank you all for your understanding and sharing the vision that became this book.

A very special thanks to Dr. Stephen Sinatra M.D., F.A.C.C., F.A.C.N., C.N.S. whose wisdom and support drove me forward to complete this book with integrity. It may anger some and bring joy to others but it is the truth.

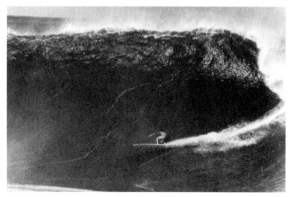

Felipe Pomar, the first world Champion of Surfing, rides a giant wave at Waimea bay 1968

TABLE OF CONTENTS

INTRODUCTION

Contrary to popular belief stuntmen are not crazy and doctors are not Gods; rather, both are calculated risk takers that hold life and death in their hands.

As a boy, I dreamed of flying. As a young man I strapped on wings and flew like the birds, becoming one of the first to step off the cliff into the new daredevil sport of hang gliding. It wasn't long before hang gliding caught the attention of Hollywood and I found my calling: stuntman. Risky, fast-paced, action, beautiful women...it had all the "highs" and lows of Hollywood to satisfy my love for living on the edge. It was a perfect fit.

After 35 years of professional stunt work, mostly in Hawaii doing shows like *Hawaii Five'0*, *Magnum P.I.*, *The Six Million Dollar Man*, *Jake and the Fat Man*, and a host of others, it was actually a non-stunt accident that turned out to force me into the most pivotal 180-degree turn I would ever experience.

I awoke from what I thought was a bad dream on Sunday, January 6, 1986. As my eyes slowly began to focus, I realized I was in a hospital room attached to an intravenous drip. My bad dream was no dream at all. I was in excruciating pain.

Now I was fully awake. The doctors were telling me the bad news. My leg was broken in 56 pieces. The tibia plateau was shattered like an eggshell. It would take three pins, twelve screws, and two plates to put Humpty Dumpty back together again, followed by a bone graft from my hip to glue it all together. Talk about pain. I did not know what hurt worse, my hip or my knee. The doctors said that my career as a stuntman was over and that I would probably never surf, snow ski, or fly my hang glider.

Twenty-four hours before, I had had it all—the best job on the planet as a professional stuntman and actor. I was respected in the surf, in the air, and on land wherever I went in Hawaii.

It was gone. I lay in that hospital bed in pain with my leg in the air and thought about how I had abused my body with the 70's and 80's "flying high" life style. It was clear to me why I was there. I had taken for granted the most incredible gift we are given, the human body, created in His image. I had abused it with drugs and alcohol and pretended I was six foot six, two hundred and fifty pounds, and bullet proof. Now, with clarity, I faced reality: I was a mere mortal being five feet ten inches tall, one hundred and fifty pounds, and made of glass.

The doctors' prognosis: Without surgery I would possibly be able to walk with a cane, or my alternative was a full knee replacement. My world came crashing down and the reality sunk in: My career was over. Either option meant I would never again be allowed on the set as stuntman.

As I listened to well-educated, brilliant men tell me that I would never again do the things in life that I loved and valued, I was stricken with a horrible feeling deep in the pit of my stomach, so deep it touched my soul. The sweat poured from my body as I felt an emotion that I could have never understood before. Hopelessness. I am a man of action, and out of desperation I imagined one last dramatic act—committing suicide!!! Taking the coward's way out.

Then came a ray of hope from a good friend who introduced me to a little-known medical technology that led to my full recovery and a new career as a doctor to the doctors.

Unlike stunt work, my recovery and the new career working with advanced micro-current technology did not happen quickly. It was a year of intensive self-imposed physical therapy and daily treatment with the Electro-Acuscope and Myopulse machines before I was back in full action. After that year, however, I was back in the stunt business, running triathlons, and thanking God for a second chance. It was a comeback with power, electrical power.

During recovery, I treated horses with the equipment to make ends meet. There were also a few dogs, a pig, and even a fighting chicken along the way. The results were phenomenal. To my continued amazement, they all got better, and fast.

Eventually the owners of the animals started showing up. They wanted the same results they saw happening with their pets. I just wanted to get back to stunt work and was a bit concerned about the legality of treating people with some little-known medical equipment in a horse stall.

Nevertheless, that's the way it happened, and eventually I did get back to Hawaii and back to stunt work. But someone else had a bigger plan, because people just kept showing up wanting to be treated. They'd say, "Go see John in the stunt trailer or the horse stall, for he can fix anything." Then one day in 1990 the director of a hospital showed up. Two weeks later, his hamstring was better than ever, he was able to do the things he loved again and even ran a marathon. I was overseeing an Electro-Acuscope and Myopulse rehabilitation program at Castle Medical Center in Hawaii.

After twenty-four years overseeing tens of thousands of treatments, I saw clearly effective protocols emerge. I studied Chinese medicine and got a massage therapy license along the way, and began to teach others how to work the machines and how to get the same consistent results. I've been advised not to use percentages without supportive documentation yet; the results that I have personally seen with this technology, when used correctly, is 90% positive.

In the past 24 years, I have owned and operated two medical clinics, overseen 40,000 treatments performed by myself and my students, and provided nearly one hundred trainings as founder and owner of Thorp Institute of Integrated Medicine, Inc. to distribute this technology. My clients range from the meek to the mighty, including many famous celebrities as well as doctors and alternative medical professionals. My business is making a real difference: healing pain, giving people hope, giving people jobs, and giving practitioners effective tools.

I am a very, very blessed person. But it is not enough. Maybe it is because people just keep showing up, or maybe it is because I believe that this is now my real calling, my life's purpose, but I just can't rest until this treatment is available to the masses. It is just too effective, too safe, and too simple, and it is time that more people know about it.

So now, once again, a 180-degree turn is taking place, from stuntman to the doctor's doctor, to author and speaker, a committed husband and father. This is my life story. Some of the names have been changed to protect the innocent. This book was written not just to heal my soul but also to spread the word about an effective way to heal pain and repair body tissues. May it help many, including you.

You will notice that each chapter is preceded by a quote from Rudyard Kipling's poem "If," written for his son in the late 1800s. This poem was given to me at one of the lowest points of my life. It resonated so clearly with me and brought understanding to why so many of us head down a self-destructive pathway due to our own low level of self worth and lack of guidance. I have included it at the end of the book as a gift to all of you and a constant reminder to me.

With Love and Light,

John Thorp

CHAPTER ONE

If You Can Keep Your Head When All About You Are Losing Theirs And Blaming It On You

My First Stunt

The surgery had gone well; four-years-old and in the hospital to repair a ruptured hernia. After I was sliced open and sewn back together again, my mother drove me home to make me comfortable before she left for the corner drug store to pick up my pain medication. The only thing on my mind was my next stunt, and the silly surgery felt like nothing more than a nuisance, an annoying crimp in my schedule. The doctor warned me not to do anything but rest, but I was feeling good and anxious to get back to my anti-gravity equipment. Although I was left alone for only a few moments, that would be more than enough time for a test flight.

I could not walk upright due to the bandaging, but found that bending dramatically at the waist allowed me to maneuver to the closet for my flying apparatus, my dad's big black umbrella. It was now or never. Looking over the Ivy covered banister, I thought the Ivy and grassy landing strip below looked more than soft enough. I slowly climbed up to the top of the banister, pushed open the umbrella, then jumped and looked up to find that, amazingly, the umbrella was holding my weight–I was flying, I was flying!

Then, in a split second, it was over. The umbrella's ribs dramatically collapsed and sent me crashing down flat on my back. My bandages were no longer white, but rather a dark red. When I lifted up the moist wrappings my guts were shockingly revealed, now hanging out after the fall had ripped open every one of the fresh stitches.

My mother found me sprawled out in the front yard with my destroyed flying craft and almost passed out when she saw my oozing wound. "Oh my God, what have you done?" she screamed. "I was flying."

She scooped up my young body and raced me back to St. Joseph's Hospital. She had tears in her eyes as she apologized to the doctor, "I only left him alone for a few minutes." The kind-hearted doctor comforted her, "It's all right Mrs. Thorp. You have a very adventurous young man who got lucky today. He'll survive this." I smiled, knowing they would have to sew me up in order for me to fly again. That scar remains as my first badge of courage, many more would follow.

My Mother's Victory

I was born on August 13, 1951, the second child of two loving parents, Al and Eva Thorp. Surrounded by a wealth of attention and care, I am told I was the happiest of babies. My early smile beamed even as my sister took me door to door dressed as a baby girl to introduce me to all our neighbors as her new sister, apparently undeterred after receiving a baby brother despite her fervent prayers for a little sis.

Our home, Burbank, California, in the early 1950s was the perfect place to raise kids. Our street, Pepper Street, was loaded with families with young children free to roam in the security of the sprouting green yards of suburban America. I was a chubby little guy, full of laughter, with a belly button that stuck out like a doorbell, and the neighborhood kids took great pleasure in taking their fingers to my belly and singing out, "Ding-Dong." I can still remember and name every house on the street and who lived in them. It had all the makings for an idyllic youth, but it all came crashing down in a hurry.

I have very few memories of a mother who was not dying. After a routine physical, she was given a crushing diagnosis: incurable breast cancer. The year was 1953, I was two, my mother 32, and the doctors gave her only a year or maybe two years to live. We went on with a dark cloud hanging over us, always looming, tainting the innocent joys and celebrations of childhood. Our small family put up a resilient exterior, but at the core we all bore the cross of impending death palpably residing on our doorstep.

My earliest memories are of a dying mother, but not of a mother who ever felt sorry for herself. She felt terrible that she would leave behind her loving husband and two young children, a mental battle she fought every day, but despite suffering, both physically and emotionally, she held her head high with her unwavering faith. This impenetrable faith, a faith that would carry her well past the doctor's predictions, sustained our family through the hardest of times.

The story of my family began happily in Lancaster, Pennsylvania, a rural town where my father and mother were born and raised and fell in love at first sight after being introduced by mutual friends. When they moved west, both of their families remained in Lancaster. I will always cherish the grand train trips we took back to the Pennsylvania countryside when I was a kid. My mother and sister and I would board the train from Union Station in Los Angeles, stop in a bustling Chicago after three days, and then arrive in the calm fields of rural America two days later. We had many wonderful childhood adventures like this; however, underneath any fun and excitement we still lived a private and quiet nightmare. Our mother was always unquestionably dying.

After a radical mastectomy came a hopeful period of remission, but soon the cancer was back. Doctors removed the other breast and then began carving into her like some kind of grotesque biology experiment. She suffered greatly from the agonizing pain, a pain beyond description, and her moans in the middle of the night are forever etched in my memory.

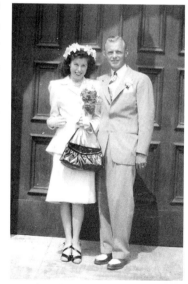

Still, as the cancer progressively ate away her delicate body she refused to take her painkiller medications, mostly disorienting dosages of morphine. Enduring the physical pain so that she would be there for us mentally, she overpowered her suffering with her faith and only gave into the pain when she slept. The haunting moans would

Al and Eva Thorp on their wedding day

come only after she lost consciousness. Otherwise, not a sound came from her in complaint.

She refused to succumb to her killer because she knew she had unfinished business. She fought for more time to prepare us for when she was gone, time to teach us how to take care of each other, support each other, and, most importantly, to love each other. She held on to fill us with lessons of a love that has no death, lessons that would have to provide for the lifetime of days we would live without her.

She was always trying to ready us for her passing, no matter how difficult a reality it was to face. I can remember her telling my father that she wanted him to begin looking for another wife. "Stop it! I don't want anyone else," he would reply, tearing up. "You have to fight," he would cry as he broke down and stormed out of the house. He loved her completely.

She would often ask us to promise to watch out for my father, repeating over and over that we must make sure he would find someone to look after him. "He is such a good man. I don't want him to live alone," she would plead. Everything she had dreamed for in life had come true, a loving husband, two healthy children, her dream home—and she was losing it all, forced to leave her family without a wife and mother.

My mother tragically suffered for ten years, but in dying, she taught us everything about living. She wanted to instill enough of herself in us that she would never leave us, and as the cancer got worse, she even moved her hospital bed into my bedroom. "Just because you will not be able to see me in this physical form of the human body does not mean that I will not be with you in spirit," she repeatedly told me. "I will never leave your side and will always watch over you. I'll be your guardian angel." Then she would remind me with a sly smile, "Don't think you can get away with anything because you think no one is watching. I'll be watching. I will also protect you, and there is nothing you cannot do in the light of God."

"I know Mom, you said that yesterday," I always responded and assured her I would be fine, but I also watched my older friends with their mothers and it hurt that I would not have the same privilege. We prayed and prayed but there was nothing we could do. My mother died. She died in the bedroom that my father had built for me. I was eleven.

Our young minister, who she had swiftly befriended and mentored in her final years, wept by her bedside. The room was unlit but I will never forget the glow. I did not see any fear in my mother's eyes that night or in the days preceding her death; instead they shined so brightly I knew she was seeing God and the light of the world to come. The suffering was over.

At her funeral, with wet eyes, the minister began her eulogy: "Eva Thorp put a faith such as mine to shame. She never blamed her God for this terrible thing. Christ made his presence known in her from an early age and bestowed in her a faith we can only pray to find. There is not anyone here who didn't feel her power or could ignore the power of her faith."

When the minister repeated the words she often spoke about how our God suffers with us, my young mind was made up that my God would not have to suffer with me. He would rejoice with me, now a White Light Warrior set on awakening the spirit that lives inside each and every one of us. My mission would be to carry on the rock of her faith and her unconditional love.

In those final days of her fight, when she had moved her hospital bed into my room, I would often awake from powerful dreams and ask my mother to explain them. My recurring dream was that I could fly, and it would always begin with me alone, running down my street, flapping my arms until I felt the pressure of the wind lift me into the sky. I would soar above the schoolyard with the children playing below and shout at them to look at me. "I'm flying!" I would scream, but they never looked up. Later, on the ground, I would tell them that I could fly, but they never believed me. Trying to show them that I could indeed soar, I would take off running down the street flapping my arms; however, no matter how hard I tried, I could not fly if they were watching, and they just laughed at me. I would awake frustrated and distraught.

My mother would hold my tear-streaked cheeks in her hands while giving a simple explanation for what I took as a crushing failure: "Johnny, you are just trying to show off. You know you can fly, so who cares if others know? You never have to prove anything to anyone else." She would give me a look I knew well and say, "If you can dream it, you can do it."

A part of me died with my mother that night of her passing, but another part of me was born. As a child I dreamt of flight. As a man, because of my mother's gifts I would be led to take a leap of faith, to strap on wings and fly like the birds.

A Man's Integrity

As a young boy, I would lie in my father's arms, fascinated and magically transported as he told me the stories of the scars on his hands. The story of the long scar on the inside of his right index finger was always my favorite. As it happened, an enraged stray dog was about to lash into him. His collie mix, Gray Dawn, jumped in to save him from the vicious attack. My young father could not help but repay the loyalty of the rescue, and in attempting to pull the stray off from Gray Dawn, the razor teeth ripped open the flesh of his finger. Each scar held a similar story of pain or courage, and it was here, cuddled up next to my father, that I learned of integrity.

My father was a big fight fan, and the privilege of staying up late with him to watch the Friday night fights was a bonding highlight of my young life. Propped up next to him on our couch, my little sponge of a mind was absorbing everything, nothing sinking in deeper than my father's belief in an honorable fight. Eventually, deeming me old enough, he spent hours teaching me to box. He taught me to defend myself and imparted the stern rule that I could only hit somebody who hit me first. This would be a difficult rule to uphold, but one which was followed—out of respect for my father, for his virtues, and for his honorable counterblows to life's sucker punches.

My father took plenty of hard shots in his life, none more staggering than the loss of my mother, the love of his life. He was left heartbroken and alone with the daunting responsibility of raising a teenage daughter and an eleven-year-old holy terror of a son, a responsibility from which he never shrank. Perhaps he was emboldened by the resiliency honed in his youth, having grown stronger each time he had picked himself up off the mat.

Although only five feet six inches, Big Al (the title awarded by his friends at an early age) easily towered ten feet tall in determination. Overcoming the limitations of his size with zeal, my father was a dedicated athlete and participated in numerous sports, lettering in basketball and tennis, and went on to play both sports at Millersville State Teacher's College. Although he graduated with an education degree, teaching and athletic competition would prove insufficient in satisfying his broadening desires and interests. He had earned his private pilot's license while still in college and soon directed his focus toward flying commercially. However, life would throw him a combination of blows in the form of astigmatisms in both eyes. He failed his physical, and his dreams of commercial piloting were crushed. Undeterred, he continued to fly privately and would proudly take his family for rides in his little Piper Cub. I remember my grandmother telling of how he had shocked her with his acrobatics the first time he got her in the plane, returning her to the earth with a sickly green skin tone. My father was set on infusing his life with adventure and challenge.

When World War II came along he joined the Navy. After fighting to keep the world free and traveling the globe, he knew that he could not go back to a mundane life in a sleepy town like Lancaster. When an intriguing job opportunity arose, making airplane propellers for the Sensenich Brothers in California, he could not pass up the offer. He would be the first and only member of his family to leave Pennsylvania, but he was not about to cast aside this golden ticket to head west. Unfortunately, as life never fights fair, the job offer came shortly after he had met and fallen in love with the beautiful Eva Miller. He begged and pleaded with his lovely Eva to accompany him, but he could not convince her to leave the comfort of her home and eight brothers and sisters. He left for California in 1946, alone.

Although immersed in a California rumbling with the excitement of booming growth and industry, my father was afflicted. No matter how hard he tried, he could not shake the love bug. Hopelessly in love, he wrote letter after letter to his beloved Eva. She, also sharing the same affliction, began writing back. Knowing without a doubt that he had found his soul mate,

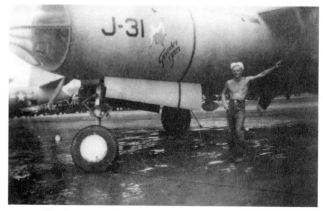

His happiest days, my father posing next to a World War II aircraft

he refused to give up and eventually convinced my mother to come to California. He saved every letter she wrote him. They were married soon thereafter, and a year later my sister was born.

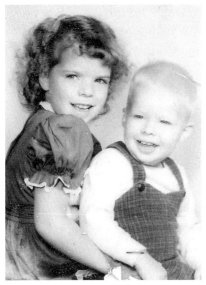

In a show of respect for the family left behind, they named their children after a combination of relatives. My aunts Betsy and Josephine were the namesakes for my sister Betty Jo, and when I came along two and a half years later my uncles John and George were to be honored. However, my father said he just could not name me John George, so they used my uncle's middle name, Stuart, instead. In August, 1951, I was christened John Stuart Thorp.

My sister, age 3, and me, age 1

A few years later my father was offered and accepted a new position with Kelly Johnson's "Skunk Works," the official alias for Lockheed Martin's Advanced Development. He held top security clearance and kept busy working on secret spy planes designed specifically for flights "behind the iron curtain" of the Soviet Union. Many of his projects were housed at a place he only referred to as The Ranch, which I later learned to be the infamous Area 51. I asked him one day if they really had flying saucers out there. All he could tell me was, "Son, I'm working on aircraft that do not look like any aircraft to me."

Only later would I learn the impressive details of his work. The Skunk Works had predicted that their initial spy plane, the U-2, had a limited operational life over the Soviet Union, and the CIA agreed. So the Skunk Works received a contract in late 1959 to build five A-12 aircrafts at a then staggering cost of $96 million. Building a Mach 3.0 plus aircraft out of titanium posed enormous difficulties, and the first flight did not occur until 1962. My father worked heavily on the SR-71 Blackbird, an improved two-seater version of the A-12, which first flew in 1966 and remarkably remained in service until 1998.

As for those mystery machines that did not look like any aircraft he had ever seen, it turned out that he was speaking of the now famed Stealth Fighter and Bomber. He would proudly recite how if a bird landed on the wing of the Stealth, the radar would pick up the bird but not the aircraft. Many of the groundbreaking projects he helped launch over forty years ago are still active today.

Although he was unable to reveal the actual magnitude of his work or the personal weight upon his shoulders, I cannot recall one incident where he did not tell the truth, as he knew it. His judgment was unbendable. No matter how hard I tried to twist things in my favor, I was usually reined in by his wisdom. And, believe me, there were plenty of times when I did my best to bend it.

Guts

When my father joined a bowling league shortly after my mother's death, I was somewhat entertained with keeping score for him and his buddies. However, I was absolutely captivated by the passing, kicking, and especially the hitting of the Sun Valley Falcons who practiced in the park across from the bowling alley. After begging my father for weeks to let me join this local Pop Warner team, he finally agreed. I would have to prove myself, not only because of my size, but because I was the sole blonde-haired kid on a team primarily comprised of Latino boys from the barrios of the Valley. They would soon learn that this little tow-head was not afraid of anyone.

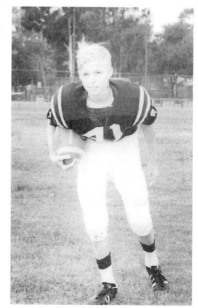

Most of the kids on the team were in the same barrio gang, and Mario, their leader, tried to intimidate me from the beginning with his taunts and dirty play. I would simply dust myself off and run back to the huddle unfazed. One day he finally took a swing at me, and I will never

"Guts" age 11

forget the look on his face when I did not back down. Mario was one tough kid and often left me a bloody mess, but no matter how battered I was, he could not keep me down. It only took a few fights for him to realize there was much easier prey. Mario may have gotten the best of me physically, but I won the mental battle when the guys recognized my toughness and eventually accepted the skinny kid from Burbank as one of the team. The Falcons had their token white boy.

I think I was often saved from more severe beatings from Mario by the coaches breaking us up. But it was during these fights that they first witnessed my tenacity, inspiring coach Garrett's nickname for me: "Guts." Any new kid on the team usually took me for an easy target and would try to pick on me first, but everyone else knew that was a big mistake. I was more than willing to sacrifice my body and ready to demonstrate what it really meant.

In the fading twilight, whistle by whistle, Coach Garrett was losing his patience. On the sound of each blast, with speed and zero fear, I would bust off the line to throw myself into the biggest obstacle found and then get back up, anxious to do it all over again. My fighting spirit needed an outlet and found one in football. Now completely dissatisfied with his team, Coach Garrett stopped the practice.

"You MUST sacrifice your body to glorify your soul," he shouted. This had become his motto. Then he pulled me out of the group, had me demonstrate how to block and tackle, and finally said, "Look, Guts doesn't weigh anything and he can still take any of you big guys out."

Our team went all the way to the playoff title game that year, which meant that everything must be done by the rules, and the rules stated clearly that there was a minimum and maximum weight. We would be weighed in full uniform, but even with the pads and helmet I was easily ten pounds under the weight limit. My father and I started scheming, and come game day we were all set to carry out our plan. After apprehensively stepping onto the scales and making the minimum weight, I dashed back to the men's room, removed the five-pound weights hidden in each of my thigh pads, and threw them out the window to my father waiting below. It was the only time that he ever bought into one of my dubious plans, but, more than likely, he was a proud accomplice that day as he watched me intercept two passes, and the Falcons won the title.

"To sacrifice your body is to glorify your soul." Coach Garrett's words have stayed with me in life and throughout my football career. I proudly wore a football letterman's jacket all three years of high school, except for one week when I had it suspended for smoking cigarettes around the corner of Burroughs High. I had proven I was willing to sacrifice my body, but I was also quickly learning how to sacrifice obedience for the sake of a thrill, perhaps a foreshadowing of events to come.

The Making of a Champion

I had discovered the thrill of speed, and with the help of my dog, I was moving fast–really fast. My collie mix, Missy, and I had been perfecting it for weeks. I would sit on my homemade skateboard and have her pull me up and down the street. The tricky part was when we got to the corner, where we needed to slow down. Missy always sped up as the sharp corner approached, and nine times out of ten I had to bail out to prevent blasting into the intersection. More than one motorist had to skid to a stop as Missy made the harsh 90-degree turn and I did not.

We were moving faster than ever this time and, once again, Missy rounded sharply, slinging me into the middle of the intersecting street. This time, however, I noticed an advancing car a second too late; too late for me to bail and too late for the car to stop. With my little wheels rattling, there was no choice but to hold on tight and commit to shooting past the car.

The driver surely must have thought he was about to kill this crazy kid passing right by the front bumper of his car. Even I was amazed to

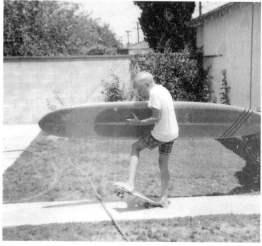

Jumping the back yard hose on my skateboard with my first surfboard

be alive after making it to the other side. He quickly jumped out of the car to check on me, but I was already running, ditching my board.

I'm afraid to say that this narrow escape only helped foster a confidence that I could pull off anything. I always felt a slight edge over everyone else in those early days, a sense of security coming from above, from my guardian angel. This protected feeling fearlessly propelled me into the dawn of skateboarding.

I fashioned my first skateboards, the Missy-propelled death traps, from two-by-fours and old metal roller skates, the adjustable ones that fit over any shoe size. I would separate them, nail them to the two-by-four, and put an apple crate on the front to fashion instant transportation, with a storage compartment and all. I was learning to surf at the time, and found that the apple crate quickly got in the way of letting the skateboard act like a surfboard, so it had to go. Then the hard rubber roller derby wheels came along in the early 1960s, a technological advancement that really made a big difference in performance. My first resin-laminated skateboard was made in shop class, and there was no stopping me with the combination of the new roller derby wheels sailing over the pavement.

My days were filled with one thing: practice, practice, practice. I soon had all the tricks down. Jumping over picnic tables, lying flat in the coffin position, walking the board, popping wheelies, 360s, and even 720s; I mastered them all. Taking my skills into competition, it was the finished handstand that got me crowned Valley Skateboarding Champion.

I felt on top of my game but quickly learned that a challenger will arise whenever you think you are at the top. It was not long before a buddy of mine, Danny, started chiding me. "Yeah, you can do tricks, but can you ride fast, downhill?" he said.

"Sure," I said. "What hill?" He pointed to the steepest hill in Burbank, and the race was on.

It was a long, hot walk to the top of Barham Blvd. There were not any sidewalks then, so we went for it right down the center of the street. Standing on the boards, our speeds increased dramatically. As a car pulled up next to me, I yelled at the driver, "How fast are you going?"

"Thirty-five," he yelled back.

Thirty-five on a skateboard, and there was no way to stop, which left the only option of barreling forward until slowing down enough to jump off. At about 40 mph my wheels went into a high-speed wobble, inevitably sending me tumbling. Rolling for over 50 feet, I came up significantly less intact, with my pants and shirt shredded and hamburger for skin. A bloody mess! Danny did not fare much better. Expecting a welcome cushion, he bailed out into some high bushes but failed to see the large cactus growing behind. We spent the next four hours picking stickers out of Danny and crafting a story for our parents to explain our mangled clothes and frames.

Eventually, instead of just going balls to the wall, we built longer and better boards to handle the speed, which made it possible to traverse the steepest sections while remaining in control. My thrill-seeking ventures were becoming grander in scale, but I was learning, admittedly the hard way, to keep each risk firmly grounded within the confidence gained through hours of practice. More important, perhaps, was my continued reliance on an intuition surely instilled from above by my guardian angel.

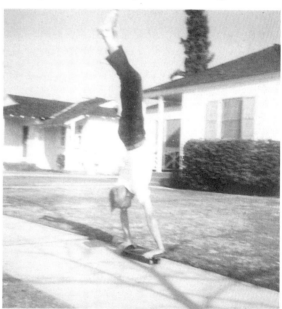

"Only contestant reversing equilibrium with a finished handstand, John Thorp won first"

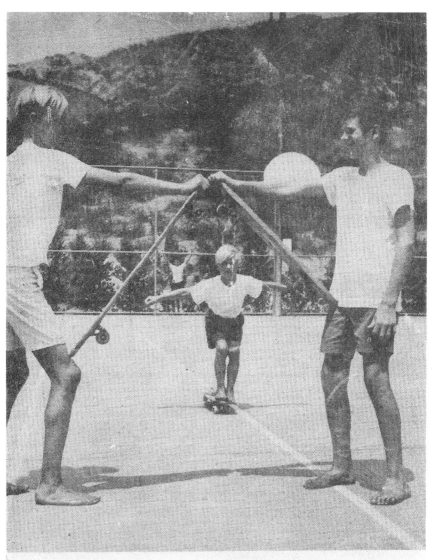

SKATEBOARD CHAMPS -- "Pud" Howland, 10, center, who took two firsts and a second in the Valleywide skateboard championships held Friday at Brace Park, Burbank, perches on the very front of his board as he skates through a bridge formed by John Thorp, 14, left, and Gary Bennett, 12. Thorp tied for the free-style title, while Bennett won the senior title and two other championships. Other winners included Steve Glance, Mike Bennett and John Davidson. The tourney will become an annual event at Brace Bark. --Stevens Studio

CHAPTER TWO

If You Can Trust Yourself When All Men Doubt You, But Make Allowances For Their Doubting Too

Sneaking Across The Border

Skateboarding was a rush; the speed, the falls, and the notoriety. But honestly, it was really just something to do when we couldn't get to the ocean. My true passion was surfing, surfing myself blue with every available trip to the water. Luckily, my father recognized this desire and took me surfing almost every Saturday. The perfect point break of Malibu was our common day trip, but we ventured to many of Southern California's pristine surf spots as well. Best of all, my dad would take the family on week-long summer beach vacations.

We spent a week at the beach in Oceanside when I was 14, and then again the following year. It was here that I met the hotshot locals surfing the prime North County San Diego waves. The respect of this older crew was quickly earned by not dropping in on them like the rest of the visiting kooks. Not being a shoulder hopper, my takeoffs were either perfectly at the peak or even on the other side. Many a crushing wipeout accompanied such late takeoffs, but once again, a little guts served as a ticket into an elite society. Impressed with my kamikaze style, they took me under wing and granted me an honorary place in their local surf tribe.

After I journeyed south to surf with the Oceanside guys whenever possible, they extended an invitation to do some surfing with the team around San Diego over spring break. My dad conceded to my determined requests with one condition: a promise not to cross the border into Mexico. After quickly swearing that Mexico was not an option, I was off to San Diego. When a big swell came in, so did the crowds. The guys were buzzing about an article in Surfer magazine that featured a completely empty spot with perfect waves known as K-38, but it was located in (yep, you guessed it) Mexico. With San Diego's top spots mobbed, it was a unanimous decision to go searching for the huge empty waves of Baja, California. Initially intent on staying true to my promise, I eventually caved after they assured me we would be back before my dad ever knew we were gone.

They hid me under the mattresses in the back of the van as we passed through the border because, as a minor, I needed a notarized letter from my parents allowing me to cross. To further avoid suspicions, we drove inland and crossed the border in Tecate instead of Tijuana. The border guard briefly shined his flashlight into the back and then waved us through. Having just been smuggled into another country, I couldn't imagine how life could get more exciting! That is, until I saw the waves.

The surf was epic, six to eight foot peeling rights. We surfed spot after empty spot, all to perfection. So, of course, when it came time to go home, no one was ready to leave. Spring break was about over, and my dad would be extremely worried if he did not hear from me. I could not do that to him and pleaded with my buddies to go back. They simply shrugged and said, "Tough luck, the surf's up and we're not going to miss it."

They had lied to me, so screw 'em, I thought. Having blown almost my entire travel budget on fireworks, I set off alone with only 15 cents, a can of fruit cocktail, and a plan to hitchhike back to the border with my board under my arm. My dad would kill me if greeted by a collect call from Mexico. I needed to cross back into San Diego before using my last 15 cents on the phone call. I waited patiently by the side of the road in Ensenada with my thumb out for hours. Finally, a farmer with a big friendly smile and a truck full of chickens pulled over. I called out, "Border," and he pointed to the rear of the truck. I jumped in and was happy to be on my way home. At least I thought I was heading toward home until I realized that we were headed away from the ocean. We were traveling too fast for me to jump off, so I rode it out until he stopped in a little village. There, the driver smiled, waved, and left me in the dust with my surfboard, my 15 cents, and my trusty can of fruit cocktail.

Across the dirt road was a Volkswagen bus with California license plates parked at a beat-up shack affixed with a large sign advertising what appeared to be custom upholstery. Surely this was a surf buggy that might be good for a ride home. I hunkered down to wait for them to come out. My stomach spiking with hunger, I was just about to open my can of fruit cocktail when a black '55 Chevy ominously pulled up next to me out of a cloud of dust. When the windows slowly rolled down, a mean-ass, ugly-looking Mexican dude greeted me with a scowl and slurred a broken, "Get in the car, boy."

"Thanks, but I'm waiting for my friends," I quickly replied.

"Get in the car, boy," he growled back.

"No thank you."

Then, in a very gruff voice he said, "You want to live, boy?" and reached for a shiny object on his dashboard, unmistakably a knife.

I was off running, surfboard and satchel swinging. That ugly *vato* proceeded to drive slowly behind me, laughing the whole time. It wouldn't take long for me to run out of gas, but I wasn't going down without a fight. Like in a bad dream, I stole quick glances back at the car on my heels. That's when I saw two surfer-style guys come bolting from the upholstery shop. They flew into their Volkswagen bus, which quickly headed in my direction and eventually pulled past the '55 Chevy. They signaled for me to jump in. As I ran toward the van and away from the slimy predator, he sharply swerved his '55 Chevy from hell in his best effort to run me over. The blessed doors of the VW swung open just in time, and I leapt inside to safety. But that crazy bastard didn't give up, remaining determined to run us off the road. He must have gotten bored because he eventually pulled back, and he disappeared just as he entered, in a huge brown cloud of dust.

After driving out of that waking nightmare, we finally found time for a breath, introductions, and the sharing of stories. As one would suspect, my new friends Mike and Sam were not out at the barren ends of Baja for a killer deal on upholstery, but rather were carrying out a somewhat dubious plan to smuggle several pounds of marijuana across the border inside the seats of their VW. The story got even juicier after learning the cause of their hasty exit from the upholstery shack. While the shop owner was working on their van, his immodest daughter took the liberty of flashing them a look at her breasts. She was then promptly extorting them for their dollars when her father came upon them gawking at his topless daughter. With only half of their upholstery job finished, they decided to flee from the very pissed off Mexican father, carrying on to the border undeterred.

When the border was in sight, Mike figured it would probably be safer for all concerned if I would walk across alone. They did not need the added scrutiny brought on by an underage surfer kid lacking documentation, nor was I anxious to be sitting on top of several pounds of dope while crossing back into the United States. We parted ways with blessings of good luck, and I began my walk to the border.

The guards took one look at me, dust covered, with only a surfboard and a can of fruit cocktail, and immediately hauled me in for questioning. I went with a story about being separated from my family while camping, and how they were waiting for me in the lot just beyond the border. After some seriously suspicious looks, they let me pass. Mike and Sam did not have it so easy. Walking through the gates, I saw that the border agents were stripping the poor VW, my salvation, to the bolts, and my rescuers were being busted. It had not been my day to die, and not my day to be incarcerated either, another bullet dodged.

Although frazzled, I was feeling good to be back in the USA, and when I started hitching again, a nice family picked me up in a big boat of a station wagon, big enough to wedge my surfboard inside. The only problem was that they were only going as far as downtown San Diego. I did not know the area very well, and the only place I could think of that my dad could easily find was the zoo.

The sun was nearly set, but we arrived just before the zoo closed its doors, so I was able to use their phone to call my dad. I started in on a story about how all my friends had gone down into Mexico, but that I had refused, staying behind instead to surf in southern San Diego. But when he started telling me how proud he was that I had done the right thing, I cracked. The guilt was too powerful, and I broke down and told him the whole nightmare I had just survived. I was tired, cold, scared, and all I had was this damn can of fruit cocktail. In tears, I asked him if he would come get me. I do not think he was in any rush to pick me up, so I sat in front of that zoo, half-frozen, for almost four hours. All he found when he arrived was my head sticking out of a huge umbrella, which I had pulled out of the picnic table and within which I cocooned my body. It was a very quiet ride home, but my father said one thing that I would not forget: "You will never understand what it is like to worry about someone until you have a child of your own."

Just as easily as I had promised my father, my surfing buddies had promised me their word. It would take a long time to regain my father's trust, and I had learned the value in wisely choosing my company while pushing the envelope. This was not my day to die, but I was starting to wander dangerously closer to the edge and starting to realize that it mattered who was standing out there with me.

Facing The First Gun

Not every adventure has a formal beginning and end, choices and repercussions, or an elaborate truth to be mined. Some encounters with reality are brutally stark; they explode into our lives and exit just as suddenly.

Most of my high school days, with the exception of my south-of-the-border excursions, were pretty typical. I went to John Burroughs High School, played football, and was on the swim team. I worked a couple of normal teenage jobs, one at Jack-in-the-Box and the other at 7-Eleven. It was at 7-Eleven, while working the late shift, where I once again saw how quickly normal could transform into nightmare.

Two men entered the store toward the end of my shift. The two happened to be black, and to be honest, that was unusual in Burbank at that time. John Burroughs High had only one black and only a handful of Latino students. Burbank was simply a very white town. Beyond their color, something did not feel right about them and my suspicions were heightened. I watched them carefully as they browsed about the store, until one came toward the counter with an ice cream. Admittedly relieved, I thought, "Just a couple of guys looking for a snack."

He put his ice cream on the counter and asked for a pack of cigarettes. After reaching under the counter to open a new carton of Marlboros, I looked up to find the barrel of a nine-millimeter staring me in the eye.

"Take what you want. It's not my store."

They were after the money in the safe on the floor, but I did not have the combination, which only made them angrier. "So this is it," I figured. "They are going to shoot me."

They asked me again to open the safe, and I said, "Take all the money in the register but I really don't know the safe combo."

"Open it!" they screamed at me, and I gladly popped the register drawer. One held the gun on me while the other reached over and grabbed the cash and warned that they would be watching and would shoot me dead if I did anything after they left. They backed out of the door while I stood frozen in shock that I was still alive.

It is strange how you feel after something like that happens to you. I stood still, not knowing what to think, what to do. Wondering if they are still lurking, you just don't know what to do or how to make sense of it all. Once I felt comfortable that they had fled, I called the police and they came over to conduct a standard interview before moving along into the night.

Surely a fluke of an event here in Burbank, I kept my job without fear of further threat. But to my amazement, a week or so later, the same exact two men came in the store once again. I made a quick exit out the back door, called the police, and promptly ended my career as a 7-Eleven checkout clerk. There were definitely more rewarding ways of endangering my life. This was the first time a gun was put to my head; it would not be the last.

Death Traps and Speed

Just when you think you have gotten away with something, the unexpected happens. My car began to feel very loose and then the rear end started to fish tail. It smelled as if something was burning, but I did not have a clue what had exactly gone wrong. At 120 mph, everything happens fast. The next thing I knew, the car was careening out of control and I struggled with all my power to rein it in. I frantically pumped the brakes, only to find that I had none.

Momentum is not easily curbed, and this unrestrained momentum projecting me heedlessly down a California highway at well over 100 mph was actually set in motion years earlier in the summer of '67 with the purchase of a slow-rolling, surf-mobile of a Volkswagen bus. My father would help with the purchase of my first car if: one, I would pay for the insurance; two, I would share it with my sister. Thanks to the treacherous late night shifts at 7-Eleven, I could easily cover the insurance, but I had to strike a deal with my sister to earn her vote for the Volkswagen. My offer was to take her to and from her job as a swim instructor at the Encino Swim School, which would give me the chance to go surfing in between. After she told my father she was on board for the bus, we paid $500 for my first set of wheels.

I customized that bus into my own private bedroom and often slept down at the beach to awake to the serenity of the glassy, early morning surf. You could not beat it for beach side accommodations, but the bus put a real crimp in my early love life. Many of my girlfriends' fathers forbid them from dating me. Surely the sight of the personal love den on wheels pulling into their driveways must have left them wincing in anguish and alarm. I cannot say I blamed them. The van was perfect for my surf voyages, and although my increasingly lengthy surf missions made it difficult to uphold the deal with my sister, my sister found other ways of getting to work and soon the bus was all mine.

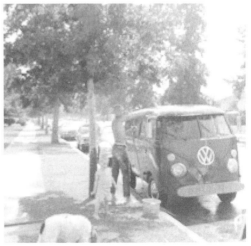

The bus made it through the summer; however, the engine blew up while returning from a

My first ride, a 1958 VW bus

ski trip to Mammoth that winter. That is how I met Bella, one of the best Volkswagen and Porsche mechanics in the Valley. He quickly rebuilt the motor, and I sold the bus the next summer for $1100, actually doubling my investment and earning enough to buy a '57 Porsche Cabriolet convertible. A girlfriend's uncle had just brought it in from Germany, and, lucky for me, had no idea of its value in the USA. He sold it to me for what he had paid for it in Germany, $900s. I painted it and put on new wheels and tires, immediately tripling the value. Although not as practical as the bus for surf trips, it was perfect for attracting the girls. I was 16 years old and living the Porsche-driving high life.

I was still determined in surf pursuits, and my surfboards ended up awkwardly strapped to the windshield and tied down to the luggage rack, which actually worked quite well. The real negative was that this required keeping the top down. As the weather got colder, the rainy trips to and from the beach nearly became unbearable. I loved the girls and loved that car, but surfing, warmth, and dryness won out in the end. I traded the Porsche for a late model VW van and went back to living on the beach at any and every opportunity. The van obviously provided well for the laid-back surf life, but concealed under the hood was the key component that would propel me toward that fateful night on the California highway.

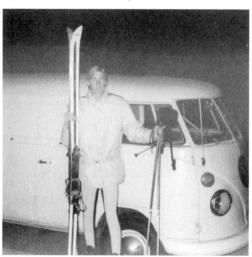

My VW bus with a secret weapon under the hood, a Porsche engine, perfect for racing up to Mammoth and along Van Nuys Boulevard

We fitted the VW with my high-powered Porsche engine. Bella, my secret accomplice, souped up the motor. That van could really fly. With the fastest van in town, and, as a member of the local VW van club, I would parade my van up and down Van Nuys Boulevard every Wednesday night. When punched, that Volkswagen could just about do a wheelie, which earned it quite a reputation on the Boulevard.

If the need for speed was already flowing in my veins, it was the Porsche engine that surely got it churning faster. I eventually found a more fitting shell for that engine while visiting a show room featuring the Ford GT and learned you could easily purchase a cheaper fiberglass replica of this famous body and assemble the car yourself. People were using both Chevy Corvairs or Volkswagen chassis and motors to do this. I cut a deal with Bella for a 1600 VW motor for my VW van to free up my Porsche engine, and he found me an intact chassis in a wrecked Volkswagen. We put on new shocks, de-cambered the suspension, and added low-profile racing rims and tires. Bella rebuilt my Porsche engine, adding double-barreled carburetors and an exhaust system that boosted the horsepower to a whole new level. We had a feeling that this freakishly powerful motor was going to give me one of the fastest cars racing about California's sprawling highways. All we needed now was that beautiful GT body.

I sold my van for just enough to purchase the GT. Since I was cutting corners in the budget every chance I could, after days of pleading my case to my father he finally agreed to co-sign for me to rent a truck large enough to haul the custom body from the San Luis Obispo factory to Bella's shop in Burbank. With a thermos full of coffee, my good friend Brad Fisher and I set off to make this dream car a reality. We had 24 hours to get the body and return the truck, and after a few big halts and some little jerks we soon had the multiple gears of the big rig down and were barreling down the road, a couple of teenage truckers.

To keep each other awake we told stories, and on the dark highway our themes turned to horror and fright. Then, as if conjured up, a mysterious streak of white flashed across our windshield. We wondered if we were seeing things before it came again, and then again. Eventually we deciphered the shocking streaks to be a giant white owl diving at us. Seemingly attracted by our bright lights, he continued his sudden dives, scaring the crap out of us each time. Just when we thought the owl had moved on, he came sweeping directly at us and smashed with full force right into the windshield. The resounding thump, leaving us screaming and three feet out of our seats, surely seemed to be the end of the owl, but we kept hearing a flapping sound. We looked at each other, bewildered. As the sound continued, we turned on the cab light to search for the source. The piercing eyes of the owl were staring directly at us from the cab's back window.

Screaming again, we swerved to the side of the road. We got out of the cab and found the owl to be dead but stuck down deep between the cab and the trailer. We drove a few miles further and asked the attendant at the remote gas station if he could help us extract an owl. He turned out to be a Native American that was none too happy with us for killing this sacred animal. We appeased him by honoring his request to honor the owl with a little prayer of reverence. After getting a little gas, we were off again without any problems, staying awake for the rest of the trip. Our eyes were open wide.

Perhaps I should have taken note of this omen of the owl, but I was too close now to abandon the dream for speed. At sun up, with the help of six men, we loaded the fresh-from-the-mold GT body into the back of the truck. My only disappointment was in their failure to mention that a paint job did not come with the agreed price. I was stuck with the color of their fiberglass, a hideous army green. Once we got it back, Bella allowed us to build the Green Beast at his shop and helped with things we could not figure out. Brad and I spent the majority of the summer building that car piece by piece.

The first test drive was in the parking lot next to Bella's shop. I punched it off the line, only to send the front end right off the ground like a dragster, which sanded off a good part of the rear end of the car. Having repaired plenty of surfboards, I knew how to rebuild the damaged body. A heavy sandbag did the trick for keeping the front end down, and the power of being slammed back into the seat on the following test drives was like nothing I had ever felt before.

It was time to give it the real test, a drive on the freeway. But as soon as I turned to go down the on-ramp, I heard a loud crack. The steering system lost all resistance, leaving the wheel spinning around in circles in my hands. The steering shaft had snapped, but luck was with me as I skidded to a stop just before entering the freeway. We pushed the car off to the side and wasted little time in getting to the junkyard for another steering shaft. One thing about building a car from scratch is that you know how to fix everything on it. Determined to get the Green Beast on the freeway, I spent most of the day laid out flat on my back on that on-ramp until finally getting the new steering shaft bolted in.

I slowly headed back up the freeway ramp, and once I was sure I could steer I put the pedal to the metal. Everything worked perfectly. I pulled off at Coldwater Canyon and headed down Mulholland Drive for the city's unofficial road racing stretch. With the motor in the rear and the hundred and fifty-pound sandbag up in the front for ballast, she clung to the road like a cat, purring smoothly with the double carbs and Bella's specially designed glass pack straight exhaust pipes. I came up on a little Mini Cooper S and hung on his tail for just a moment before flying past him on the inside and destroying his any attempt to stay with me. What a great feeling when his lights grew further and further back. My next chosen victim was a Porsche 912, who saw me coming and bolted. But it was not long before his lights, too, were fading in my rearview mirror.

Thursday nights on River Road were race nights, complete with the works, starter flags and all. We could normally get away with ten or twelve races before attracting the LAPD, and we had too many cars tearing off in too many directions for them to get us all. A week or two lay-off after a police raid, and we would be at it again. The Green Beast was blowing minds and blowing away the competition, going undefeated for weeks. Our first defeat came to a set up 911 S after I got a poor start. And, to make matters worse, I looked into my rearview mirror and saw the red flashing lights behind us. Our only way out was the on-ramp to I-5. We took off again, still racing as we left the police far behind in the dust.

This is when my car racing momentum reached terminal velocity. Just when you think you are racing away to freedom, the unexpected clamps on the brakes. But, funny enough, it was the very lack of brakes that slowed my racing days. The strange burning smell, the loss of control, and the realization that I was without brakes sent me fighting with all my strength to tame the Green Beast I had heedlessly unleashed and which was now wildly barreling down the interstate. Barely missing cars, swerving back and forth across five lanes of traffic several times, I pumped the brakes once again, but the pedal went to the floor. The next thing I knew, I was spinning and then going backwards down Interstate 5. The next thing I remember was hitting the embankment, sending dirt and ivy flying and blinding me as I just barely missed a light pole. As I came to a halt I was shocked that the car was still in one piece. The rampaging Green Beast had torn out about 100 yards of shrubs and plants and came to a stop, cock-eyed at a 45-degree angle. I got out and checked my vitals, amazed that I was in one piece. My car, on the other hand, was missing a rear wheel, and the brake drum was sanded in half. Well, that explained the burning smell.

Within seconds, the first cop arrived, with sirens blaring and lights flashing. I expected the worst, an irate cop set on street racer vengeance, but he was astounded after witnessing the entire catastrophic show. Initially speechless, he eventually commented on how my wheel had shot off down the freeway and that he had no idea where it ended up. We both admired the sanded-off brake drum and partially sanded-off rear tail section, the only real damage to the body. A minute or so later, another equally astonished cop pulled up on a motorcycle and eagerly offered to help find my tire.

I waited next to my car with the first cop as the motorcycle cop went looking for my runaway tire. In all his years, he had never seen an accident like this. I still expected the riot act to come, along with severe consequences. But as we sat and looked at the skid marks not more than one inch from the light pole, he simply shook his head in amazement and said, "That was one hell of a light show. The sparks from that busted brake drum lit up the road better than any Fourth of July fireworks, and all without hitting another vehicle." He looked at me with a sly smile and said, "You are one lucky son of a bitch."

He did not write me up. I could consider it my lucky day, but I would still have to pay for the replanting of the obliterated ivy and the tow truck to wench me up and tow me home. I was thanking him profusely when the motorcycle cop pulled up from the other side of the freeway, calling out excitedly and holding up the rubber circle, "Hey man, I found your tire."

It cost me $150 for freeway repairs and another $250 to tow the Green Beast back to Bella's shop. The following day we found a break hub and were back on the road. If the dead owl was not a strong enough sign that this car was bad news, those skid marks inches away from the light post surely drove the message home.

I ended up selling the Beast for $6,500 to an adventurous young girl. She saw the sign in the window and fell in love with the look of the car even though her father forbade her to purchase it. She came back a day later, paid me cash, and said she was going to hide it at her girlfriend's house until her father calmed down about her buying what he referred to as "a sure death trap." I couldn't argue with that. The deal was made and I kept my lips sealed.

Grapefruit Knee

With street racing, pushing the limits meant not only matchless speed but also unparalleled risks, including crushing impacts, jarring collisions of steel and concrete, and eruptions of fuel and flames. With little hesitation, I sold the death trap that was the Green Beast, but my hunger for speed and danger remained. Downhill racing on a ski slope was the perfect transition, faster than surfing and more forgiving than cars if you blew it. Or so I thought.

During my final year of high school my friends and I spent as many winter weekends at the mountain as possible. Planning to move to Mammoth and devote my life to downhill racing, I could not wait until graduation. I followed through and moved north the winter of 1969, landing a job at the

Mammoth Mountain Inn as a parking lot attendant. Skiing all day and parking cars at night; it couldn't have been better.

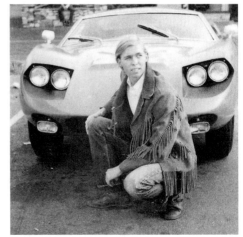

Just after my arrival, the mountain was hit with one of the biggest storms on record, creating well over a 50-foot base of snow. At the bottom of the cornice run, a huge ramp called Hair Jump emerged after the storm. If you hit it right you could go about 30 feet straight up, hopefully

"The Green Beast," my Ford GT, the car that almost killed me

clearing the flat spot on top and landing on the down slope on the other side. Of course, I decided to see just how high I could go. I started my descent from a much higher point than anyone else had attempted, and sped down so fast there was little doubt that I was headed for one of the biggest launches of the day. And boy did I launch. Easily climbing 35 to 40 feet up, I began to fear that venturing to this altitude was beyond my capabilities. It was surreal, soaring so high above the ground, but then shockingly sobering after realizing I was not going to clear the flat spot. The landing was an explosion of skis, poles, and flailing limbs. Then everything went black.

When I awoke, a few skiers that had witnessed the soaring flight and violent return to earth were already tending to me. I immediately attempted to get up but came to an unsettling realization that I could not move my right leg. When I looked down, it felt like I was dreaming again. I was in disbelief of what I saw on my own body. With the precision of a scalpel, the edge of my ski had severed my kneecap as cleanly as any surgeon could. I had never seen a cut so deep, yet was even more amazed by the reaction of the human body to such trauma. The tendons and ligaments were neatly severed, but, surprisingly, there was a considerable lack of bleeding.

It would take a couple of very skilled surgeons to put me back together again. As luck would have it, two esteemed young surgeons who recently returned from Vietnam had opened a practice in Mammoth. Dr. Eckerdt and Dr. Steadman served as medical carpenters, performing their magic in reconstructing my knee. Dr. Eckerdt used a miraculous new technique that

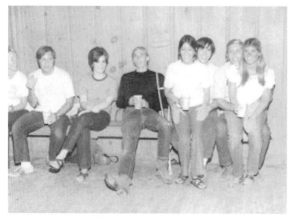

Down to one crutch,
but not the last time on crutches

he had developed sewing up our soldiers in Vietnam, and I surely benefited from the knowledge he gained from his days knee-deep in the rice paddies fighting to save the lives of hundreds of men. I lay in the hospital in Bridgeport, California, struck with a new perspective. I was here by my own doing. I knew I was a full-blown adrenaline junkie, feeding the growing addiction that held potentially very painful consequences.

I knew very well what I was doing, but it could not be stopped. Not even my leg in a barrel cast could stop me from skiing. My girlfriend at the time, was also addicted to speed. She had recently competed in several National Standard Races (NASTAR) and was becoming a rising star. Unfortunately, she too lost a bit of her sparkle when she returned from a race in Steamboat Springs with a cast on her ankle. We were quite the pair, with our two casts.

One day after I had recently gotten out of my cast, my girlfriend was out shopping while I stayed behind and built a big fire, our only source of heat in the little cabin we shared on Old Mammoth Road. I had dozed off in front of my roaring flames, as snug as a bug in a rug, and was lost in my dreams when I resurfaced to reality to what sounded like somebody yelling. I rolled off the old leather couch, still half asleep, and heard the yelp once again. I opened the door and found my poor girlfriend completely stuck in the snow. It had snowed heavily and her cast and crutches made the already precarious path, which was about fifty yards from the road, close to impossible to use. She had been out there for almost an hour, too embarrassed, or should I say too stubborn, to call out. In her mind there was nothing she could not do, and to call for any assistance was to admit she needed my help. When I found her, she was frozen to the core, teeth chattering. How could my heart not go out to her? I grabbed her, hugged her close, and carefully lifted her into my arms. The snow was deep and my leg was still very week, but cautious step by cautious step we made our way to the cabin door. We were just about there when the snow gave out from under my foot, sending her cast down right on top of my reconstructed knee.

I heard an awful tearing sound, the sound of all of my inner stitches ripping apart. Excruciating pain soon followed. Now we were both stuck but at least closer to the cabin than before. We lay defeated and pissed off for a few minutes, but then we looked at each other and could not help but laugh at how absurd we must have looked, embracing the breakdown.

We eventually dragged ourselves in and collapsed by the fire. By the next morning, the pain had subsided. I was feeling optimistic and figured a hot bath might do me good. Oh, boy, was I wrong.

Relaxing in the tub, I watched in awe as my knee suddenly swelled to the size of a grapefruit. My girlfriend walked into the bathroom and let out a gasping scream at the sight of the grotesquely ballooning joint. We did not know what was happening, but knew we had better get to the doctor before it exploded. After even my baggiest of pants failed to fit over my knee, I yelled for her to bring me a blanket. I'll never forget the look on her face as she wrapped me in the blanket and shrieked again that it had gotten even bigger. With her hobbled condition we were completely immobile. Good thing we had a phone. She called two fellow Mammoth racers and they came over to help carry me to the car, then into Dr. Eckerdt's office. He took one look at my knee and said to grab a bucket.

"We are going to drain this thing," he said calmly and moved the huge knee around a bit. "You sure must love Bridgeport Hospital, because that is where you are going again."

I spent another week in the hospital after Dr. Eckerdt repaired his own handiwork. Much to my relief, I would ski again, and even jump again, perhaps even better than before. However, I was setting a strange trend with everything happening twice.

Boy Scouts and "My Son The Bum"

I was in the Boy Scouts as a kid, mostly to make my father proud after my older triplet cousins had all achieved the highest rank of Eagle Scout. To be an Eagle Scout meant you were the best of the best, a top honor. Star scout was the highest rank I would ever reach, and I would come to develop my own ideas of honor.

Two of my older friends, Mike and Joe, did go on to become Eagle Scouts, pursuing the path of the best and brightest right off to the early days of the Vietnam War. One day, Joe's younger brother came over to show me Joe's most recent letter home. Sent along with the letter and pictures was a gift, a wooden beaded necklace with a beautifully carved peace symbol. Behind the symbol hung a human ear. I will never forget the sickening sight of the little hairs on the withered ear, the ear of a Vietcong soldier now ornamented to prove and celebrate a kill, apparently an honored gift in Joe's mind. The pictures displayed my buddies standing on a pile of dead bodies, smiling proudly like scouts playing king of the mountain. They did not look like kings to me, but rather like boys caught up in the horrors of war. I did not see the best of the best but deranged victims of a senseless power struggle.

Soon my friends started coming home in boxes. Sadly, it was not long before I was at Joe's funeral. I stoically watched the ceremony, the 21-gun salute, the presentation of the flag to his parents, and the draping of his coffin. None of it seemed to represent the young man that I camped, surfed, and grew up with. I went to Malibu that afternoon, paddled out, and said a prayer for my friend. Out in the water, on the periphery, I gazed in toward the shore and knew in my heart that I was looking at a world gone mad, and I finally broke down and sobbed. The ocean, with its swells and currents, was my only comfort, and I rode wave after wave, for once feeling in control. The ocean is a great place to release; everyone has red eyes. No one knew I was crying. But I knew and will never forget that day.

In 1969, the military draft was governed by the lottery system, where numbers were drawn from a hopper to determine who would go first. My number was high, so it was not long before I received my papers to report to the Army recruitment station for my physical. If I passed, I would be sent off immediately. These were desperate times, and people were doing all sorts of things to get out of the draft. I considered fleeing to Canada, but I just could not run away. I turned to my father for advice, but it seemed like my father would rather be handed a flag than save his son. He would only say, "I went to war, now it's your turn."

I felt more like a symbol than a son as I left that morning for my physical. I packed my overnight bag and my toiletry kit because if I passed, I would not be going home. They stripped us down to our underwear and herded us around like cattle, poking and prodding. The guy in front of me had tried to starve himself for an exemption. He was at least six foot four and could not have been a hair over a hundred pounds, nothing more than a skeleton with skin. His Fruit of the Loom underwear hung off his bony ass, and every time they would pull out a needle, he would pass right out, collapsing to the floor. Certainly, they would not take this walking dead man. But me, I was not so sure.

I looked down at the huge scar wrapping around my knee, a scar I was once confident would keep me out of this crazy war. I had called Dr. Eckerdt and asked if he would write me a letter, but he refused and said that actually he had fixed it better than new. He added that he had even seen me win a few races with that "bad knee," and if I could ski on it, I could fight on it. I was left to figure this out on my own. When it came to the part where they asked you to get down and squat, a brilliant thought came to me. I had been the star of a school play, and if there was ever a time to act, this was it. The sergeant came over and said, "Get down and squat."

"Look," I said, pleading to him that I could not get down because I had a knee replacement. "Here is the scar to prove it!"

"Where is your doctor's letter?"

"I didn't get one," I replied.

"Then get down and squat," he yelled. I started to squat but then keeled over, grabbing my knee and rolling around on the floor, acting as if I was in excruciating pain. He helped me up and sent me on to the next station like nothing had happened. My act did not seem to impress him.

I went through all the other bells and whistles, and when we came to the final table, the walking dead man was just ahead of me. When they asked him to get on the scale, he was shaking like a leaf. They slid the weights, and the sergeant looked up with a smile, saying, "A half-pound over. We will beef you up. You're in."

Shit! If they took the walking dead man, I did not have a chance. I got on the scale. The sergeant weighed me and passed my chart to another soldier, who took his time reading through it. He asked to see my doctor's letter regarding my knee, so I repeated my story about my knee replacement and apologized for not having a note. He looked at the scar, looked me right in the eye, stamped my paper and handed it back to me. I couldn't believe it. I was 1Y, which meant I was out. I yipped and yelled, barely remembering to limp out.

It was not my day to be sent off to die. On cloud nine, I returned home to show my father my new draft rating.

"So what does this mean?" he asked.

"It means I'm out," I could not help but beam back.

"Well, are you going to school? If you want to stay here at home and go to school, I will support you. I'll give you everything you need for college, just like I did for your sister."

"That's not for me dad. I'm going to Hawaii."

"If you want to go be a beach bum be my guest, but you will not get a dime out of me. If you want to be a bum, be a bum. My son, the bum," he said, repeating it to himself while shaking his head.

I never looked back. Hell, I didn't think I would live past 21, with all the madness erupting in the world around me. The country was clearly messed up, and with all my friends coming home in boxes the one thing I knew for sure was that I wanted to make the most of my life. I would show him I was no bum. He lived his life his way, and now it was time for me to live mine, my way.

CHAPTER THREE

If You Can Wait And Not Be Tired By Waiting

Insanity 101

My buddies and I decided to drop acid and go surfing. It sounded like a good idea at the time. The sunset, the surf, a perfect six to eight, the north shore of Oahu absolutely glowing; no better time to glow ourselves. We had gotten our hands on the famous Ozzlees's Sunshine acid, the very stuff lighting up the Grateful Dead and much of the Northern California coast in the late '60s. We were instructed to take a half a dose each, but looking out past the surf to the shimmering horizon, surely feeling six-foot-six, two-fifty, and bulletproof, we each took down our own little orange barrel. We smoked a joint and paddled out to the advancing energy walls, anxious to greet the unknown beyond, feeling ready for the adventure to the hidden dimensions of our own minds. For this coming trip, however, I do not think I was equipped.

Finally living full time in Hawaii, I was enjoying the life of my dreams, actually expanding the very limits of my dreams with each new physical and mental expedition. My Hawaiian dream began with a search for the perfect wave, bringing about my first voyage after I graduated in '69. I came back for the ski season at Mammoth, but as soon as the snow turned slushy, I was on a plane to the islands again. It was a good life, ski for six months and surf for six months, but it was not long before the ski trips got shorter and shorter and the islands became my home. At Queen's and Three's, two of Oahu's world class breaks, I shared waves and began hanging out with surf legends like Leroy Achoy, Reno Abilero, and Felipe Pomar. Leroy was a good friend of Joey Cabell, who owned the Chart House restaurant. Leroy ran the valet parking concession for Joey, and when one of Leroy's parking attendants abruptly had to go home to Kauai, he asked me to help. Just like at Mammoth, I could park cars at night and play all day, charging epic break after epic break. What a life.

Afloat in the line up, waiting for the Sunshine to kick-in, everything looked a little more beautiful than normal, but that was to be expected. We were all still expectantly waiting for the real magic to rain down. I had done acid a few times before, but never this much, and this stuff was supposed to be the best. My first acid trip was somewhat fittingly during my high school graduation ceremony, what a group of us saw as our very own defining leap forward. We started coming on during the commencement exercises, and, to be honest, we barely got through them. Trails brightly streamed off my diploma when the principal handed it to me, his face morphing into floating cartoon features. I could not help but burst out laughing as he shook my hand. Right after the ceremony, high as kites by this point, we rolled right on to the bus headed for our all night grad party at Disneyland. We laughed at the characters, we laughed on the rides, we laughed at each other; we could not

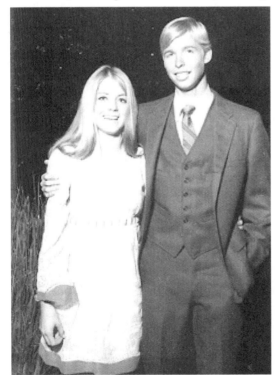

stop laughing but also could not find our bus at the end of the night.

Our parents loved that one! I imagine they were not laughing when the principle called and reported us missing. Ah, the memories rolled back to me as we paddled out into Hawaiian perfection.

We had a great three-hour surf session, but when we paddled in, all agreed that we had not felt much beyond the joint.

Grad-night at Disneyland. Do we look like we are on acid?

"Let's find the guy that sold us this shit and get our money back," declared my good buddy Rick.

We went our separate ways and it was agreed that whoever found the guy that had burned us with this bunk shit would get our money back. I headed home, a little bummed out, but slowly it started to become quite obvious that we had not been burned at all. In fact, as I started to come on it was blatantly clear that class was now in session, the bell was ringing, welcoming me to take a seat in Insanity 101.

First, my face went completely numb, and when I looked in the mirror, it shifted into all kinds of strange contortions. I called Rick and asked if he was feeling anything. He said that he could not move, but that his walls were moving. Instantly, my walls started moving too. Coming closer and closer, closing in on me. I had to get out, and I figured I would try to walk it off with a stroll down to the international marketplace. The streetlights gave off the most radiant halos, absolutely fixating my attention. Until I saw the cars. One by one, every car on the road transformed into a cartoon car with a big, smiling face. Then they started jumping out at me, funny at first, but then it got scary. The faces lost their smiles, and I was sliding, sliding down the slippery slope of paranoia.

Fighting to stay up, I proceeded to the market's Fun Zone and put a quarter in the pinball machine. The first ball I sent up never came down, and I wondered if I ever would as well. The points racked up exponentially as the ball never even came close to the flippers. I was clearly blazing now. The ball shot and bounced in all directions, lighting up random pockets and corners, and such was the state of my mind. Thoughts ricocheted off one another, lighting up my brain. My mind racing at full blast, I could not think a full thought. Every thought tripped open ten more thoughts, which seemed to trigger ten more, half thought upon quarter thought, upon eighth thought. Oh my God, I was going crazy.

A friend lived in an apartment nearby, and it seemed like a safe place to be. Antagonizing cars still leaping out for me, I dodged them on my way down the sidewalk. I finally reached his apartment building, and the numbers melted right off the door as soon as I looked at them. I knocked, and, thankfully, a pretty little hippie girl let me in. A few people sat around smoking grass, having a mellow little party. I joined them, trying not to give myself away, but my mind was going full blast and now even the people were melting. A little later, we were all sitting on my buddy's big waterbed, somehow being supported by the termite-weakened floorboards. As I was fixating on a potential crash through the floor into the apartment below, we suddenly started melting into the waterbed. Lost in some crazy trip of her own, the hippie girl had been unconsciously playing with her hairpin, repeatedly sticking it into the bed. Just like the *Wizard of Oz*'s Wicked Witch of the West, I was melting in the water that, in reality, was now actually soaking everybody on the bed. I was already on the verge of freaking out completely, but when the management called about the downstairs tenants being leaked upon, the thought of the cops sent me flying. I attempted to descend the staircase, but found it futile, because I was now stuck on an escalator going backwards. Finally, back on the street, the damn cartoon cars came again.

Would the ball ever drop? At this point, I did not think so, but somehow I made my way to Rick's apartment by one in the morning. Rick, a little sleepy and obviously back from his own trip, let me in.

"I'm on a bummer Rick," I cried. "I don't think I am ever going to be the same again." I told him about my paranoia, the cars with faces, the waterbed, the escalator, the never-ending pin ball game. He just laughed.

"Sleep it off on the coach," he said. "Boy that was some really good shit. And think, we thought we got burned." He handed me a little blue pill and said, "The antidote."

Popping the downer without even a drink of water, I eventually started to come down. Rick went to bed, and my brain began finding a more comfortable pace, when a blue light came through the window and engulfed me. Immediately overwhelmed with the utterly calming feeling of understanding, I became a radio receiver picking up God's voice, a transmission from the divine, loud and clear.

"Only when man stops killing other living things and only eats what was given to him by me, will there ever be peace on the planet. As long as man kills, he will be killed."

Everything began to make perfect sense. Everything settled into its right place. I was being given the answers to the problems of the world.

"Violence becomes violence. Peace becomes peace."

I decided that in case my insanity returned, I had better write my dad a letter and explain everything, make everything right with us. I was overcome by the intense desire to come clean with every lie I had ever told him and to tell him I loved him and was sorry for all the problems I had caused. I had not talked to my father since abruptly leaving home after escaping Vietnam, but my first instinct in this moment of clarity was to erase the distance that had built up between us with an honest letter.

I found some paper and a pen and began composing this letter divinely guided from the Main Man himself. I wrote how I was the one who stole the coins from his collection, replacing them with wrong-dated coins that he later discovered. I wrote how much I loved him, but I might never think a sane thought again. I continued to tell him about every drug I had ever taken and how this letter might be my last documentation of what little sanity I had left. Then it dawned on me that insanity was just another point of view. I immediately felt better with that revelation, but if I did, in fact, go crazy in this moment of perfection, I needed to come clean with it all to my father. After completing the soul-baring letter, I calmly walked outside and mailed it. Everything looked beautiful.

Upon waking up the next morning, the strange paranoia returned, and then reality struck. I remembered writing the letter, and then, worst of all, I remembered mailing it. Oh shit, my dad was going to think I had finally done it and cracked. This letter was going to kill him. He already thought I was a bum, now he would see me as a liar, a drug addict, and a crazy bum. I ran down to the mailbox and waited for the mail carrier, confronting him as soon as he made his way up to the box.

"I mistakenly mailed a letter and I need to get it back," I pleaded. My letter was right there on top when he opened the box, and I reached out for it.

"Son, you can go to jail for that. You are messing with the U.S. mail," he snapped as he grabbed my arm.

"But my letter, it's my letter, I can prove it!"

"It's ours now."

I begged him to no avail, and the letter was sent. My father was the kind of man that saved every letter my sister or I had ever written him. We had our differences, but I knew he was a good man. He did not deserve the worry this letter would cause him.

A few days later, my sister called. I had followed her through school inescapably labeled as Betty Jo Thorp's little brother, both an honor and a curse. She was the queen of everything, even crowned homecoming queen at San Jose State that year.

She was the good one, and my father immediately called her about the letter. She then promptly called me to say that Dad had read her the letter and that he had broken down in tears.

"This is all I have left from my drug addict son the bum," he told her. He was so hurt. He kept that letter to his dying day.

One thing I can say about my father is that I never doubted his love for us. Even though it may have been tough love, it was the purest of all love, unconditional. When we finally spoke again, he reminded me, "Only when you have a son or a daughter of your own will you ever know what it is like to worry whether they are safe."

The life I had chosen and the alternative paths I had taken worried my father greatly. It may have been unorthodox, but it was my way, a breaking and challenging of walls of perception and barriers of fear. I was desperate for my father to understand these pursuits, yet I would have to be patient to reveal there was something bigger, an overarching plan and philosophy. Until that day, I would have to continue to find reassurance in intuition and faith.

Nothing But Integrity and a .45

Doc was close to death by the time help arrived. I was covered in blood, mostly Doc's but plenty of my own, so the cops came right over to me.

"I saw it all," I said.

The cops escorted me home and asked if I would repeat my account of the incident in court. I most definitely would.

"It could create some real problems for you," they warned.

"Six to one, that was not a fair fight. Screw 'em!'"

The following day my roommate, Ric, decided it might be a good time to take a vacation, and he packed his things quickly. Someone had told him some Hawaiian heaveys were going to kill his roommate. He left me alone in our apartment, my Colt 45 on my knees, waiting for them to kick in the door and kill me.

My father and I may have been thousands of miles apart, both geographically and in our relationship, but I never felt closer to the sense of honor he imparted during those Friday Night Fights next to him on the living room couch in Burbank. My path was patently different, but entrenched in the very same integrity that my father had used to plow his own way, and for this I could hold my head high, which wasn't too bad an idea since my eyes had better be scanning for whoever or whatever was coming for me. My guts had gotten me into another mess, and I was wondering if this time guts would be enough to get me out of it.

I had met Doc while parking cars at the Red Vest. Rick, my buddy with the antidote, called one day and said that his roommate was moving back to Florida, leaving an opening at the Red Vest for a valet. He also offered me his roommate's bedroom, and, best of all, their apartment was directly behind the Red Vest. I met some interesting characters while parking cars there, none more memorable than a black pimp named Doc. Although he never would admit he was a pimp, he was into some shady businesses, pimping surely being one of them.

One day he said he was going to open a little restaurant inside the nightclub across the street, the Red Noodle. We had become friends, and he asked for my help, of course offering to pay for my time. After finishing my lunch shift at the Red Vest, I showed up to help with his opening night. Doc's restaurant was located in a back section of the club that had been previously used for storage. The club's bouncers, a handful of the scene's biggest Hawaiians and Samoans, had grown accustomed to using the rear restroom that was now located in Doc's new restaurant. Since the restroom was behind the counter where the cash register was located, Doc decided to close it off to all but his personal employees.

When the first Samoan bouncer came back to use the restroom, he was not very pleased to be denied the use of it by Doc. A few minutes later he returned, this time with the entire Hawaiian and Samoan crew of 300 pounders who made Doc seem small in comparison. They immediately blocked the door, and the offended bouncer took a free hit at Doc. Possessing a well-built, 200-plus pound frame, chiseled on the toughest streets of Harlem, Doc was capable of fighting back. And fight back he did, knocking the hell out the big Samoan. But then all hell really broke loose as all six ganged up on Doc, kicking the shit out of him until he was barely conscious. With nobody else around to help, I jumped on the back of one those monsters and pulled him to the ground. Another bouncer grabbed me by my throat and raised me up, leaving my feet dangling like a rag doll. I cracked him between the eyes, which slightly loosened his grip on my neck. He slammed me up against the wall a couple of times and muttered, "Cool it brah! It's not you who we want."

I continued to struggle with this burly dude until he tossed me aside as if I was a pestering child. One of them was blocking the door so no one could come in or get out as the beating continued. They picked up the now unconscious Doc and threw him out into the back alley, coldly threw him right into the big rolling trash bin, without a shred of concern or remorse. As they cleared out, they all glared at me on the ground, one of them saying, "You didn't see anything, if you know what's good for you."

I immediately went outside and dragged Doc back inside to the bathroom, the trivial source of this senseless brutality, and I began trying to clean him up when one of the bouncers returned.

"What are you doing, you fucking Haole," he yelled at me, and I knew I was in for it. But just as he went for me, the cops walked into the room. I have never been happier to see a cop in my life. When the police started asking questions, nobody said a thing. I was sickened as witness after witness denied seeing the attack. How could they stay quiet after witnessing such a vicious beating?

I could not stand by and keep my mouth shut, not only for Doc's sake but also for what was right. I told the cops everything they wanted to know, and now I was left with nothing but my integrity and my Colt 45. For two days I waited and watched, but, possibly thinking I was a little too crazy, they decided not to mess with me. They never did come crashing through the door, and I followed through and testified. Without my testimony the case held little merit. On a daily basis both Doc and his attorney, David Shutter, promised to take care of me monetarily after they received the settlement. But when it was all over they never offered a dime. I did not testify for the money, however, or even the gratitude. The empowering feeling from standing up and doing what was right was simply enough. Doc did take me out to lunch to thank me for bravely doing the right thing and said that he would never forget it. I never saw or heard from Doc again.

Unknowingly, this was my introduction to the local Hawaiian Mafia. At the trial, the only thing the Samoans and hawaiians could say was that I was one crazy Haole. Standing up against them actually gained their respect and eventually made me one of their limited Haole friends.

Somehow stepping through another perilous window, narrowly escaping with my life, what had not killed me was indeed making me stronger. And at 19 years old, I was left wondering what other challenges might possibly be out there for me. What else was waiting beyond the limits of even my own dreams? What I did know was that I was healthy, confident, and beginning to better understand the divine guidance that blessed us all if acknowledged and accepted, a validating voice from within now only growing louder.

First Encounter From Above

On a hazy morning in late 1972, three young men bounced along the Oahu dirt road in their rusted-out surf car, their sites firmly set on the peaks ahead. They each silently marveled at the cliffs, which dramatically shot 1,300 feet straight up above the Waimanalo coastline. They had noticed an arrangement of towers up on the very top, so they figured there must be a road or at least a path of access to them. After following several dead ends, they found a gate locked by a chain with several padlocks. Undeterred, they climbed the fence and followed the paved road that indeed led them directly to the top, where they found a spot more perfect than they could have even imagined. For this clear path to the top, they could thank the U.S. government. Unbeknownst to them, further down the road actually serviced a military compound and an old missile site here at the top of the Ko'olaus.

The Ko'olaus is a mountain range jutting up out of the Pacific Ocean, created by a series of ancient volcanoes. The range starts just after Sandy Beach, rising from the ocean to the Makapuu light house and extending over 25 miles through Waimanalo, Kailua, Kaneohe, Haiku, Valley of the Temples, Waialua, and ending at the sleepy village of Kahuku, home of the famous Kahuku sugar mill. Its cliff face runs the entire length of the northeast side of Oahu. It is here where the powerful trade winds blow straight in and then straight up the face of the incredible cliffs, the consistent flow creating the perfect lift.

That same morning, my girlfriend, Kim Scott, who later became my wife, was lying on the beach at Waimanalo. Kim and I had met the year earlier, at Manhattan Beach, California, where I was visiting my sister. It was love at first sight. But when I met her very young and single mother things really got exciting. Remember, this was the hippy days and the attitude of "make love not war" of the late sixties and early seventies was in full swing.

Her mother made us feel everything was just perfect, no matter what age we were. There were components slightly similar to the movie The Graduate, infamous at the time, about a college kid having a relationship with his girlfriend's mother. My feelings for the two of them were confusing, to say the least. To be clear, I never actually made love to Kim's mother, but we did everything but, including the favorite drugs of the late sixties and seventies. I was a kid in a candy store with a drop-dead beauty on each arm even though they were mother and daughter. I left Manhattan Beach to return to Hawaii, and it was not long afterward that Kim's mother allowed her to come and join me. She was just fifteen, and I had just turned twenty.

We were lying on the beach below these very cliffs when we noticed something that we had never seen before. A large object was floating above us. At first glance, we thought it was a parachute, but then we realized it was a glider of some sort and there was a man attached underneath. The strange glider peacefully circled above, descending closer and closer, and then flew directly over us and landed on the beach a hundred yards away. Absolutely blown away by what we had just witnessed, Kim and I immediately walked over to get a closer look at this crazy flying contraption. Little did we know that this encounter would change my life forever.

When I approached the pilot, it was like looking in a mirror. He was a man about my size, with eerily similar long blond hair and blue eyes. If you looked at the two of us together, you would say we could be brothers. He greeted Kim and me with a warm smile, extending his hand and introducing himself as John.

"Me too. My name, that is, John," was all I could say as I enthusiastically grasped his hand. Already in awe of what I had just witnessed above, within just a few minutes I felt like I had known him all my life. I was excited now and began asking him all kinds of questions, which he calmly and efficiently answered while he methodically rolled up the wings of his flying craft. This was my introduction to John Walbert and to the exhilarating new world of hang gliding.

It was not long before his two companions pulled up in the rusty, beat-up surf car, complete with a couple of hang gliders folded and tied to the top. The two men jumped out yelling and screaming, ecstatic over what their buddy had just accomplished. John introduced me to Harvey Baumgartner and Ray Hook, two more hang glider pilots, now bursting over John's epic flight. They broke out a six-pack of beer, and we all sat around celebrating. We had just witnessed the first hang glider pilot to soar off of the now legendary Makapuu Ridge.

One encounter was all that was needed. I was hooked! We followed them back to their apartment on the Ali Wai canal. An assortment of gliders, fashioned from bamboo to plastic, filled their courtyard, many ripped and torn. They told me the daunting story of each broken glider's demise, and, more importantly, what they had learned from each crash.

"That glider came apart on me at about 50 feet in the air. I hit the ground so hard it knocked the wind clear out of me, broke a few ribs, and I pissed and spit blood for days," said Ray, explaining the brutal lessons leading to their glider advancements. "It was definitely time for something stronger."

His words took me back to my first flight with my dad's umbrella and its lack of strength, which led to the painful memory of being strewn out and bloodied in the front yard. As Ray continued his stories, my vivid childhood dreams of flying with the birds came rushing back to me. Those wild dreams as a kid, the ones I would cry to my mother over because I ached so badly for them to be real, were now laid out before me. They would soon be remarkably manifested into reality.

They were all going flying again first thing in the morning, and they welcomed me along. Lost in my thoughts, sleep would not come that night, my mind rolling over and over the scene of John hovering in the air above us and knowing that would soon be me. Morning finally came and brought howling winds, but when I arrived at their apartment Harvey said that I was in for a treat. The first stop would be a little alteration along the road to the Makapuu launch spot. When we arrived at the padlocked gate, John pulled out a large pair of bolt cutters from the trunk. There were several locks on the gate, but by cutting one of the chain links they could add their own lock. We now had direct and lone access to what would soon become arguably the best flying spot in the world. Proud of ourselves, we proceeded through the gate, drove the narrow paved road to the top, and arrived at a positively breathtaking view. You could see half of Oahu from up here, a view tourists would pay handsomely to access, and it was now ours.

It was a short hike to the spot where John had launched the day before. From here, the cliff was utterly vertical; if you dropped a rock, it would easily fall over 1,000 feet without hitting anything. We would soon name every portion of this incredible cliff. New records were set weekly flying on these reliable trade winds. On a good day, you could fly all the way to Kahuku. To many of us, it became our sacred home, and for those that were not so lucky and perished here, a place to scatter their ashes.

We waited, but the wind remained overwhelming, blasting at 30 to 40 mph. Harvey also explained that the wind was blowing from the wrong direction. Always instructing, he pointed out the distinct wind lines on the water moving nearly parallel to the ridge. It would be impossible for anyone to fly off Makapuu under these conditions. The easterly wind direction was bad for the cliff but perfect for the sand dunes of Kahuku. As luck would have it, the dunes would be a perfect place for me to attempt a first flight.

An hour later, we arrived at Kahuku Golf Course. The strong winds made arduous work of setting up the gliders, requiring the combined efforts of everyone, one to hold the nose down and the other two to open the wings. With the help of Harvey holding the nose down and into the wind, John demonstrated how to balance the glider. When Harvey lifted the nose up to just the right angle, John ran as hard as he could, gently lifted off, and made a 30-second soaring flight above the sand dunes. Harvey flew next, and although he did not stay in the air as long as John did, he made an utterly beautiful landing down the beach. Now my time to learn to fly had finally come. Harvey held the glider by the front wires and let the wind carry it up the dune. I hooked the seat belt around my waist and let them guide me into position. Harvey held the nose down and instructed me in how to handle the awkward glider. My heart was pounding while I tried to balance the glider. One moment it weighed nothing, and in the next instant it weighed more than one could possibly hold and slammed into the ground.

Harvey and John had made it look so easy. But I was strapped into this thing that wanted to pull me off my feet in every direction but the direction I wanted to go, which was down the face of the sand dune. Harvey yelled at me to keep my wings level. Scared shitless, all I could think of was the destroyed gliders back at their apartment. What if I go shooting straight up 50 feet and wind up pissing blood like Ray, or even worse? They say flying is easy; it is the landing that will kill you. Harvey was still yelling at me and snapped me back into the moment.

"As soon as the wind backs off I'll give you the signal," he said, and just a few seconds later he yelled, "RUN!"

I took a deep breath and tried to run, but the nose of the glider lifted abruptly, instantly yanking me straight up off my feet, and then drifting off to the right.

"Pull in," Harvey screamed over the wind.

Yanking the bar hard into my stomach shot the glider straight down the face of the dune and slammed my head into the sand and the control bar into my stomach. With my head embedded in the soft sand and the wind throttled out of me by the bar, I gasped for air as they eventually lifted the glider off me and dusted the sand from my head and face.

"Don't pull the bar in so fast. All your moves should be smooth and controlled, not jerky," Harvey directed patiently. "Use your weight to control the direction of the glider, and the nose angle will control your speed. Then push the control bar out to slow down and pull it in to speed up."

I was rapidly trying to digest all his instructions while spitting sand from my mouth and picking it out of my eyes and nose when he finally caught my full attention.

"Stop fighting the wind," he said. "You have to join it."

Still noticing terror in my eyes, he said one very important word, "Relax!" He let that sink in and then finally continued, "When I say run, run. And this time go with the wind, and if it pulls you to one side shift your weight to the other."

The wind backed off once again and Harvey lifted the nose. When he asked if I was ready, I was no longer sure if I really wanted to continue, but Harvey was persistent and repeated the question. I lied and said, "Ready!" This time when Harvey yelled *run*, I ran hard, with a death grip on the bar. When the nose lifted off, I was looking straight down at Harvey while rising straight up.

"Pull in," he yelled.

Remembering what happened the last time, I gently pulled in. The glider corrected, and flew. I flew above and past Harvey when suddenly it dawned on me that in all the excitement, nobody had told me how to land. Getting closer and closer to the ground, I heard Harvey shouting to push out. I eased the bar out and began to slow down as I approached the water, skidding to a stop on my butt just short of the surf.

Harvey was jumping with joy as he followed down the beach, and he helped me up just as a wave rolled in and soaked our pant legs.

"That was great. Next time, just put your feet out and you will land perfectly."

We carried the glider back up the dune, where John stuck out his hand.

"Welcome to the club," he announced.

I wasn't exactly sure what I had done and if it could be done again. Nevertheless, it had sent me to cloud nine. Harvey gave a little more encouragement and offered me a few corrections. He said to lean my weight to the right and head parallel to the beach this time, not straight into the surf. I was still in fear mode as we got the glider pointed in the right direction again, but he lifted the nose so I could see him and said with the biggest of smiles, "Same as you did before, only this time put your landing gear down. And when I say flare, push the bar out."

I launched again, repeating the previous scenario, but this time everything went perfectly, with a stand-up landing even further down the beach. The rest is history. On the ride home, Harvey assured me that we were ready for the next level, so if the wind stayed the way it was today he would take me to a 100-foot hill over in Kailua along Pali Lookout. I had survived my first flight but was wondering if my luck would hold out. At over 100 feet, was it wise to depend on luck?

Flying The Pali Lookout

In 1795, after already conquering Maui and Molokai, King Kamehemeha I, the Hawaiian Island's unifier and first king, won the pivotal battle for Oahu by driving more than 400 of Kalanikupule's soldiers off the cliff of Nu'uanu Pali, sending them to a gruesome death 1,000 feet below. According to legend, King Kamehemeha continued to use this windward facing section of the cliff as his judge, jury, and executioner for any and all in opposition to his rigid authority. King Kamehemeha and his followers would throw the accused from the cliff, leaving their fates in the hands of the winds shooting up the face of what is now Pali Lookout. If innocent, a strong wind would propel them back up to the ledge; if guilty, the winds would accordingly fail to prevent the ghastly plunge to certain death. On the day of the trial, a prisoner would pray desperately for the salvation of a powerful wind.

Committed to learning to fly or to die trying, my judgment day had now arrived. I do not fully understand and cannot exactly explain what was driving me into Pali Lookout's fickle hands of fate, except that, somehow, it felt like destiny. I had returned home from the previous day's flights at the sand dunes a new man. After anxiously sharing my adventures with Kim, I endured another fitful, sleepless night, impatiently waking every hour on the hour in anticipation of first light. With only the faintest shades of dawn approaching, I was en route to the guys' apartment, and I sat mesmerized in the driveway, staring at the gliders, until Ray eventually wandered out wiping the sleep from his eyes.

"You are up bright and early," he said.

"Harvey said to get here early before the wind gets too strong," I countered. Ray nodded and went to go wake him. Thirty minutes later, Harvey and I were on the road to Pali Lookout.

We unloaded the glider off the top of the car and shared the task of carrying it, evenly distributing the considerable weight upon our shoulders. We would not be going to the very top of the lookout, which was just fine with me. One hundred feet was more than enough of a test. Harvey swung his machete, chopping our way through an overgrown trail, until we came to a small clearing on the Kailua side of the Pali Highway. This was the spot, Harvey announced, and he told me of the many flights he and Ray enjoyed here. He pointed out another clearing a couple of hundred yards below and said, "That, over there, is your landing zone."

Twenty minutes later, the glider assembled, I positioned the plastic seat under my butt and strapped the seat belt around my waist. An incredible amount of adrenalin pumped through my veins, combining with fear to create a mysterious alloy of pervading calmness. As a pioneer in an untested, possibly deadly sport, my survival meant unwavering trust in my own reactions and an unflinchingly honest assessment of my own courage and ability. The rest was up to the wind, God's breath of life. Like the prisoners awaiting a divine verdict nearly 200 years before me, I offered a prayer.

Harvey positioned the glider into the wind and held the nose down, no different than he had done for me at the sand dunes. Only this time we were readying for a takeoff over a hundred feet in initial altitude. Also, the highway was just off to my right, so I definitely did not want to drift in that direction to have my fate abruptly decided by an oncoming windshield or fender. This was outright insanity, but my feet continued to walk the glider to the edge, and I pushed those thoughts out of my mind as Harvey gave his last instructions and asked if I was ready.

"Ready," I yelled out, once again a fearful but bold lie. It is tough to muster a "ready" when affirming your willingness to leap to uncertain injury or death.

Yelling above the strong winds and the flapping Dacron sail, Harvey called out, "The next good cycle of wind will be it." I could feel my synthetic wings filling with air when Harvey screamed, "Go!"

Charging forward, my feet quickly escaped the earth, climbing upward, higher and higher and higher. "Oh shit!" I yelled in panic, but within seconds the fear receded as my survival mechanisms took over. The prior day's instruction thankfully came flooding back, and I reminded myself, "Relax." I enjoyed the view and noticed a line of halting traffic as the cars passing along the highway below caught site of a flying man. Then I helplessly watched my projected landing zone pass along right underneath me. The glider was still a hundred feet in the air. The fear returned. Maybe this was the day I was going to die. I flew away from the highway, toward the jungle, and began rapidly skimming the treetops when I pushed out to slow my descent. I felt the lift fill my wings again and take me climbing away from the dense green below. Then everything got strangely quiet; that reassuring whistle of flight and the flapping of the Dacron sail were absent. I had pushed the control bar out too far, sending the glider into a stall. The nose dropped, my speed alarmingly accelerated, and the jungle raced closer at a frightening rate. I somehow managed to evade a penetrating collection of banana trees, and before hitting what I assumed to be the jungle floor, I once again pushed out the control bar, perfectly this time, and landed softly in a thick bed of vines, branches, and towering green shoots. Slowly, the glider and I started sinking deeper into the jungle until it completely swallowed me up, covered and out of sight from everyone that witnessed the wild flight, including Harvey.

Pummeled by wave after endorphin-filled wave, I was hooked and awakening to a new, incredibly addictive feeling. Born again as a true adrenaline junkie. Blissfully amused by the screeching tires of motorists pulling over to question if they had really just witnessed a man soaring out of the sky, only to disappear just as abruptly into the enveloping jungle, I sat for ten minutes until hearing Harvey yell for me.

"I'm OK!" I called out and was immediately greeted with the hooping and hollering of Harvey's relief and excitement. Good thing he had brought along his machete, because he had to chop his way through the thick jungle for several minutes before he reached the entangled glider.

"Wow, John, that was unreal," he exclaimed. "You should have seen all the cars that almost crashed watching you fly."

It took us over two hours to chop away the jungle's twisting hold. Then, after a grueling trek back to Harvey's car, we found two of Honolulu's finest graciously waiting in their patrol cars for the crazy pilots of Pali Lookout to emerge. We had not broken any laws, other than maybe trespassing, and since nobody had complained, they were just glad we were not injured or dead, in which case they surely would have had a real mess on their hands.

"Don't let us catch you two up here again," one of them warned. "This is private property, and I am sure the landowner would not be happy to know you were crashing into his land without his permission. Plus we don't want to be filling out any reports about any dead hang glider pilots." They got back into their cars and pulled away shaking their heads.

We headed directly to the liquor store for a six-pack celebration. Harvey had me beaming as he continued to express his excitement over how well I flew and how far I had gone, a new record off that spot for sure since I had been in the air for at least a couple of minutes. When we got back to the apartment, Harvey made sure everyone heard about my flight, appearing equally adrenaline-charged from the morning's adventure. Most importantly, nothing was damaged on his glider or, thankfully, on me. Any landing you walk away from is a good one, a certainty I would come to know very well.

I felt like I had just walked out of the very shadow of death. Before all of nature, history, and even King Kamehemeha, I had been pardoned, exonerated by the divine order of the wind. I felt more alive than ever before.

Flying Anna Bananas

A few days after my perilous flight at Pali Lookout, we were at it again, the next stop another 100 foot mountain in Kailua. This time, however, replacing the thick jungle below was a broad cow pasture. The hill, already soared many times by John, Harvey, and Ray, was dubbed Anna Bananas after the bar located directly across the street from the takeoff spot. They had all enjoyed long flights here, many over five minutes, and John had once stayed in the air for almost 20 minutes. This would be the perfect place for me to attempt a soaring flight.

One thing about this sport was that you were always rewarded with an incredible view; the distraction was welcomed as we lugged the bulky glider up the narrow trail. With the glider set and ready, I scanned the distance. This place looked good. The pasture was wide and long, plenty of room to plan a landing. Feeling confident and beginning to understand what to look for in the wind and surroundings, I felt good. The wind was steady, at a consistent 10 mph. Harvey held the nose up, the wind filled the sail, and he yelled to go. The takeoff was successful.

I leaned to my right, and the glider flew to the right. I corrected to the left, and the glider straightened out. Above a gathering of cows running away from my encroaching shadow, I pushed out the control bar gently to extend my glide. This time landing on my feet, it felt like I was becoming a hang gliding pilot. Once again yelling and screaming, Harvey ran down the hill to greet me. I think he was more excited than I was about the successful flight and landing, and I thanked him profusely for not letting me give up. We each made a couple more flights and called it a day.

Several of the patrons at Anna Bananas had watched us fly, which made us the stars of the day and the drinks were on the house. What better way to end a perfect day than enjoying a free beer.

When we got back to the apartment, Ray was putting the finishing touches on a new glider. He said that he wanted to build four identical gliders for all of us, for our team. If I wanted to buy one, the offer to join the three of them was on the table. Six hundred dollars later, I was on the team.

We sat around one evening to brainstorm what we should call our fledgling hang gliding group. We settled on DOVE. Development Of Vertical Expression became both our label and our aspiration. Going higher, real fast, was the pursuit, and we soon realized that if this rising team of aviators was going to push the limits and survive, it would take stronger and lighter gliders and a team effort to design them.

The design approved by all, we quickly ordered the aircraft aluminum (5/8" thickness), rip stop Dacron for the sail, and 1/8" wires with stainless steel swedges (double swedged for safety). With Harvey, John, Ray, and I at the core, and with the help of a few others who lived near or at the apartment building, we transformed the complex into one of Hawaii's earliest hang gliding manufacturing plants. Our dream manifested, the four of us stood like proud parents over the four matching blue and white gliders lining the courtyard. They looked beautiful. With the leading edges measuring 16 feet and the nose angle at 90 degrees, these gliders were heavy and built to handle the forceful trade wind flow. At least we hoped so.

Flying Hanauma Bay

Harvey was trying to convince me that it did not matter if the glider broke at 100 feet or 1,000 feet: "You could already have killed yourself at any of the spots you have flown," he said. You were dead either way, so what was the difference between a few hundred feet? I could not argue with his logic but cannot say it provided much comfort either as we drove every morning to scout the top of Makapuu. So far, the conditions had not allowed us to repeat what John accomplished that day Kim and I sat awestruck from the beach below. To be honest, I let out a sigh of relief every time we got to the top and found the wind parallel to the ridge. There was no doubting my commitment to hang gliding, but no matter how much you could prepare for Makapuu, that cliff and its 1,300 foot sheer drop still scared the shit out of you.

Just when I thought I had escaped to live another day, Harvey said we had another option, Hanauma Bay. John and Harvey knew the lifeguards there and had a key to the gate. Hanauma Bay, located just east of Honolulu, is a marine embayment formed within a volcanic cone. With its aquarium-like crystal clear waters, the bay is one of Oahu's premier snorkeling spots, making it one of the most popular tourist destinations on the entire island. At one time accommodating over three million visitors per year, the bay has suffered somewhat from overuse. Portions of the reef were dynamited in the 1950s to make more room available for swimming.

Our takeoff spot was up on the rim of the crater, at about 400 feet. John, Ray, and Harvey had all successfully flown from this spot, but John had a painful reminder of the treacherous conditions often surrounding this ancient volcano. Flying a prototype bamboo glider off the top, he crash-landed halfway down, breaking his leg; however, he was quick to dismiss the injury to poor judgment. He expressed full confidence in the bay's flight potential under the correct wind direction.

Today the wind was blowing in perfectly, and the lifeguards granted us permission to fly at sunset after most of the tourists had left the beach. We ascended the narrow paved road in a caravan to our takeoff spot, unloaded our gliders and started setting them up one by one in a true team effort. We tied the noses down to the tent stakes we had pounded into the ground and waited for the tourists to leave. At five o'clock, the lifeguards waved a big red flag, our sign that it was now safe to fly.

John would be the first off, Ray second, and if they both had good flights, Harvey would launch me. I watched both John and Ray make perfect flights, although the wind was so light that they basically took a direct sled ride down. Harvey told me once again to relax. "Just take your time," he said, "and when you are getting close to the ground, start your flare."

The adrenalin began to flow along with the butterflies now, making a mess of my stomach. Harvey and I went through our routine, and in a few seconds my glider was airborne. I leaned to my right to follow John and Ray's flight path when an unexpected patch of turbulence almost ripped the control bar out of my hands. I yanked the bar back in toward my stomach, and when the glider responded pushed it back out so gently that the glider began to rise again smoother than ever. The air was calm now; the wind in my ears was like nothing I had ever experienced before. I shifted my weight to the left and glided steadily toward the beach. I thought I had followed John and Ray's path perfectly but was soon running out of beach below. My only option was to try to turn back toward the water's edge and hope that I could land before going out over the Pacific. But I had no such luck. I glided over John and Ray to make an otherwise perfect landing in knee-deep water. Once again, any landing you walk away from is a good one, even if you are knee-deep in the ocean, so you wouldn't catch me complaining.

We looked up to see Harvey pick up his glider, point it into the wind, and launch himself with only a few steps. He made beautiful "S" turns and quickly joined us with a perfect landing. As we celebrated with beers at the beach and talked over the day's flights, John noted my corrections for turbulence and said that tomorrow might be the perfect day for Makapuu. The turbulence, he explained, was caused by the wind switching, coming more from the northeast, the ideal direction for Makapuu. As we headed back to Waikiki, the wind continued to change to perfect off-shores, so it looked like tomorrow would indeed be my day to soar from Makapuu. Everything was evolving rapidly and challenging my comfort zone, but flying seemed to be in my bones. Plus, what was a few hundred more feet?

Soaring At Makapuu

Once again, I was at Harvey's first thing in the morning, but this time I found everyone up and busy preparing. Apparently I was not alone in anxious anticipation. Harvey introduced me to Byron Akiona, who they had brought on board to act as driver and to assist in launching the last person. We packed up the gliders and tied them securely to the roof of the car.

The gate was unlocked when we arrived, a situation we had not previously encountered, and we drove ahead fearful of finding an obstacle other than the wind that might prohibit us from flying that day. We had not traveled far when we came upon a Honolulu Electric crew working on the power lines. They were far up the pole, and we drove by acting like we owned the place. We got to the top, scrambled out of the car, and, like mountain goats, were at the summit in seconds.

The view was breathtaking as always, but, more importantly, the wind was blowing right up the face at a perfect five to ten mph. We set up the gliders on the level below the summit, and Harvey stayed above to call down the wind conditions. Just as before, John would be first, Ray second, I third, and then Harvey last, launched by Byron.

John picked up his glider with his head protruding through the triangle control bar, and like an awkward duck began climbing the 15 feet up the volcanic path to the summit. In deep concentration with every step closer and closer to the edge, he turned to us and confidently told us to stand back. The wind was light enough for an unassisted running takeoff, and when Harvey yelled back that the wind was coming right up the face, John took a couple more steps and was gone, diving out of site for just a few seconds. Then, in awe, we watched him rise above us and make a turn down the ridge. He flew back and forth effortlessly, yelling down at us the whole time. Now this was flying, the flying from my dreams as a child, and as I watched my friend playing in the wind I could hear my mother's voice saying, "If you can dream it, you can do it!"

Ray was in the air in a matter of seconds as well, soaring with John above the ridge. They made it look so natural, and it is hard to describe the separation from reality I experienced while watching them, knowing I was seconds away from freeing the destiny long embedded in my soul, seconds away from flying like the birds. I knew all of my previous flights were in preparation for this moment; all my life's defining moments had brought me to this summit. There was no turning back now. I held the glider up, made sure my wings were level, and waited for Harvey's word. "It's perfect," he yelled, and I took a deep breath and ran off the edge.

The nose of the glider rose abruptly and then there was dead silence. It is amazing how fast the human mind works as it replays your prior experiences, because in less than a second my mind computed what that silence meant, and it could only mean one thing. My glider was in a stall. My mind flashed back to the sand dune when everything went quiet and to the painful consequence of slamming head first into the sand. Once again,

I overreacted and pulled in too quickly to regain my airspeed. Thankfully, I was still over a thousand feet above the beach, descending rapidly but with plenty of time to prepare for a landing.

I looked back and up and could see that John and Ray were still soaring hundreds of feet above me. Sadly, now out of the lift area, it was too late for me to make it up to join them, so I had no choice but to go for the landing zone. I practiced a few turns and the glider reacted perfectly. I began to calm down and enjoy the incredibly peaceful feeling of flying. There was no way I was going to make the landing zone, but the good news was that the tide was low, leaving plenty of sand for a landing further up the beach. At about a hundred feet above the ground I heard the laughter and sounds from the people below, taking me back again to my childhood dreams where no one would look up to notice me flying. In this reality, everyone was looking up. Cars were pulling over; people were climbing out and pointing to the sky, saying, "Look! Look!"

My concentration returned to the sand rapidly approaching. Twenty feet, then ten feet, and just before my feet hit the ground, I heard Harvey's familiar words resounding clearly in my head, "Push out!" I came in with a perfect, stand-up landing on the sand, and the people immediately surrounded my glider to bombard me with questions and adulation. I could get used to this, I thought, but underneath the heaps of adoration, I knew I had blown it by pulling in too quickly. And that was why my glider was resting here on the beach, and John, Harvey, and Ray were still up in the sky. With envious eyes, I could only watch as they continued to soar silently above.

A few minutes later, Byron pulled up in the chase car and was relieved to see that I had made it down safely. We loaded my glider on the car, and as we pulled away I waved goodbye to all my adoring fans. Because I overreacted, I had missed the landing area by over a quarter mile, and if it had not been for Byron watching where I went down it would have been a long hot walk with a very heavy glider to get to the landing zone. There was still a lot to learn.

An hour later, John, Harvey, and Ray all performed perfect landings at the designated landing zone. Byron went for some beer, and the four of us sat around sharing our flight stories as we all had something to celebrate.

Harvey and Ray had stayed up longer than they ever had before. John had climbed up onto the control bar and flew the glider while standing up, a trick no one had ever seen or even heard of before; and I had made my first flight off of Makapuu,

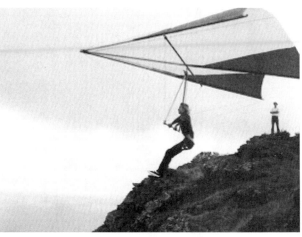

Flying off Makapuu Ridge in my first hang glider

flying further, longer, and from a higher altitude than I had ever flown. We enjoyed a couple of beers, feeling like intrepid astronauts having just landed on the moon.

Kim greeted me at the door with a kiss and a big hug. When she asked how it went, all I could say was that I was still alive. I explained to her how I had screwed up and was unable to soar with the other guys, but she reminded me to be proud that I was now one of the elite few to ever fly off Makapuu ridge and then hugged me close and asked if she could come along tomorrow. We made passionate love that night, and as I lay in bed watching her sleep as the rain fell on Waikiki, I could only feel gratitude for the incredible experiences of the day, for this life I was living. Once again, the thought crossed my mind, "Will I live through tomorrow?" But I also wondered will I have soared?

CHAPTER FOUR

Or
Being Lied About, Don't Deal In Lies

The Body Does Bounce

The next morning we were back at it again, up at the top of Makapuu to scope the conditions. The wind was much stronger now but the direction was still good, so it wouldn't be a long wait for another chance to soar. Having never flown in such strong wind inspired a few doubts, but I launched anyway and I was finally flying like the birds. All four of us were soaring together, and we maneuvered gracefully about each other in the fierce wind, becoming the first formational acrobatic hang gliding team in the world.

With every opportunity, we strapped on our wings and flew past our limitations. In a time of radical new ideas and when everyone seemed to be searching for a distinct identity, we had found our own through the unique experience of hang gliding. My life felt like the makings of myth and legend, but as with most mythology, there were always a few hard lessons to be learned.

Without flying or surfing, a day was incomplete. "Sorry if I am acting like a jerk, but I did not get my adrenalin fix today," was a common excuse I delivered to Kim. Looking back, I can admit it was all about one thing: me. I was a jerk, a selfish guy. All addiction is detrimentally selfish. It would

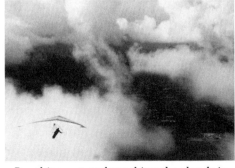

Reaching out and touching the clouds in my comet

not be long until I discovered the particularly painful consequences of a flying addiction.

There were many days when the winds were just too strong, too light, or coming from the wrong direction for Makapuu, which kept me constantly searching for new takeoff spots. One day, driving around alone, I stumbled upon a place with great potential on the side of the Kalanianiole Highway. Just past Waimanalo was a drop-off over a new housing development. I looked at the takeoff and thought, "If I could just clear those new home foundations, I could fly all the way to the valley below."

I unloaded the glider from the top of my car and quickly set it up. I waited for just a few minutes to see if anyone would pull over to assist me in my launch, but I had no such luck. I would have to do this on my own. I strapped myself into my seat, rocked the nose of my glider upward, and, feeling the wind in the sail, I ran. It was a perfect takeoff, and the glider soared easily above the housing development below. I banked to the right, got some more lift, and flew over the new terraced foundations, with altitude to spare. Then, out of nowhere, I hit the unseen rotor and downdraft that was out there waiting for me. I frantically tried to push out but slammed dramatically into the last housing foundation, butt first. I hit so hard that it felt like all my blood rushed to my feet, and my feet were going to explode. The last thing I remembered was that I bounced, doing a front tumble and landing upside down tangled in my glider, submerged in the jungle at the bottom of the ravine. A pleasant darkness followed as the pain was replaced by unconsciousness.

I lay at the bottom of that ravine for over two hours before Harvey thankfully happened to be driving by and saw my unattended car on the side of the road. He pulled over to see where I was and may have kept on his way if not for spotting a small part of my blue and white sail sticking out of the jungle below. Harvey came to the rescue, machete once again in hand, cutting his way through the brush to pull me out. I could barely move, let alone climb back up the embankment, but Harvey managed to get me back to my car. The horrifying paralysis steadily faded, and, luckily, I was able to walk the following day.

One lesson was clear: the body does bounce. More importantly, it was becoming harder and harder to deny that there must be somebody looking over me. I hit the ground way too hard to simply walk away, and if it was not for Harvey driving along that road I probably would still be hanging upside down in the Hawaiian jungle, my remains an archeological lesson, a modern day Icarus, sharing his fatal flaw of thinking he was a god and could fly to the heavens. As Icarus got closer and closer to the sun, his wings melted, and he fell from the sky and died a humble mortal death. I too had now suffered, but ultimately hoped to make the necessary corrections to escape his harrowing fate.

We were not the only ones flying hang gliders in Hawaii in the early '70s. The popularity of the sport seemed to explode, with pilots coming from all over the world to fly the renowned cliffs of Makapuu. Incredibly talented people, men and women who understood and shared our passion for flight and freedom, soon surrounded us. A community of winged warriors, we launched our bodies from the tops of just about every windward facing cliff on the Hawaiian Islands, often soaring from Maui's Haleakala volcano at sunrise and then off Makapuu's cliffs at sunset.

On a full moon, we would set up camp at the top of Makapuu. We would build a campfire, drink beer, cook steaks and corn on the cob, and then fly off into the brilliant moonlit sky. It seemed to me that everyone in those days had his or her heart and soul in the right place. Life was good.

In a sport where one mistake could kill you, this valiant group of pioneer pilots and their gliders were holding up surprisingly well. There were a few broken leading edges and bent control bars, but no one had been seriously injured or killed. Nevertheless, miscalculations were inevitable. Although they only resulted in minor injuries, they increasingly exposed the glaring risks we took on a daily basis.

One painful incident, the product of a simple miscommunication with my launch man, occurred as he held my wires, preparing to launch me from the cliff. Believing he heard me say to go, he dropped the nose of the glider prematurely, and I was flung into a nose-down takeoff that slammed me into a boulder and bounced me into the air. My back rear flying wire got hooked on my swing seat's metal hinge. This caused the glider to make an instant right turn and sent me streaking out of control down the face of the cliff. "Oh, shit, this is it!" I thought once again.

I have already mentioned my guardian angels; this was another one of those times when they must have been there. The wind hit me perfectly and lifted me up and over the cliff edge. I landed, standing on my feet, on the lower level where everyone was setting up. Either the boulder I hit, the swing seat straps, or possibly a combination of both dislocated my right shoulder. My glider was mostly undamaged, just a groove in my swing seat hinge from the wire. Nothing a hammer and a metal file could not fix. A quick trip to Castle Hospital's emergency room fixed my shoulder, and a few weeks later I was as good as new and back in the air. Saved by those watching above or by merely a random wind gust, I knew I was lucky, and I seriously worried that sooner or later, for me or for someone else, this luck was going to run out.

Carl Burman, one of the top tandem pilots on the islands, had a crash very similar to mine. His nose was too high on takeoff, causing him to stall and crash his glider back up on the top. He walked away uninjured but broke a leading edge of his glider. Instead of waiting for a new leading edge to come in from the mainland, Carl felt that he could fix it on his own by splicing the edge together with an aluminum aircraft sleeve. He had seen others repair a leading edge this way and was confident it would work just fine.

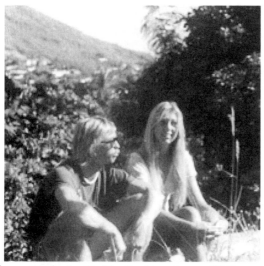

My first wife, Kim Scott, and me - 1974

A few days later, on a full moon night with perfect conditions, Carl felt it was time to test his repaired glider, which was fine with me except for one thing. He asked Kim to fly with him. Since I had not become a tandem pilot yet, Kim was forced to fly with others and had gone up several times before with Carl. Kim and I argued all afternoon about the condition of Carl's glider, and before leaving for work, she had to promise me she would not fly with him. Kim had recently become my wife. My sister and brother-in-law had recently become lay pastors. They came to visit, and, appalled by our "living in sin," had marched us down to the courthouse for an official proceeding. Admittedly, I saw our marriage as nothing more than a formality, but I did love Kim and was not about to lose my girl to Makapuu.

She was very angry with me, saying that if I always went flying when I wanted to, why couldn't she? I told her to wait until Carl took a test flight and tried to explain my uneasiness about the larger piece of aircraft aluminum he had used. I questioned if it would flex properly or create a dangerous shear point. If Carl thought it was safe, it must be safe, she argued, reminding me that Carl was a builder and that I was just a test pilot. I left for work that night with an extremely pissed off young wife.

At about ten o'clock I got a call from Kim. I could tell she was on the edge of tears, and I immediately asked what was wrong.

"I love you so much," she cried. "You were right. Carl died tonight." The news reported that a man was killed in a hang glider accident but was withholding his name until his family was contacted. She received call after call from our friends asking if I was okay, and although she could relieve them that I was safely at work, she knew right away who it was.

It was indeed Carl, and I soon learned the full details of what happened. He had taken off just as the full moon was rising. His takeoff was uneventful, and everything seemed to be working perfectly. He made several passes over the launch spot, yelled down that everything was fine, and then flew about one hundred yards away from the cliff and cranked an aggressive turn in front of the launch platform. That is when the wing tip snapped, and, sadly, my shear point theory proved to be accurate. He crashed into the cliff and died instantly.

It took four hours before they could extract his body from the cliff with a helicopter. We were blessed in Hawaii with one of the best helicopter pilots in the world, Tommy Hauptman. Tommy could rescue people from places other pilots would not dream of approaching, hovering inches from a cliff in greater than 35 mph winds. It was tricky and we were actually lucky that nobody else was killed that night. Finally, we got our fallen brother's body into the chopper.

I held Kim tightly in my arms that night, thinking how fragile we really are.

The Rainbow Glory Phenomenon

It was not long before Kim was back in the air with another great flyer from Kauai, John Hughes. Test flying various gliders and taking them to their limits was not the right time to have my loving wife Kim on board with me. However, I felt comfortable letting her fly with John, an intelligent, highly evolved spiritual being, and, most importantly, he possessed excellent flying skills. It was always great to see the smile on Kim's face as I would pull up next to them, our gliders just inches apart. With the help of John, a true gentle giant, we shared many special moments flying together. Although Kim flew with him every chance she could, it was time to get a tandem glider, as I was anxious to directly share these incredible experiences with her and my friends.

I bought a twenty foot Wills Wings glider with an all white sail. Wills Wings was one of the first mainland hang glider manufacturers, and its creator, Bob Wills, was an early participant in our soaring flights around the islands. Bob even set one of the first world hang gliding records with a flight off of Makapuu.

John Hughes had also recently purchased a new high performance glider from Wills Wings and promptly began putting it through its paces. After about two hours in the air, John attempted a maneuver that went wrong, terribly wrong. He attempted a whip stall, and when the glider fell back through, it inverted and John tumbled to his death. We had lost another brother.

Everyone that Kim had flown with had died hang gliding, so I decided it was not a good idea for me to take her flying in my new tandem glider. Actually, Kim and I never flew tandem together. Those moonlit nights would soon claim victim after victim, making it impossible to deny the extreme danger inherent in my passion. Call it superstition, call it whatever you want, but trusting my instincts over anything or anyone else may very well be the reason I'm still here today.

The big glider got its first test the following day and flew perfectly. The sail was extremely quiet and the stability was unbelievable. With it easily passing every aerobatic maneuver, this glider would certainly be the one to use to share my soaring experiences with others. A few pilots had already started charging for tandem rides, so I decided that tandem flying would become my new occupation. To get paid to do what I loved would keep me in my passion 24/7.

My friend Byron Akiona and a few others helped me set up the big 20-foot glider. With perfect wind conditions, I was off within minutes. The glider was performing unbelievably well. It maneuvered like a much smaller craft, and most impressively had me flying higher than anyone out there. Skying out, a term we used when the lift was so strong and perfect that the altitude barrier seem nonexistent. The perfect lift, thus allowing us from the moment of takeoff, where for the first time the clouds were not a limit, it was here, above the clouds, that I witnessed something strange I had never seen or heard of before.

A perfectly circular rainbow enveloped the shadow the glider was casting against the clouds below. Was this some kind of religious experience? It felt as if my body had slipped the surly bonds of earth, climbing upward and upward to touch the face of God. The luminous halo appeared just like God's eye watching over me.

This phenomenon was a glory rainbow and had a scientific explanation. It was not uncommon for pilots to see them from their aircrafts. If the sun shines at just the right angle above your craft, whether it's an airplane or a glider, a shadow is created on the clouds below. With just the perfect amount of

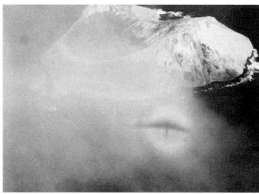

My first glory rainbow above Rabbit Island –
"I thought I was having a religious experience"

moisture and the perfect angle, this shadow on the clouds creates a glowing circular rainbow.

Rational explanation or not, the experience is powerful. Talk about meditation, this was it for me. I found transcendence in the presence of the glory rainbow. It felt like I left my body behind on the cliff, with only my mind, the wind, and the divine now directing this flight. Feeling completely cared for yet completely free, I stayed in this euphoric state for almost three hours before finally drifting back down to the reality beneath the clouds.

Getting hungry, I soared back over to my landing spot and noticed several cars were parked around my sign. Ah, customers, time to put on a show, complete with aerobatics and whip stalls all the way to the ground. After a perfect landing on the beach, the bystanders—and hopefully future customers—greeted me with applause and cheers.

This was why we took the risks, why we carried on after the tragic losses of our fellow gliders. We continued because of what we were finding up there above the clouds, what we were learning about our place in the world, and about ourselves. There was nothing I would rather do or share with others, and now I would have the opportunity to do both. Unbeknownst to me, hang gliding would soon bring opportunities and adventures beyond what I could even imagine.

Give The Kid a Shot

I was flying alone, making sweeping turns for what felt like hours over the beach at Waimanalo. It was 1975, and with years of experience already under my wings, flying was as natural as breathing. I was living my dream and could not imagine what could come next.

Having just landed my glider on the beach, I noticed a convertible full of typical tourist types all decked out in classic floral patterned aloha shirts. Two of the gentlemen approached me to shake my hand and comment on the shear beauty of what they had just witnessed. I was pleased, thinking they were a couple of potential customers, and entertained their questions about my background and the consistency of the conditions at this location. We carried on a casual conversation, they took my information, and we went about our ways. After they did not call that next week, I never really gave them another thought.

About a month later, the phone rang, and it was one of the impressed gentlemen. It turned out they were interested in more than just a thrilling vacation memory. He introduced himself as Ernie Pintoff, director and screenwriter. The other man I had spoken with was Randy Spangler, a location manager, and Bernie Ozzransky one of the head producers for the hit CBS crime drama *Hawaii Five-O*. Seeing me fly over Waimanalo that day inspired Ernie and their creative team to craft a screenplay about a hang glider pilot who witnesses a murder from the sky. He wanted to know if I was up for doing the stunts for an episode they were calling "Turkey Shoot at Makapuu." Sign me up! I was on board in more ways than expected.

The story was about a girl who witnesses the murder of her friend from above while flying in her glider. Naturally, as the only witness to the murder, the killers have to kill her too. However, the twist comes when the hang gliding girl lets her brother test her glider, and, sure enough, the killers shoot down and murder him instead. As they described each stunt, they would ask me if I could do it. With a lump in my throat growing bigger and bigger, I would unhesitatingly say, "Sure!" The most difficult stunt would be simulating being shot down while flying as the brother. It would require me to spin the glider out of control, hanging on with one arm as bullet after bullet ripped my glider and me apart. I would also have to crash the glider into the ocean, a stunt never performed before. To make matters worse, they wanted me to end the scene in the shark-infested waters off Makapuu out by Rabbit Island. They agreed to everything I requested, and it was now up to me to pull it off. This was going to be fun, not to mention profitable, but the priority would have to be safety first.

Flying over the location where they wanted to have the girl murdered would be impossible in a glider, due to the turbulent conditions and lack of a lift zone. So I suggested a helicopter could be used to get the shot. We hung the lower part of the hang glider and my normal swing seat under the helicopter, and then we rigged up another seat behind it for the cameraman, who was fully equipped with a bulky 35 mm Ari BL3 mounted on his chest. Propping his knees up against my back to stabilize himself, he could shoot directly over my shoulder and obtain the elusive aerial point of view (POV) from the glider down to the hit men. This was exactly what it would have really looked like from a hang glider's vantage point, and, needless to say, Ernie and the producers were thrilled.

I gave them my list of desired accessories and explained that they would have to buy me a new glider since we would destroy the one that landed in the ocean. They did not bat an eyelash, funding every one of my requests. So this was what it was like to work with the budget of a successful network television program. The show (running for 12 seasons, from 1968 to 1980, and holding the title as the longest running crime show on American television until the police drama *Law & Order* surpassed it in 2003) was in its heyday, and I was enjoying the liberties it provided. I was given the chance to play, but it would all still have to be carried out with professionalism.

The good Lord really looked out for me those couple of weeks as we pulled off stunt after stunt to perfection, without a scratch or a squandered minute. Pulling off top-notch, unprecedented stunts right out of the gate, I was treated like a king around the set. Each morning, they praised me for the feats from the day before, and I could not help but eat it up.

One particularly memorable and funny moment, at least to me, was during the final scene of filming. Molly, the original witness, crash landed on the beach. The show's star, Detective Steve Magarett, played by television icon Jack Lord, was supposed to jump out of the car and go see if she was okay. Doubling for the girl, I was lying under the glider waiting for the scene to play out. So here came Magarett and Dan'O, his trusted partner played by James MacArthur, racing in and skidding to a stop. They both jumped out in dramatic fashion. The only problem was that, unknown to most, Jack wore lifts in his shoes to make him look taller, and one of these lifts caught on the door base. Out came Detective Magarett, falling flat on his face. Honestly, it was the funniest thing I had ever seen. My laughter escaped uncontrollably and had me rolling on the ground in stitches. Then I realized no one else was laughing. Jack glared at me and eventually said, "John, it wasn't that funny." There was not a hole big enough to climb into.

Jack actually had a well-earned reputation for being quite hard on everyone. Jack was not only the unquestioned star and center piece, but also a co-creator and executive producer of the show, and everyone got nervous when he came onto the set. Luckily, I had developed a special relationship with Jack since the first day he saw me fly and came down to where I was putting away my glider to shake my hand. He asked me to sign his autograph book and write what it felt like to soar through the air. This was surely some absurd dream. Here was Stoney Burke, the rodeo saddle bronco rider on the 60's CBS series I had loved as a kid (Jack's first staring television role), asking me for an autograph.

Chuck Couch, *Hawaii Five-O*'s stunt coordinator, walked by while Jack and I were talking. Chuck was Jack's personal stunt double and had worked with him for years.

"So, what do think of this kid?" Jack asked him. "Would you do what he just did?"

"Not on your life," Chuck said, shaking his head.

Chuck shook my hand once again and offered another sincere, "Good job." Then Jack began to tell Chuck, right in front of me, how he really liked what this kid here did for them on the show and that they should use him if something comes up.

"He deserves a shot," Jack said. It was hard to believe he was talking about me. "He certainly has the guts, and he pulled off every stunt on time. Anybody questions why you're using him, tell them to talk to me."

A few weeks later they had me jumping out of the way of speeding cars, ducking punches and even being dressed as a girl, living the life of a stuntman. I was basically trained on the job, and every day was something challenging, different, and always exciting. I never looked back as the jobs kept on coming. They say you are either born into the industry or you get lucky. I was at the right place at the right time, but I was doing something I loved, which fortunately was something few others did. When asked to perform, with luck and my guardian angels, I pulled off every stunt. I was in, and best of all, never had to kiss anyone's ass to be there.

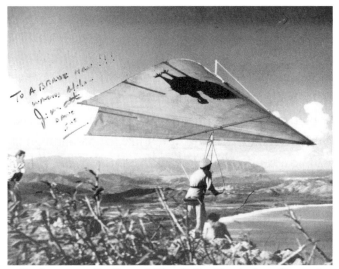

My first stunt for Hawaii Five-O, Jim MacArthur (Danno)
looks on. He wrote on the photo,
"To A Brave Man"

"Practical Jokes Can Kill You"

Hawaii Five-O kept me busy with stunt work the next season, and for the season finale, the producers brought back Ernie Pintoff, who created another hang glider episode that would feature my gliding stunts. They approached me with a script entitled "Practical Jokes Can Kill You." Many of the same characters would be back from the "Turkey Shoot" episode, and I was excited to have a reunion of the cast from my very first show.

The episode featured a daredevil prankster who landed on the top of buildings like a comic book super hero. His next big prank was landing on the top of the museum to "borrow" the ancient feathered cloak worn by King Kamehemeha. Molly (the same actress from "Turkey Shoot") and her new boyfriend ran a hang gliding shop, and Magarett pays them a visit to let them know that whoever the hang gliding prankster is, he will not have charges filed against him if the feathered cloak is returned to the museum. No big deal, until the bad guys hear about the stunt and kidnap Molly, who just can't stay out of trouble. They figure if this birdman can land on a museum, he can certainly land on the roof of the National Guard Armory and let them in to steal thousands of weapons. They threaten to kill Molly if he does not comply with their request.

Once again, the plot would demand a previously unperformed stunt. The script clearly called for me to land a hang glider on the roof of a building. Not an easy task by any means. The National Guard Armory sat directly behind the launch from Makapuu. By constructing scaffolding just above the armory building and with the help of a few camera cuts, it would look like the glider was coming in from a thousand feet above. Even with the scaffolding, this stunt could be extremely dangerous if I overshot the roof. We could use the helicopter as we did in the past for the other shots, and we assured the producers that it all would work.

Before any big stunt, the doubt starts to creep in the night before but actually creates a healthy apprehension that boosts your focus until you pull off the stunt. My every thought was especially calculated that evening before these obviously risky stunts. There is an industry saying that you are only as good as your last stunt. In the competitive business of television, this goes for the entire crew. Sadly, you are really only as good as your last job.

The grips, the lighting and rigging technicians on the set, had even nicknamed me "One Take," and my hard-earned reputation of getting the shot on the first attempt was on the line. No matter how many stunts performed, there was always a great satisfaction in hearing the director say, "Print it." Giving them what they wanted without wasting their time was sure to get you called back again, and a one-take stunt felt just like catching the winning touchdown pass. The crowd on set would go wild, and you were the star, but the thrill of victory one day could easily turn into the agony of defeat the next.

More focused than ever, I arrived at my 5:30 am call time knowing my only option was to trust in my preparation, my abilities, and myself. Like always, I showed up on time, even though I may not be called to the set until 5:30 p.m. or later. The life of a stuntman is to hurry up and wait. We would sit in our honey wagon trailers reading books, playing cards, or working the stunt over and over in our minds through meditation. Very seldom would we be out on set watching the actors doing their thing. Anyone in the industry will tell you, filming television or movies is really quite boring the majority of the time.

Finally they called for my glider stunt, and when the stuntmen appear on set, not a soul can be found in the trailers or hanging out at craft services. The actors show up, the producers get off their phone calls; everyone is standing at attention to see you risk your life to bring reality to their fantasy. Your outer appearance is one of complete confidence, even while your inside is churning with that nervous anticipation. Had you found every flaw? If something did go wrong, had you prepared your body to handle the impact? Conditioning is the key to survival, and you wonder if you had trained hard enough. Just after your last anxious thought, "Don't screw this up with everyone watching," the adrenaline begins to kick in and pushes aside all that useless self-doubt.

Before the stunt, I said my regular prayer followed by a deep breath. "Think it! Be it! Do it!" I repeated just before leaping off the edge. It all went perfectly, and I walked away one more time without a scratch. The wind was dead calm, and, as predicted, I was able to run off the scaffolding, barely clear the fence, and land on the roof of the armory. It all went off without a hitch, and once again, not a dime of time was wasted. With the help of my team, we pulled it off in one take and the touchdown pass was ours. A stunt or a stuntman is only as successful as the team cooperation.

CHAPTER FIVE

Or
Being Hated, Don't Give Way To Hating

The Restaurant Business

When I was not on set, in the sky, in the water or with Kim, I was still working at restaurants. Dealing in fine dining eventually proved no less adventurous than navigating the perilous winds of Makapuu or pulling off a demanding stunt for *Hawaii Five-O*, especially after I jumped from parking cars to sporting a white tuxedo at the door of a five-star restaurant. With money coming in from the tandem flights, it had looked as if my career in the restaurant industry was phasing out, but then I got in good with the boys at Mateo's, which sent me down a colorful path littered with uncountable precarious situations, the least of which involved the late night pirating of a Hawaiian icon's bed.

It all started when my good friend Rex Chandler, who managed a respectable Italian restaurant in the heart of Waikiki, pulled me away from my valet position at the Red Vest. The owner and chef, Matty Giordano, had grown up in Hoboken, New Jersey, with his childhood friend Frank Sinatra and had even been delivered by Frank's mother, who was a midwife back in Hoboken. Matty had spent time as Frank's personal chef, but eventually, with help from friends like Hooky the Bookie, Eddie the ex-Hit Man, and Jerry the Silver Haired Fox, he brought his traditional Italian cuisine to Oahu, opening Mateo's in 1970. When Frank or any of the Sinatra family or entourage was in town, Mateo's was naturally the hang out, and, lucky enough, they paid me to hang out with them. Actually, I was a waiter, but what a life. I could still surf and fly all day, and now, instead of riding the parking lot all night, I was rubbing elbows with a cast of characters pulled straight from *The Godfather*.

I enjoyed my time immensely at Mateo's, meeting interesting people every night, but soon one of those people would lead me away from "the family." I met Mark Rodden, the general manager of the five-star Nick's Fishmarket, and he mentioned that they had an opening at their front door. He was going out on a limb by even offering me the possibility of the position. They had never hired someone off the street into a management position, but I had already met Nick Nicholas, the owner, on several occasions, from parking cars at the Red Vest and also from seeing him around the set of *Hawaii Five-O*. Mark set up a meeting for me to sit down with Jeff Harmon, Nick's partner who was looking to lighten his load at the restaurant. As Jeff explained the simple duties at the front door, the pay and management's nightly access to the five-star menu, I could not believe my good fortune. After telling Jeff about my waiter experience at Mateo's, the deal was sealed.

I was now a hang gliding, stunt-performing kid in restaurant management. I spent a week with Nick behind the bar, a week in the kitchen, and a week on the floor to understand exactly how this prestigious restaurant worked. I loved it, and it was not long before Nick decided to take me under his wing and became my big brother, my mentor, and, most importantly, my trusted friend. This was like stumbling upon a full scholarship to the finest men's finishing school, all under Nick's careful guidance. Instilling an incredible

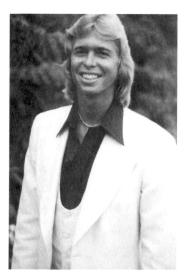

My nightly uniform at Nick's Fishmarket

confidence, Nick taught me to hold my head high no matter who I may be addressing at the front door of "his house." That is how he referred to his restaurant, and there was no doubt that this was the house that Nick built. I wanted nothing more than to bring honor upon it.

My father had raised an honest son of integrity, but I was unquestionably a little wild and somewhat untamed. Nick finished where my father left off, making me a gentleman, polishing me into a man with considerate sensitivities in relations with people, no matter what race, creed, or income level. He sent me to see his personal tailor,

Andy Mohan, who measured me up for a couple of first-rate tuxedos. "I want you to stand out," Nick said. "All the waiters are dressed in black tuxes. How about a sharp white silk one for you?"

If you did not know better you would think I owned the joint as I entertained the likes of Mick Jagger and the Stones; Crosby, Stills, Nash, and Young, Ted and the Kennedy clan. On any given night you could find mob bosses, entertainers, CEOs, congressmen, and pro athletes all mingling amongst the tables. I can't say enough about how great it was to work at the Fishmarket. Nick and Jeff really knew how to take care of their management team. They even sent me and the two other guys, Hans Van Renes and Billy Van Osteen, my partners at the door to Las Vegas, all expenses paid at Caesar's Palace, in the days of Irving "Ash" Resnick and the Jockey Club. Front row seats at the Follies Bergere and bottomless glasses of Dom Perignon led to a two-day romp with a couple of showgirls in our penthouse suite, one of which followed us back to the islands for a little more fun in the sun. There could be a book all in itself about the happenings and crew at Nick's Fishmarket.

Stealing Don Ho's Bed

One particularly adventurous night put all of us at the restaurant into a bit of a dangerously awkward position. It was the night before the Carol Kai Bed Race, an annual charity event started by the popular Hawaiian entertainer Ms. Kai that benefited a local school for children with special needs. Every restaurant and club in town would decorate a hospital bed the night before, and the following day, with usually one beautiful lady in the bed and the fastest employees behind pushing, we raced the rolling beds down Kalakaua Avenue in head-to-head elimination heats. The night before the race, when we should have been decorating our bed, we were sitting around the bar having our Pau drink with our normal afterhours crew of Marc, the GM; Billy Van Osteen (aka VO) Hans Van Renes, Eddie Campbell (aka The Soup) and Nate, the bartenders; and, of course, a few chosen lovely ladies. Nick came up to the bar, having had his share of drinks as well, and declared that since there was no way we were going to get a bed at this late hour, we would just have to steal one from someone else.

Nick had us in stitches as he began calling around saying that we were from the Carol Kai Committee and wanted to come by and inspect their beds. Most of the other restaurants were skeptical and immediately blew us off, but we finally found one that took the bait, the Polynesian Palace. This could not have been more perfect, as it was the restaurant of none other than the smooth Hawaiian crooner, Don Ho.

Don was Mr. Hawaii, extremely popular and actually one of the most powerful men on the islands. He mostly kept busy with his lucrative music recording and performing career, but his financial and personal influence branched all throughout the islands, and he had a clan of local followers who were as tough as they get. Don's boys were known for roughing up people who had wronged Don or who "didn't go along" with certain ideas of the organization, and leaving them in the cane fields. Many were retired vice cops or, worse yet, ex-Metro Squad guys. In the late '60s and early '70s, if the island's Metro Squad caught some Haole dealing drugs or ripping off a tourist, they would not take them to jail but would beat the shit out of them instead and drop them in an alley. Justice in Hawaii was served on the street, not in a courthouse.

Don's boys were above the law, and even Don had little control over them. Don would mention that someone had offended him or that an employee was not working out, and instead of being reprimanded or let go, as Don intended, the poor sap would wake up in a pig farm or a cane field. Don did not want anybody to end up in a field or an alley, but if they did, he did not want to know about it. Clearly, Don Ho and his followers were not to be messed with, and that is exactly what we at Nick's were planning to do.

When we called the Polynesian Palace and rolled out our Carol Kai Committee bed inspection bit, the girl who answered the phone was so sweet, saying of course we could inspect the bed, and letting us know it was right downstairs in the parking lot where they had just finished decorating it. She could not have served it up any better.

"Let's go get Don's bed," Nick joyously called out as he hung up the phone, leaving us all a little shocked. We all knew that nobody messed with Don, but we also knew Nick was no small fry in town either. He drove a big Lincoln Continental with "The Greek" on the license plate, and he had a limousine to pick up important guests of the restaurant and for our personal use when the restaurant was not using it. Nick's Fishmarket had a presence in Honolulu, and those of us who worked there felt as cool as it gets, so it did not take long for Nick to convince us that this would be a great joke to play on Don.

"We need disguises," Nick demanded. "Have you got your sunglasses?" he asked, looking directly at VO and me. Nick had Marc throw him the keys to his black El Camino, the only vehicle available that could handle the size of the hospital bed. So Nick, VO, and I, all laughing as we rolled out of the parking lot ridiculously dawning shades, drove off into the darkness of the 2 a.m. morning with enough cocktails in us to light up the town.

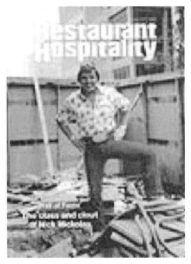

Nick Nicholas

We took one lap around the Polynesian Palace parking lot and saw the unattended bed sitting outside, seemingly waiting for us to steal it, just as the girl said it would be. We wildly loaded it into the back of Marc's El Camino and raced back to the Fishmarket. Having pulled off what we somehow thought to be the perfect crime, we unloaded the bed downstairs at the restaurant and wasted little time in stripping off all the Hawaiian flags and island-themed decorations. Feeling the need for a few celebration cocktails, we decided we would have our team redecorate it in the morning, and we went back inside to the bar. All the afterhours employees and guests flipped when we took them downstairs to show them what we had done. Don Ho's bed sat in our entryway, completely destroyed.

"They are going to kill us all if they ever find out," I said to Nick in a sober moment of concern.

"Well, let's hope they never find out," he said. "Now let's have another drink."

We were all back in the bar with the doors locked, having a good laugh, when we heard a loud pounding at the front door. Nobody moved. Then the phone rang, a very nervous night clerk calling to inform us that the lobby was full of large angry Hawaiians. They had discovered their destroyed bed and were now waiting downstairs to deal with us.

"Oh, shit," Nick said to me. "There is only one thing to do."

"What?"

"Face them. This might get ugly."

Nick opened the door with a big smile and said, "I guess we are busted!" He was trying to play it off as a big joke, but the large Hawaiians did not find it funny. Nick continued to smooth talk them, the front desk guy called the cops, some pushing and shoving ensued, and we all braced our selves for a riot. Nick truly did have the gift of gab. Somehow he got Don Ho on the phone, and thankfully Don called down his dogs, and the slaughter was off.

Generously, they designated me the one to drive the sad looking bed back to the Polynesian Palace. En route, I wondered if I would return or not. After all, ending up in a pig trough was a distinct possibility. But luck was with me and they left me alone while they removed the bed from the back of Marc's car. I went back to the Fishmarket and joined my cohorts, drinking at the bar with our tails between our legs until sun-up. We called the race organizers to see if we could get a last minute bed, but it never showed up. Nick's Fishmarket had been blackballed from the bed race.

Oh well, we were all pretty hung over the next day, and we ended up with more notoriety for our attempted theft than any competitor would receive. A feature article ran in the paper with a headline that read, "The Theft of the King's Bed." Being the gentlemen that we were, we gave the entire staff of the Polynesian Palace free dinners at Nick's for months, which more importantly diverted their hostility and the possibility of a nasty retribution. All in a day's work at the Fishmarket.

Clean Oil and a Crosswind Landing

Another adventurous enterprise that filled my days took place back in the mid '70s after my stunt career was established and I was still holding on to my position at Nick's. I ran into my old friend Barry Hilton, son of Baron Hilton, the CEO and president of the Hilton Hotel chain, and he invited me to Maui for a sailing excursion with a crew of bikinied bodies. I was always cautious about flying my plane into Maui, but I was not about to let a little wind stand in my way of a day at sea with the ladies. Actually, I faced the horribly cruel wind shear that consistently gripped Maui's Ka'anapali Airport. Having eaten many a plane, the ornery conditions left skeletal remains scattered along the runway as a precautionary greeting upon approach. I anticipated a very tricky crosswind landing.

It could easily be done, but I would feel better with a little extra weight on the co-pilot side of the aircraft. As luck would have it, the phone rang, and it was my friends Ric Marlow and Daryl Willingham. Daryl was a waiter at Nick's and Ric Marlow was a song writer infamous for writing the popular tune entitled "*A touch of Honey*". They both jumped at the chance to join me on the trip to Maui. I warned them it was a little windy over there, but having more weight would help with our approach. They did not quite get what I meant, but they would figure it out soon enough.

We met at the south ramp at Honolulu International Airport, and I loaded all our bags on the passenger side of the airplane. We took off on a beautiful day and headed for Maui. As expected, the crosswind became so strong that both Ric and Daryl had to sit as far as they could to the right side of the aircraft to compensate for the strong crosswind. I told Daryl to sit as far as he could against the window because this landing was going to be interesting. Their eyes went wide as I held my little Cherokee at a 45-degree angle and side slipped down.

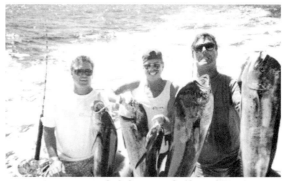

A great catch fishing with (from l to r) Barry Hilton, John Thorp & Phil Carr

"Aren't the wings supposed to be level?" asked Ric.

"Not in this kind of wind," I replied. "Hang on." They pulled their seat belts tighter as we landed on the right tire first and stayed that way until the airspeed bled off. Then the left wheel touched, and eventually the nose wheel, a perfect crosswind landing.

I heard a couple of loud sighs of relief when the plane finally came to a stop. "Jesus," Ric said. "I have never landed like that in a plane, ever."

"Welcome to small aircraft travel," I said. To me it was just another landing. Ka'anapali Airport no longer exists at that location. It was just too dangerous a place. The conditions of my flights may have been varied and at times thrilling, but I have walked away from every landing, making every landing a good one.

Trusting in yourself is having faith in your ability to adapt to the demands of the moment. One shift leads to another shift, and before you know it, a building confidence carries you through even the most precarious scenarios as if they are common and mundane. That faith opens your life to all directions, and it surely took mine to new people, places, and opportunities. My life has followed many directions. One memorable shift took its course at the hands of hot oil and toilet paper.

Daryl approached me one evening not long after our creative flight to Maui and asked if I was familiar with the Franz oil filtration system. I told him that I was and that I had used it on the GT I built as a teenager, the Green Beast. I loved the system; not only did you not have to change your oil as often, but it had a chrome oil filter container that added a custom appearance to your motor and looked great.

The Franz system used a roll of toilet paper as a filter. Its claim to fame was that if you used this system you would never have to change the oil in your car, just replace the roll of toilet paper every other week. This worked well for those backyard mechanics who had the tools and loved to monkey around with their cars, but for those who would forget to regularly swap out the roll, the paper disintegrated and was sucked into the engine block by the pistons, freezing the motor. No matter how good it looked or how much oil it saved, after several frozen motors the system's popularity plummeted.

You could still order the Franz system from the back of hot rod magazines, but they published a strong recommendation for changing the filter every week.

Daryl, always full of fun and bearing an uncanny resemblance to Fred Flintstone, loved to throw parties on his days off from Nick's at his Diamond Head beach house. This also provided all his wave hunting buddies like myself with prime parking in front of one of the island's best surf spots. He rented one of the finest places on the beach, and it was fully loaded with a commercial kitchen, including a deep fryer. Daryl loved to deep-fry his fresh fish, prawns, and chicken for these weekend barbecues, so he was familiar with the cost of good vegetable oil. Looking to cut his costs and improve his food quality, he started experimenting with filtering the oil.

Daryl rigged up an old washing machine pump and motor, mounted it on a 4" x 4" board, and connected the Franz oil filter system to it, chrome filter container and all. He tested it on the oil in his home fryer unit, and the results were amazing. At one of his parties, he showed me how he could turn coffee-black oil into golden-beer oil. Although his filter pumped a little slow and appeared too time consuming to filter bigger vats of oil found in a large restaurant, I was absolutely blown away.

He asked me if I would be interested in presenting his invention to Nick. I was glad to, but mentioned that he should try to pump the oil a little faster. About a week later, Daryl pulled me aside at work; he had solved the pumping problem and was ready to demonstrate it to Nick.

He asked me if I would be willing to invest in his company. He needed additional capital to apply for the regulatory and safety documentation needed to take his product to market, certifications from the likes of UL (Underwriter Laboratories) and NSF (National Sanitation Foundation). He also needed additional funds to apply for the patents to protect his incredible invention. He showed me the figures of a normal restaurant's oil costs, and how with this system he could guarantee to cut their oil bill in half, if not more. It didn't take me long to do the math and realize this could be a very lucrative investment. I agreed to be his first investor if he would give me all the marketing rights to sell it worldwide. We sealed the deal with a handshake. He formed Diamond Head Clean Oil Corporation, and I began forming Diamond Head Marketing Corporation.

I talked to Nick that evening, and he agreed to let us do a demonstration for him in the kitchen in the morning. He saw the value in cleaning the oil not only for the savings but also to improve food quality. Nick said, "John if this works as well as you say it does, and removes all the taste and smell from the oil and saves me money, you might just have something that could really be of value."

We arrived at the kitchen at 10 a.m. sharp, anxious to demonstrate our wonder machine for Nick. We instructed the chef, Eddie Fernandez, to heat the fryer up to its normal cooking temperature, 350 degrees, since the oil needed to be filtered hot to remove all the particulate matter. We placed one hose in the deep fryer and the other in a large stainless steel holding container. I took a sample of the oil in a clear glass jar and held it up for Nick to see the dark cloudy oil before we filtered it, and then I told Daryl to hit the button, praying it would go well.

I was a little shocked at the loud racket produced by the more powerful pump and motor, but I was pleased to see the oil coming out faster and looking nice and golden as promised. I sprayed a little of the filtered oil into another jar and showed Nick the difference. One jar looked like cloudy coffee, and the other jar was golden in color and crystal clear.

Daryl and I stood by with our cocky looks of "I told you so." Nick inspected the jar and nodded his head in a congratulatory manner. Just as Nick was saying, "It looks very good John," the machine made a loud grinding sound. I looked over at Daryl for an explanation of the commotion and was greeted with an eyebrow raised in bewilderment. Suddenly the chrome filter container blew off and hit the ceiling, spraying hot oil over both Daryl and me as we frantically tried to turn the damn thing off.

Nick was wide-eyed after watching Daryl and I dance under the hot oil, and said that we had a good idea but it appeared to be a little dangerous. I probably had 50 tiny oil burn spots covering my hands, arms, legs, face, and neck. Daryl didn't fare any better, since he was wearing shorts and a tank top as well. It was back to the drawing board to fine-tune our safety issues, but there was no argument that the oil looked incredible after being filtered.

We found our error. A filter overloaded with fried breadcrumbs had caused the pressure to build and the clamp to fail. We corrected the flaws by using a wire mesh screen over the intake hose to block the heavy particulate matter from getting through to clog the filter and a heavy duty-locking clamp to hold it shut. We tested it on Daryl's fryer, filling it with a clay-like substance called diatomaceous earth to substitute for the heavy breading we encountered with Nick's fryer. This time it worked perfectly! We called Eddie, the chef, and asked if we could come back and try it again. After we promised to clean up any mess we made, he agreed to let us give it another go. The rest is history.

I went on to sell this oil filtration device to over 20% of all the restaurants in Hawaii. Daryl had gone after Maui Potato chips and proved that his motor could handle filtering 50-gallon drums of hot oil. We followed through in obtaining the necessary safety validations with UL and NSF, and even took it a step further by having an independent laboratory use a spectron microscope to measure the particulate matter left in the oil after filtration. We proved that we removed particulate matter down to 1/100 of a micron and had been successful in removing all the taste and smell from the oil.

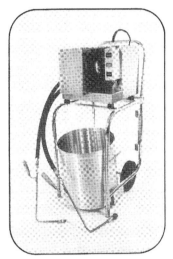

The Clean Oil Filtration System

Many restaurants were able to keep their oil for over thirty days without changing it. They were amazed that the products they cooked looked and tasted better than on the first day of using fresh oil. With our filtration system, their product was always golden in appearance and they had cut their oil bill three to four times instead of just in half as we had promised. One chef, Siggy, at Fisherman's Wharf, had maintained the same oil for over three months and figured that he would never have to change it again but could keep adding fresh oil after filtration. An unbelievable savings and improvement of food quality.

Eventually, we flew all the way to Natick, Massachusetts, to test our equipment to see if it was up to military standards. We met with the head purchasers for the Army, Navy, Air Force, and Marines; it tested to be one hundred times better than military specifications required. We received our first purchase order from Natick Testing Laboratories itself to upgrade their standards to meet our equipment's results.

Back in Hawaii, I landed contracts with Kaneohe Marine Corps, Scoffield Barracks, and several other military kitchens. Receiving glowing letters of endorsement from all the restaurants and kitchens using our equipment, I felt that we were well on our way to becoming millionaires.

I contacted my good friend and our old sailing buddy Barry Hilton to tell him about what we had created. He agreed to take me to the Beverly Hilton, where his father, Baron, had his office, and he allowed us a demonstration for the famous resort's head chef. The results could not have been better. We cut their oil bill in half and improved their food quality as we had done with every kitchen before. Barry quickly became my number one sales representative. He approached and introduced our system to all the hotels directly linked to Hilton Hotel Corporation. With the son of one of the most well-known hotel chains in America as my representative, things could not have been going better. He could get into places where it would have taken me months to find even the right guy to talk with. All he had to say was "this is Baron Hilton Jr. calling" and the doors would fly open. However, just when you think you can do no wrong, everything goes wrong.

One of the heads of food and beverage for the Pasadena Hilton was so excited about the results that he wanted to join our team and become a sales representative too. He invited several food and beverage managers from other hotels to witness the incredible results of the oil filtration machine that was presented to him by none other than the son of the president of the hotel.

He had one of the clearly novice kitchen helpers who was still straining to understand instructions in English bring out our oil filter machine. He directed the kitchen helper as he had seen me do, and was ready to collect a sample of the dirty oil coming from the drainage hole. They drained the hot oil into a large stainless steel container, and he put the suction end into the container and the opposite end into the fryer. Because we had the oil pumping so fast through the filter, we were able to clean out a fryer's vat and flush out all the crumbs through the drain hole using its already hot and filtered oil, leaving a beautifully clean fryer. Close the drain hole and you could begin filling the fryer up again with golden oil.

Unfortunately, the kitchen helper was not paying attention to the fact that the oil was coming out at 350-degrees. When the manager asked him to shoot a little clean oil into another jar, he missed the jar completely and sprayed the food and beverage manager with hot oil. They had to rush the poor guy to the emergency room with third degree burns all over his crotch. He almost lost his goods.

"John, I think we have a problem," said Barry when he called me that night. After hearing the story, I tried to explain to Barry that it was not the machine's fault that the guy got severely burned, but rather human error that led to the accident. I tried to reason with him, but the incident brought up too many liability issues involved with filtering hot oil. We lost the support of the Hilton Corporation. Barry, who was still a believer, said they simply could not take the chance of another employee getting burned, no matter how great the savings.

This was just as small setback, a slight wrinkle that could easily be ironed out. I put warnings on the machine, supplied heat resistant gloves, and created a demonstration video that would point out the dangers of the filtration process. We demonstrated how to filter the oil safely, and clarified that the hoses should never be touched while the filtration was in operation. We coated the lines with heat-protected rubber to cut down on the possibility of an individual getting burnt by the lines. Our new motto: "Safety first." With so much confidence in our new enterprise, I left Nick's Fishmarket to deal in this oil filtration business.

I contacted my old buddy Dennis McKenna, and he was interested in helping me market the machines. He had recently been doing very well in another financial planning company that he had started called Pacific Audio Marketing Corporation. He had generated several million dollars in a short period of time and agreed to finance my travels and help in the marketing of the Diamond Head Oil Filtration Machine.

We continued to sell machines to various restaurant chains on the mainland, bolstered by discoveries that the disposal of rancid oil was becoming an ecological concern. Used oil was causing problems in drains and in landfills, so if we could cut the amount of oil used, we could highlight the ecological benefits of our product as well. Not only did it cut oil bills in half and improve food quality, it also lessened the contamination of the planet by reducing the amount of disposed rancid oil, another win-win.

With all the bugs worked out, we felt ready to go after the frying powerhouses, Burger King, Taco Bell, and McDonald's. The large chains were already using filtration devices, but we could cut their oil bills in half. Most used diatomaceous earth powder to absorb the microscopic particles down to 10 microns. We were removing particles down to 1/100 of a micron.

I told everyone I met about our amazing equipment. I said that if they were interested in investing with us, we were on our way to becoming multi-millionaires; I also told them that this was an incredible investment opportunity. I attracted the attention of a woman who was the head of the restaurant association of Houston, Texas, and had connections with Burger King and McDonald's.

Nick had already expanded his restaurants to Chicago and Houston, so when I was in town to help Dar Robinson, one of the top stuntmen in the world, with his show at the Astrodome, we arranged to meet at Nick's Fishmarket for a demonstration of the instruments. That morning at the restaurant, I was pleasantly surprised to be awarded a certificate of merit by the Houston Restaurant Association for not only improving the quality of the food in the city's restaurants but also cutting down on the waste product that was contaminating rivers and dump sites. We filmed the event, and at lunch that day the head of the restaurant association made me an offer I did not think we could refuse.

She offered us $500,000 for 50% of my marketing company and 50% of the manufacturing company, putting her in equal control of both elements. If she was going to get involved, she wanted to make sure that the quality controls were handled by her. I would still own 50% and Daryl would own about 45%, since he had sold hundreds of thousands of shares of stock to raise money to get the needed approvals and put the finishing touches on a filtration paper. Our plan was to give them the machine and sell them the filters.

I called Daryl with the great news, but he refused, straight out. He said she was trying to steal the operation from him and that he was not about to relinquish control. I tried to explain to him that this was the infusion of funds we desperately needed to take us to the next level. Daryl was broke and had used all the investment money merely to survive. The few machines that I sold per month could barely keep the doors open, and I was putting every penny I made from the stunt business as well as my entire salary from working at Nick's to fund my travels, printing of brochures, and the general expenses of bringing a new product to market.

She had the funds to approach all the large chains, and we would still maintain a huge profit margin for doing little or nothing by letting her team run with the ball. Daryl had never seen $500,000; nor had I. This was the opportunity of a lifetime, but no matter how it was explained to Daryl, he refused to take the offer. He refused, and I had to walk away. The wind behind our sails was gone, left in search of the next direction.

Jupiter and The Source

Between my new restaurant, hang gliding, and showbiz families, I was revolving in very diverse and dynamic worlds. With equal speed, people burst in and out of my life, and every day brought a new lesson, learned either firsthand or through friendships with other dream seekers. My life was in some way enhanced or altered by every soul I encountered during those early days on the islands. Few souls were more intriguing than Dennis McKenna.

Dennis McKenna entered my life during the days at Matteo's. I was working in the reserved section of the restaurant making a table-side Caesar salad for a VIP when another waiter came back to tell me that there was an interesting character sitting at pro baseball player Bo Bolinski's table, and he was asking to meet me. He had been talking nonstop about hang gliding all night. Overhearing this conversation, the waiter had mentioned to them that one of the best hang glider pilots in the islands was working there tonight. This prompted the request for the introduction. We went through the normal pleasantries, compared our pasts, and shared friends and acquaintances in the world of hang gliding. It was immediately clear that he was new to the islands and a novice when it came to flying. Nevertheless, he had brought his own glider and was anxious to visit the local flying spots. He beamed a big smile when he heard about our flying club, known then as "The Pacific Trade Wind Sky Sailors."

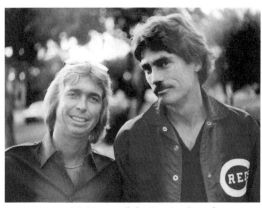

Dennis McKenna (aka Jupiter) and me

Over the following years we became good friends. Dennis soon decided that Hawaii was the place to be, and moved there. He rented an astonishingly beautiful circular home in Lanikai, complete with a spectacular 360-degree view of the Mokaluas, the island chain resembling Egypt's Great Pyramid and Sphinx that sat a half-mile off shore. The place was soon the bachelor pad of all bachelor pads, more of an after hours club that often pumped well into the morning. Dennis and I were birds of a feather and flocked together with beautiful women, good pot, and every now and then a little pure cocaine. We would go down for a swim, and on the way back stroll along the beach looking for more beauties to join the perpetual party. "See that house on the side of the mountain?" was all we had to say and the party was back on.

One quiet afternoon when I called Dennis to see if he wanted to go flying, a sweet female voice answered his phone. Nothing uncommon about that, but oddly enough she said that nobody named Dennis lived there. I recited the number to her and she said it was correct, but that no one by that name lived there.

"Is this the house in Lanikai?" I asked her in confusion.

"Oh yes, it is so beautiful here," she joyously answered back.

Now I was really puzzled. It had only been a few weeks since my last visit to the house. Dennis had said he was going to check out the big island for a bit, but he should have been back by now. Quizzing the young spacey voice on the other end did not result in many answers.

"Stop playing games," I said, beginning to lose my patience. "Dennis McKenna lived there two weeks ago, and I would certainly know if he had moved."

"Oh," she exclaimed, something finally clicking. "You must mean Jupiter."

"Jupiter?" I echoed. "You've got to be kidding. Well, let me speak to Jupiter."

Sure enough, my friend formerly known as Dennis got on the phone and said hello, sounding as happy as could be.

"What the hell is this Jupiter stuff?"

In 1969, a man by the name of James Baker opened one of the nation's first organic restaurants on the Sunset Strip in Hollywood. Over 30 years ahead of his time, Baker and his family ran the extremely popular Source Restaurant, serving organic vegetarian food to celebrity regulars including John Lennon, Marlon Brando, Steve Allen, and Warren Beatty. A highly decorated WWII Marine veteran and martial arts expert in his 20s, Baker moved to California to become a Hollywood actor but fell in with the Los Angeles-based Nature Boys, an eclectic group of beatniks living according to nature's laws. Baker was an avid student of philosophy and religion, even practicing as a Vedantic monk for a time, before eventually becoming a devoted follower of Yogi Bhajan, a teacher of Kundalini Yoga and a Sikh spiritual leader.

Baker would eventually part ways with his Yogi in the late '60s to fuse his experiences with Eastern religions and Western mystical traditions into what he called the Source Family. He became Father Yod, and later Ya Ho Wha, the leader of a group of young people devoted to his teachings and philosophies. They all helped run the lucrative restaurant on the strip, men becoming sons and women known as either daughters or mothers, but all goddesses. Many young women were attracted to his loving communal lifestyle and found themselves in his bed. He was still legally married at the time, but in his mind he was free, and his offer was open to anyone who wanted to "come along for the ride." And many did, following him to Hawaii after he moved to the big island with his 13 new wives.

He had a dream of a new age community and sought his own truth. He believed in complete honesty, hard work, and organization. Tolerant but strong, he once had a few problems with a couple of jealous men who attacked him, and when he defended himself, his unlucky assailants actually died from the injuries he swiftly and deftly inflicted upon them. Arrested for manslaughter but acquitted on self-defense, he had to register his hands as lethal weapons. But Father Yod was a determined man of peace, and his communal living experiment initially seemed to be working out well for all involved. He and his followers lived in harmony and continued to create the psychedelic music they had started in California. Soon his sons also had a few angels or wives of their own, and a total of 52 little spirits came down to bless the family, all born the *au naturale* way. The Source Family was unquestionably going strong in Hawaii.

That is when the Source Family and Ya Ho Wah discovered my good buddy Dennis and converted him into Jupiter. After he explained it to me, my only question was, "Can I call you Jupe?"

"Hey, I have two beautiful women that I call my angels and they are taking good care of me," he answered seriously, but could not help but laugh. "I am happier than I have ever been. You have to come by and check it out." He further explained that once they saw him fly it was a done deal; he was immediately accepted into the Family and rose right up the ranks in their esteem.

Not long after, Dennis called me for a large reservation at Nick's Fishmarket. I was introduced to Jupiter that evening when he showed up to the restaurant dressed in a blood red tunic, flowing pants (all handmade), a big belt buckle with a strange insignia, and several of his beautiful angels on his arm, one breast-feeding her little spirit baby. Needless to say, they created quite a stir at Nick's that night. Both Nick and Jeff knew that Dennis was a hang gliding buddy of mine, but I still had to explain to them what these zany looking people were doing in their restaurant. I started going into how they were the new generation of spiritual devotees, but we all agreed that with no make-up and with hairy armpits, they just looked like a bunch of hippies, not exactly fitting the mold of our regular groomed and dressed-to-the-nines patrons. Unlike other hippies, however, they had no problem paying their bill and had even arrived in their sun colored Mercedes Benz that they used to tour around the island. The famous restaurant in Hollywood had obviously paid off well.

Once seated, Dennis honored me with the introductions, all their names granted by Ya Ho Wha. Rain, Tantalayo, Mercy, Heh, and, of course, Jupiter all carried themselves proudly and never turned away from the stares, looking deeply into the eyes of the gawking diners, who then nervously looked away to leave the group in peace. This tribe was different and proud of it.

Nick, with that big Greek smile of his, just chuckled and let everyone know that they were my friends. From that point on, any longhaired or hippie looking people that came through the door at Nick's were referred to as John's friends. I became the designated ambassador to the counterculture, which was not so bad. This was the early '70s, and many of these people labeled as hippies were members of famous rock and roll bands in search of a good time, with plenty of money to find it. I took great care of them at Nick's, and they took very good care of me, financially as well as with some of the finest herbs and other treats that a touring rock band might be known to ingest along the road. Tolerance was working out well for me. Everyone who I greeted at Nick's was given the same five-star service, and I carried that attitude outside of the restaurant too. If Jupiter wanted to spend his days with angels, who was I to stop or judge him. We were all having fun.

Then one day while working, I got a call from a good hang gliding buddy, Duff King. He wanted to know if I had heard about a bearded guy in a long flowing robe who had plunged a hang glider off the cliffs at Makapuu and crashed at Kione Beach Park. I did not know a thing about it. The word was that someone had attempted Makapuu on his first flight ever in a hang glider. He would call me back if he found out more, but from what he had heard the guy had survived and amazingly was doing just fine.

Hearing about the long robe triggered thoughts about Dennis. I wondered if it might have been him or one of his tribe. I tried to reach him at his house but did not get an answer. A few hours later, Duff called back, and it turned out to be none other than Ya Ho Wha himself who had crash landed with only a few bruised bones in his back but without any serious injuries. My thoughts also went to the threat this posed for our hang gliding club and the potential loss of access to our flying spot. This incident could make for really bad press and might even cost us Makapuu.

I finally talked to Dennis, who told me that Ya Ho Wha had broken all the rules, had taken his glider without his permission, and had taken several members of the tribe up to the top of the cliff. A hang gliding pilot, Mercury, who was also a member of the Source Family, launched him. Dennis was not there himself but told a story of Ya Ho Wha making a couple of nice S turns before making a safe landing with only a few scratches from putting his legs out to brace himself. He was "in the light." Dennis and I disagree on the points of what is safe and what is a crash. If you do not walk away from it, I call it a crash.

The story that Duff had heard was that Ya Ho Wha had blasted off the top of Makapuu and zigged and zagged wildly out of control until he ended up in a twisted heap in the Beach Park below. But the report of the lack of injuries was the same, and all described it as quite a scene down in the park. A gathering of huge Hawaiian and Samoan locals stood over this long-haired, bearded man tangled-up in a wrecked hang glider asking them where the angels went that had guided him down.

Now this tribe loved the sacred herb (marijuana)-enhanced morning ritual, and Ya Ho Wha had a tiny stash of coke for special occasions, but that was it, and Dennis swore that Ya Ho Wha was not on anything the day he flew, other than maybe a little pot. Most hang glider pilots enjoyed a puff and a beer before takeoff, which was not at all uncommon in those days.

Dennis said that Ya Ho Wha spoke in their native tongue to the Samoans surrounding him after the fall. Supposedly, Ya Ho Wha had lived in Samoa and had saved the life of a Samoan princess. As his reward, her father gave her to him, further adding to his legend. My account of the crash and the following events comes from Dennis, who I trust was giving me the straight scoop to the best of what he had heard or witnessed.

Ya Ho Wha's women and Mercury showed up at the park in their yellow Mercedes, loaded their Father into the car, and bolted. The only visual injuries on him were the scratches on his legs, so he refused the hospital.

Later Dennis would notice a big donut-sized bruise around his butt. This was not caused by the impact, according to the Source Family, but from when Kundalini went off, whatever that means.

Supposedly, he hit very hard, right on his butt. Dennis gave me updates on his condition, and they all thought that he was going to be just fine. They figured he was resting and healing, so they were all quite stunned when he died nine hours later.

Nobody outside the family had known that he had passed when I went over to visit the following day. Dennis greeted me at the door, and explained it was time for Ya Ho Wha to become a spirit. From the door I smelled the strange odor of frankincense and myrrh and saw his candle-surrounded body lying on the floor with the women rubbing oils all over his semi-nude limbs. Dennis said that Ya Ho Wha was shifting into spirit.

"Is he alive or dead?" I asked.

"Neither," Dennis answered. "He is reviewing his past Life Rivers. Please come in and share this beautiful experience."

The intensity of the scene and the smell was strong enough from outside, so I decided to pass on joining them. Dennis eventually admitted that he might be dead on the earthly plane. I told him that my prayers were with him and his friends and left them to their life river ceremony.

A few days later, the headlines in the paper read that one James Baker, aka Ya Ho Wha, was killed while flying a hang glider off of Makapuu, and a week later, there was also a full-page story about his life. Funny enough, Ya Ho Wha had often stated that we are all stars in the making. Sharing the front page with the article on his life was a separate article reporting that an unidentified new star had been identified one week earlier, the very same day Ya Ho Wha passed. Believe it or not, it is hard to deny that Ya Ho Wha's life was shrouded with transcendent endeavors and inexplicable mysteries.

Almost a year to the date of Ya Ho Wha's passing the Source Family's Mercury set a new world record of 13 hours aloft in a hang glider. Unfortunately, on his very next flight, flying under the full moon to celebrate his record and honor the anniversary of the passing of Ya Ho Wha, Mercury died off of Makapuu. The family would give him the same ceremony they gave Ya Ho Wha, allowing him to review his life river and move peacefully into spirit as well, but the word got out that another Source member had been killed off Makapuu, and that his deceased body was in the family's house. The police got involved, and after a peaceful standoff, some of the members were arrested.

It was not easy for people to understand the new ways and beliefs of this group, but eventually the charges were dropped and the mandatory autopsy, required by state law after an accidental death, was granted a postponement until after the three and a half days the family's ceremony required for the soul's passage to spirit. The Source Family's belief in a transition at the end, where one reviews his "life river" before ascending, sounds very similar to the Christian belief in the three days Jesus waited to rise again after being crucified on the cross. We never know how we will find the way to truth or in what shape and form it may find us.

Our hang gliding club maintained access to our hallowed launch spot. After the two deaths, there were no other wild attempts by any Source Family members to review their life river by means of a leap from Makapuu. The family eventually went its separate ways, and Dennis left Hawaii with one of his angels, Tantalayo, to manage her band. Many of the others branched out into music recording and performing as well. The Source Family really did create some beautiful and at times angelic music. It was too bad the only music being recognized at the time was disco, just another sign that Ya Ho Wha and the family was possibly too far ahead of their time, perhaps even for themselves.

More Risks and Records

Why would a person take huge risks, push himself or herself to do something nobody else had ever done, to break a record, to attempt the impossible? Because some people, those who choose to define their own existence, who stay in their passion, and who trust themselves as their guide would rather not ride at all if they cannot enjoy the ride to its fullest.

Bob Wills and John Walbert were two men determined to experience all they could in life. Bob set many of the first daunting flight records off of

Makapuu, and John was often the first to break them. This was a cycle they carried out for years as the records they set came and went. It would never take long for Bob to get wind that someone in Hawaii had broken his record, and he would be on a plane within weeks to set a new one. He eventually set an astounding record of seven hours in the air. Someone else stayed up for eight, and then Bob was back and stayed up for eleven hours. All his records would fall, and sadly so would Bob. Tragically, both Bob and John were eventually killed flying hang gliders. I wonder if they are breaking each other's records in heaven.

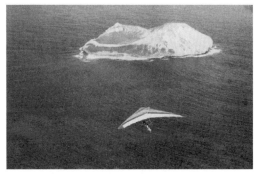

Soaring high above Rabbit Island

Carrying on the torch, our friend Mercury stayed up for 13 hours. Someone else stayed up for 18 hours, but then my good friend Jim Wills set the record that still stands today off the cliffs of Makapuu. Jim stayed in the air for an amazing 34.5 hours, which even broke Charles Lindbergh's previous record of 33 hours of flying without sleep when he crossed the Atlantic in the Spirit of Saint Louis. Few people have ever heard of Jim Wills, while Lindbergh lives on in history and legend.

Jim, a talented jeweler living in Honolulu, was a man of incredible, as we would say, Will Power. He was also the first man to do an inter-island crossing in a motorized hang glider. I escorted him on his final leg.

I had recently earned my private pilot's license and was invited to join a couple of other pilots in purchasing a Piper Cherokee 150. This newfound freedom of flying airplanes improved all of my flying skills.

After a sunrise take-off from Honolulu Airport climbing up through the clouds where no hang glider could fly, I remembered the days with Harvey as I cleared the Pali Lookout. In a few minutes I was circling above Jim as he was taking off from Olamana golf course. I followed him along the Ko'olaus and then over the 100 miles of lonely blue ocean to Port Allen on Kauai. He had a perfect flight, with about half a gallon of gas to spare. I landed and then watched Jim make a perfect landing on the little deserted landing strip at Port Allen. My time with brave souls such as Jim, Bob, and John continually reminded me of my mother's words, "If you can dream it, you can do it."

Setting records was one thing, but we all knew what was next: competition. This was a sport that had no margin for error, and I was afraid competition would push people past their abilities prematurely, so contests were not for me. Too many ashes had already been scattered in reverence off the launch spot of Makapuu, and we were not eager to scatter anymore. Unfortunately, that would not be the case.

At last count, 22 people have been killed while trying to fly Makapuu. The hang glider pilots that still fly the world famous cliff are an elite few. For all the souls of my dear friends lost up there while challenging their mortal limits, I hope you are eternally soaring.

Finally, I would like to give credit to those other early aviators that were also gravitating to this adrenalin pumping sport. This is a list, to the best of my recollection, of the early hang gliding pilots from Hawaii: Clive Armatage, David Bettencourt, Steve Claybourne, Dr. Bill Harris, Steve Leader, Sam Nottage, David Goto, David Darling, Jon and Guy Lindberg, Steve Rahefield (passed), John Hughes (passed), Carl Burman (passed), John Walbert (passed), Ed Ceasar, Bob Thornburg, Paul Bates, Hank, Byron Akiona, Woody Brown, Jim who broke his face, Blyth, Julie and Pete Brock, Linda Tracey (passed), Mark Bowles, Mark Rodriques (from Kauai), the little blonde girl, Kitty, who always crashed, and Paul Courtney, the youngest of us all.

The Legend Of Buzzy Trent

Dove Hang Gliders held its first Exhibition at Oahu's Ala Moana Shopping Center. We even constructed a hang gliding simulator, which consisted of a glider hung from the rafters so we could demonstrate how to make all the maneuvers and controls. We had a good turnout, and the response to the simulator was great. While giving one of my instructional talks, I noticed a bedraggled individual dressed in army fatigues, his pants cut off at the knees. He was hanging out toward the back of the crowd. To be honest, I thought he was homeless.

He waited to approach us as we were packing things up, and he asked us if we could teach an old man like him how to fly. He seemed really eager to try the simulator, so we helped him into the harness and could see that he was in great shape. In fact, he was built like a rock. I showed him how to control the glider and shift his weight, and he was amazed at how simple it was. I warned him, "Flying is easy; it's the landing that will kill you."

After the demonstration, he stuck out his hand and introduced himself, "I'm Buzzy." When I asked him if he surfed and he said he did, it dawned on me that this was my childhood hero of the surfing world, Buzzy Trent. I had a poster of him riding a thirty-foot wave that hung above my bed when I was nine years old: "Buzzy Trent Rides a Makaha Bowl Monster." It was a pleasure and an honor to be face to face with this surfing legend, and I told him as much. "Ah, it wasn't anything," he replied.

He said he had been coming out to Makapuu to watch us fly for the past couple of years, and he really wanted to know if he could do it. I assured him that there were guys older than him flying and that it was not about strength. He was still in such great physical condition that I did not have any doubt that we could have him soaring.

"So when can we get started?" he asked. I countered, "We could get going as early as tomorrow if you want to meet me out at the sand dunes at Kahuku." He did not hesitate to accept and even offered, "If you teach me how to fly, I will teach you to surf some big waves." We had a deal.

I arrived at the sand dunes the following morning and Buzzy was already there waiting. He was like a little kid, full of questions and willing to help anywhere he could. He helped me set up my training gliders and was soon climbing into a harness and hooking himself in. I gave him some last minute instructions and that was all it took. He made it all the way to the water's edge on his very first flight. When I ran down to congratulate him, he had a smile on his face and was jumping up and down; a sixty-year-old man exuding the innocent joy of a ten-year-old kid. Flying has been known to do that to a person.

He carried the glider back to the top of the dune, no small feat, and repeated this trick at least thirty times. There was no doubting that this was a very special human being. I was amazed at how his body moved and reacted like a twenty-year-old's.

"Well, what's next?" he asked. I told him the next step was a launch at around the 100-foot level, my old training site of Anna Bananas in Kailua. This hill could give him about a minute or two in the air. I arrived at Anna Bananas the next morning about a half an hour earlier than I had told Buzzy, but once again he was already waiting. I unloaded the glider from the top of my car, and Buzzy was quick to throw it over his shoulder and head for the narrow trail up to the summit. I was only carrying the harness and had difficulty keeping up with him. This guy was an animal.

When we got to the summit, we found the wind was already picking up. This might be a little too much wind for a beginner, but there was no talking Buzzy out of it. We got him into the harness, made sure he was hooked in correctly, and moved to the front of the glider to prepare for a wire launch. I lifted the nose of the glider and, as we always did with trainees, looked directly into his eyes to gauge his mentality before the flight. This was the face of an intensely focused human being.

After some last minute instructions, we waited for the wind to smooth out. I barely got the words out of my mouth, "When it feels right, run," before Buzzy took two tiny steps he was airborne. I yelled at him to pull the bar in to counteract the strong lift. He was going straight up and had not begun to penetrate into the strong wind, but he reacted to my command perfectly, moving forward and away from the strong lift zone.

Then the turbulence, caused by the buildings in front of this cow pasture, hit him and threw the glider into a sharp right turn. He corrected immediately by shifting his weight in the opposite direction. Buzzy was a natural. He continued to correct his positioning, and, before he knew it, he had flown a few hundred yards out into the pasture. With the high winds, he flew past the landing zone and landed right in the middle of a small pond with a big splash.

By the time I got to him, he was dragging the glider out of the water, soaked from head to toe with a smile on his face that could not be washed off. "Wow! That was great," he said as I approached.

"You did great, Buzzy," I congratulated him. "That was probably one of the longest flights at Anna Bananas."

"Let's get up there and do it again," he said. The wind was picking up even more. Due to his lack of experience, I didn't want him to get hurt.

"I don't think you have enough experience to handle the turbulent conditions," I said. I tried talking him out of another flight, but he begged me to let him try it one more time. He wanted to achieve a stand-up landing instead of landing in a pond.

I finally agreed to let him try it one more time, but if the wind got any stronger, we would call it a day. It took every ounce of strength I had to keep up with this mountain goat as we climbed back up the narrow path. He seemed to get stronger as he went along. The wind direction was good, but the velocity for a beginner was definitely risky. Since there was no talking him down, I would have to play the cash card. "If you break my glider you're going to have to pay for it," I informed him, but that did not faze him.

"Don't worry," he said. "I'm going to buy a glider as soon as you can get one for me." He was adamant that he could do it. "Hell, if I can handle thirty foot waves I can handle this hundred foot hill," he argued. "Come on John, just one more flight."

I finally agreed, helped him into the harness, and secured his hook-in. I repeated the same maneuver of holding the nose while he steadied himself into the wind. Either Buzzy or the sudden gust pulled the nose of the glider right out of my hands, and he went straight up and a little sideways as I yelled to pull in. He reacted and pulled the bar all the way into his stomach, but even with the correction, it was not going to be enough to gain penetration. The nose continued to climb. Then another gust lifted the left wing and sent the glider into a hard left turn. Buzzy tried to correct, but it was too late. He cleared the top of the hill, going down-wind in a classic blowback. He crashed into the bushes behind the place he had taken off with a loud thump.

I looked down into the gully below, and did not see any movement. I began running down toward the upside down glider. Still no movement. The brush was so think it was difficult to get to him. I finally reached the glider and found Buzzy sitting with a dazed look on his face. He had hit hard.

"Are you all right?" I quickly asked.

"Yeah, I'm fine," he said, "but your glider isn't." The aluminum control bar was wrapped around him like a pretzel. "Don't worry, John," he offered. "I'll pay to get it fixed." I was just glad that he was okay.

He asked what he had done wrong, and I explained that when you fly in high wind conditions, you must keep the bar in until you get airspeed. He did not have any airspeed, so he stalled. Basically, he did a hammerhead stall right behind where he took off. It was a good thing the bushes were there to break his fall. Buzzy had cheated death one more time.

It took me a few days to get the glider back together. I called Buzzy to let him know what he owed me. He had gotten some money from his wife, Viola, to buy a new glider and wanted to know how long it would take one to get here. It would take a few weeks, but in the mean time, if he wanted to fly he could use the glider I just repaired. He thanked me profusely and wanted to know when we could go flying again.

We agreed to meet the following morning at Anna Bananas, and if he could show me a couple of good landings, I would check him off for the cliff at Makapuu. I did not want to be the man who ended the legend of Buzzy Trent, but there was absolutely no stopping this man once he was started.

The Big Wave Trade

The wind shifted during the night before I was to fly with Buzzy and was now coming out of the south. Kona flying days were really very limited, since the Kona wind only blows about 25% of the time. We appeared to be out of luck, but Buzzy mentioned that he knew of some trails on the Waianae side of the island that could take us up to a cliff directly facing the south. He had lived on the Waianae side for 30 years and knew every back trail from his days hunting pigs. I had always wanted to fly that side of the island, but Waianae was not a very friendly place for an outsider

Haole. He assured me that he knew everyone there, and we would not have a problem.

I picked him up a few hours later, and we headed for the cliffs of Waianae. I could launch Buzzy but would need someone to help me if the wind was too strong. I had tried to find a driver for us who could also launch me, but I did not have any luck, so it was just Buzzy and me on this adventure.

We got to Waianae by the late afternoon, and once again I got my heart pumping following this mountain goat up the side of the mountain. By the time we got to the summit, there was probably only an hour or so of daylight left, so we quickly set up the gliders and moved them into position facing into the smooth Kona winds. The conditions were perfect, about 10 to 15 mph at the most, and clean. I gave Buzz his pre-flight instructions and explained to him that once he was airborne he should turn parallel to the ridge and stay in the lift zone. I held the nose of his glider until he was ready, lifted it into the wind, and within a few steps he was flying again. Like a duck to water, I thought, as he carried out my instructions perfectly.

I was anxious to join Buzzy, but without a launch man, my timing had to be perfect. I moved my glider into the same spot Buzzy had launched from, rocked it back to lift the nose into the wind, and completed a perfect unassisted takeoff. Catching up with Buzzy, I yelled for him to follow me back into the bowl, where there would be plenty of lift. We stayed in the air until sunset, and both made perfect landings at a local elementary school. Buzzy was hooked, even professing that flying was possibly the most exciting thing he had ever done.

Buzzy called a few days later to say that the wind was gone but the surf was up, way up. Buzzy did not surf much anymore, but it was his turn to fulfill his end of the deal, and he wanted to take me into some big waves. It was my turn to learn, and I would be learning from one of the bravest big wave chargers in surf history. Buzzy never had much interest in the competitive side of surfing, choosing to focus on the battle between him and the sea instead. Known for his obsessive training, even pioneering the carrying of boulders along the ocean floor, Buzzy sat deeper and farther out than anyone else, fully confident he was prepared for the ocean's unpredictable and occasionally vicious nature. He was the prototype for the modern big wave rider, monstrously fearless and adeptly capable.

We met the following day at Haleiwa and found the surf pounding in with over 20 foot sets. Buzzy looked out at the smashing swell and explained that the really big waves were out at the reef known as Cloud Break. We paddled almost a mile out into the ominously dark blue sea, and I was just able to get through the inside break, which was running about 15 feet. Buzzy kept reminding me to stay calm. He asked how long I could hold my breath. I used to sit in front of a clock to time myself. "About two minutes."

"Piece of cake," he said. A big wave could hold you down for a minute, but not much more. He said to relax and count when a wave took you down deep. Almost directly after he delivered these prophetic words came absolute horror as my straining eyes made out a feathering spread of pitching waves right on top of us.

We paddled like invading warriors; This was the pre-leash era, when leashes were not even a thought. Buzzy barely made it over the first wave, but I did not. Wrapping my arms and legs around my board in a death grip I hung on for dear life. All to no avail as I was sucked over the falls, free falling for about 30 feet, exploding upon impact ripping the board from me and then plunged to the depths, the power of the crashing wave pressed me nearly 50 feet down. I reached the surface just in time for the next one to hit me and drive me back to the dark depths once again. This sickening cycle carried on for about 15 minutes, and I was starting to feel like I was going to black out.

I thought I had weathered the set when another daunting row of waves was upon me. I fought to stay in the white water, knowing if I didn't I would be sucked back out to sea in the rip tide.

Somehow making it to shore, I found my expensive new surfboard in two pieces. Buzzy found me chucking up my guts after he paddled in to check on me. I learned a whole new respect for big wave riders that day and decided that 15 foot Hawaiian waves would be my limit. Needless to say, that ended my career as a super big wave rider at Cloud Break.

As I regrouped on the sand, a single scene from the frightful ordeal kept replaying in my head. Upon one resurfacing I had caught the utterly surreal image of Buzzy emerging out of an exploding lip of raging water on a monster wave. He made it look easy, like a casual motion of the element-taming titan. However, I worried Buzzy's go-for-it attitude could get him into trouble in the hang gliding world. His years of experience as one of the first big wave conquerors created a fearless attitude in his domination of the sea. But you can't dominate what you can't see—and that is the wind.

Buzzy Learns The Hard Way

Buzzy began hitting spots all over the island, and I began to hear rumors that Buzzy was flying in the strongest winds and ending up in all kinds of strange places. On one of those high wind days Buzzy attempted to fly off Lanikai, but the wind was way too strong and he couldn't even set up his glider. He decided that Anna Bananas would be a place that was sheltered enough for him to fly, and when Buzzy wanted to fly, we all knew he was going to fly. He was well known for surfing when no one else was out, but this maverick mentality could get him killed in the hang gliding world.

He arrived at Anna Bananas about an hour before sunset, quickly carried his glider to the top, and was set up in minutes. The wind had to be gusting to around 40 mph, but Buzzy was unfazed. He waited for the perfect moment, and took-off. He was able to soar Anna Bananas for about half an hour, a feat few had ever done before, but he was pushing his luck and was about to learn a very painful lesson.

The lift area was right in front of a water tower that sat on top of the hill. Just as Buzzy made a pass by the tower, he was hit with some violent turbulence, and it forced the glider straight down, smashing him into the top of the tower and nearly ripping his leg off at the knee. He lay unconscious for nearly an hour. When he finally came to, he had nearly bled to death. He tore his t-shirt into strips, which he resourcefully used as tourniquets to stop the bleeding, and somehow hauled himself down the mountain and drove to the emergency room at Castle Hospital. They were able to reattach his leg, but it would take several more surgeries before Buzzy would walk again. To say he cheated death one more time was an understatement, because how he lived through this was anybody's guess. Buzzy definitely had a few guardian angels surrounding him. This injury extended his life because it kept him from flying again.

I ran into Buzzy often as he walked along Kalanianaole Highway. On my racing bicycle and Buzzy walking alone, I would always pull over and we would talk for a bit before he would unfailingly invite me over to his place for a cup of coffee so we could exchange our grand stories of surf and flight.

In September 2005, after an absence working and living on the Mainland, I was back on Oahu and checked in the phone book for all of the Trents. I found Anna, Buzzy's daughter, and she gave me his new number. His new wife explained that he was alive, but had recently suffered a stroke from which he was still recovering. She said he did not like to talk with people anymore. I told her my name and asked her to tell Buzzy that I was on the phone. Sure enough, he picked up. I was honored that he took my call.

Buzzy passed away in September 2006, and he will be forever remembered as one of the greatest big wave riders of all time. Buzzy always lived in his passion and inspired me to continue to do the same, reaffirming my belief that when you understand that life is way too short you will keep enjoying it till your very last breath. Thanks for the surf lesson Buzzy, but you taught me much more about keeping alive the burning fire of passion and joy well past the days of youth.

For those of you that have no idea who Buzzy Trent was besides being my dear friend and mentor, here is a little history. He will be deeply missed.

(An Article by a Honolulu Newspaper)

> Buzzy Trent was a fearless adventurer who fought bulls in Tijuana and boxed before gaining fame as one of the legendary pioneers of big-wave surfing. "Buzzy took on challenges that stimulated his adrenaline in sports that most would be hesitant to take on, primarily surfing and hang-gliding," said friend George Downing, himself a renowned waterman. "When he was asked to take on a challenge, his answer was when, not where."

Peter Cole of Sunset Beach said Trent, his lifelong friend from grammar school in Santa Monica, Calif., was an exceptional athlete who could run 100 yards in 10 seconds in high school. Trent was an all-state football player whose career was cut short at the University of Southern California by a leg injury suffered in practice. Buzzy had reminded me several times that Jan. 12, 1958, was one of the greatest surfing days of his life." "It was gigantic, 25 to 40 feet," he recalled. "At the end of the day, Buzzy said to me, 'My life is now complete.' "Trent and Downing were in a class by themselves, the first big-wave masters of Makaha, said author and former surfing champion Richard "Ricky" Grigg. "George had the ocean knowledge, he was the general, and Buzzy had the guts to lead the charge," said Grigg, a University of Hawaii professor of oceanography. "Together, they formed a great team that conquered big waves." Grigg said, "Trent was known for his power and high trim and had the willpower, stamina and true grit to take wipeouts head on."

Trent took up hang-gliding while it was still a relatively new activity. Wearing only shorts, Trent once hiked up the slopes in Waianae to hang-glide and was blown several thousand feet high. "He almost froze to death."

He always used to tell me, "If you're out surfing, take risks, but calculate it first and then go for it." Goodwin Murray Trent Jr. was born in San Diego and raised in Santa Monica. His grandfather, John Parkinson, was a Los Angeles architect who designed several of the city's historical landmarks, among them the Los Angeles Coliseum, City Hall and University of Southern California campus.

Goodwin Murray "Buzzy" Trent Jr. died Sept. 6, 2006 at Hale Ho Aloha nursing home in Pacific Heights. He was 77. His ashes were scattered at sea.

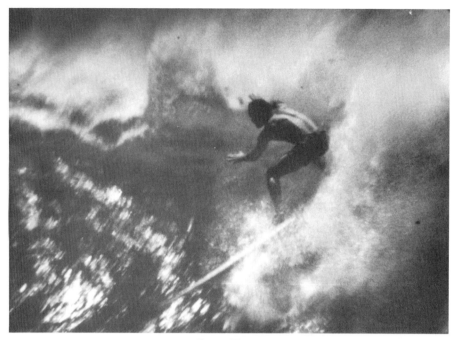

Buzzy Trent
A true legend in Surfing 1929 - 2006
Photo compliments of Anna Trent Moore

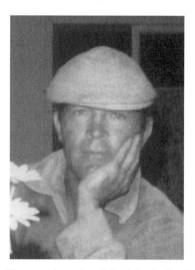

A figure like Buzzy Trent epitomized the ideal of calm in a crisis. The more that was on the line, the more methodical his approach, and I cannot deny the influence this intense man and surfing legend had upon my psyche under stress, especially in the ocean. It may very well have been his mentoring that pulled me through the treacherous scenes still waiting for me.

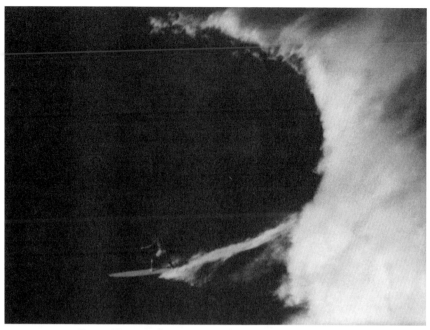

Buzzy Trent Rides a Waimea bay monster wave 1962.
Photo compliments of the Bud Browne Archive and Anna Trent Moore

CHAPTER SIX

And
Yet Don't Look Too Good, Nor Talk Too Wise

It Is The Easy Ones That Get You

The other brave and talented waterman who led me into such tests in my life is my buddy Randy Craft, one of the best sailors in Hawaii, and later in life one of the teachers of the legendary Buckminster Fuller. He lived right on the water in front of a great surf spot. One day I stopped by his house to see if the waves were firing. The surf was completely blown out, but Randy convinced me that the huge ocean swells could be surfed, not on a surfboard but on his new boat. In a matter of hours, I would once again be fighting for my life and my cool.

Randy had recently become the Hawaii representative for a new catamaran called a Prindle. Prindle Cats were built in Australia and aimed to compete with the popular Hobie Cat, made by the surfboard company in Oceanside, California. Randy had just received his new Prindle Cat and was anxious to launch it. His crewmember had not shown up, and with the wind gusting over 35 mph, there was no way he could sail the boat alone. Fate would have it that I would show up at just the right time, and thinking it sounded like fun, I decided to give it a go.

We headed out past the breakers, and the wind really picked up. We were flying. I had never experienced this kind of speed in a sailboat. I was already in the trapeze, my toes barely rapped around the hull, stretching out when Randy hiked, out hanging from his own trapeze seat to keep the boat from flipping. A huge ocean swell was heading our way, and Randy nodded his head in the direction of this mountain of water.

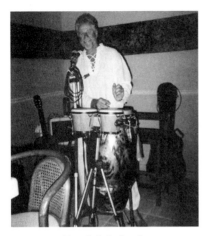

Randolph Craft

"You wanted to go surfing," he yelled. "Here is the wave of the day." He tried to line the boat up to the incoming wave, but just as he did we were hit with a huge gust of wind. The boat flipped so quickly that I was catapulted into the mast, a jarring collision that instantly dislocated my shoulder. Randy landed flat on the lower pontoon with such force that he feared he had broken his back. Whether he had a busted back or not, I still wanted to punch him, but my dislocated shoulder made it a little difficult.

He swam over to where I floated, holding onto the rigging, and tried to calm me down. Here we were almost three miles out to sea, the boat upside down and our bodies bent all to hell, and we were screaming and yelling at each other. It became quite funny as we both realized that all our emotions were not going to get the boat upright, and we laughed at our predicament. Bucky's words resonated in our minds, "boys it is cooperation, not competition that gets the job done." We immediately choose cooperation.

After several painful minutes of pulling, Randy was able to pop my shoulder back in place. The sun was starting to set and our next stop would be Kauai if we did not get the boat flipped upright. Despite a dislocated shoulder and a damaged back, we somehow managed to right the boat. We were still miles out to sea, but now we knew we could get to shore. We could have spent days at sea before anyone would have found us, but we were smiled upon from above, got back in just after sunset, and lived to sail another day.

The Prince Of Decadence

In this same period of time I came into contact with Bunker Spreckels, surfing's divine prince of decadence. The millionaire playboy stepson of Clark Gable, Bunker was a natural performer, surrounded with beautiful starlets and an abundance of drama. We trolled the islands in search of waves and women, indulging in a fantasy lifestyle of sex, drugs, and rock and roll, but we eventually started talking about cleansing our souls. When it came to drugs I chose to drink or smoke, but Bunker had moved into harder stuff. I did my best to shift him from some substances that I just could not deal with to those that seemed at the time to offer more harmless fun.

Addiction was such a scary thing for me. When I knew I was hooked on cigarettes I gave them up for good, even though it wasn't easy. All addicts are just one day away from returning to their habits.

One habit I never acquired was shooting anything into my veins. I hated shots. Bunker and I had long talks about our personal demons. He told me he wanted to be clean and traded his drug of choice for a little pot, a few drinks, and some wild women. An even more effective antidote was to get into some big waves and then find some great women. Besides waves, drugs, and women, Bunker loved the film industry. He talked about working with me on a hang gliding and surfing documentary which we would call "Return Flight to the Land of Endless Summer." Bunker and I were dreaming big. He had succeeded in staying clean for over six months when he flew over to my house on Oahu for a dinner party. He showed up that night a complete wreck, nodding off at the table. Six days later authorities found his body in a cheap hotel room on the north shore of Oahu. You are deeply missed my brother.

Dying For A Breath

I first met Bo at Nick's Fishmarket in 1977 when a mutual friend, Ric Marlow, introduced us. Ric is an actor, singer, and composer perhaps most famous for writing the Grammy Award winning song "A Taste of Honey." He was also mentioned earlier in the book regarding our epic flight to Maui. Ric was married to a beautiful South African girl named Irene, and she and Bo grew up as neighbors in Cape Town. Bo had just arrived in Hawaii with his new wife, also South African. Ric told me all about Bo's background and his reputation as a treasure diver and great white shark hunter. The story Ric relayed was that Bo had flown for the South African Air Force and had quite a background as a fighter pilot. His plan in Hawaii was to live off the ocean like he had done in South Africa. Ric felt that Bo and I had similar interests and that we would hit it off.

Bo is a very likable guy, a guy's guy: surfer, diver, fisherman, hunter, martial artist, and, from what I was told, one heck of a fighter pilot. His fighter pilot days far behind him, his move to the islands was supposed to be a semi-retirement. However, his plan to live off the ocean did not quite pan out in Hawaii. Unlike the relatively untouched South African waters, Oahu is pretty nearly fished out.

I had just earned my private pilot's license and was doing a lot of inter-island flying. A hundred miles over water in a single engine airplane was nothing for me at the time. Bo went flying with me on several occasions. The idea of having a jet fighter pilot as my co-pilot was very comforting. Strangely, he never did ask to take-off or land the plane. Every time it was suggested he would say, "She is your bird, you take her in."

We shared a great respect for the ocean, a shared passion that cemented our friendship. He had a great fishing boat and we fished the outer reefs at the banks about 20 miles off the northeast shores of Oahu. Bo's boat, christened Snake Eyes, was a 24 foot Bertram and was powered by two inboard Volvo motors. He had rebuilt the boat by hand, so the good news was that if something broke, which it normally did, he knew how to fix it.

One day Bo invited me to go diving with him. I had done plenty of free diving with a mask and snorkel but had never had an aqualung on my back. Bo assured me he was a master diver. We met at the China Wall in Hawaii Kai, and he had all the gear laid out on the cliff side when I arrived. He explained how to use the regulator, and repeatedly stressed how important it was to remain calm since a panic would consume all your air in a flash. He was helping me place the tank on my back as we sat on the cliff side when I noticed that my regulator was missing a gauge to check the remaining oxygen level.

"Don't I need a gauge?" I asked.

"Naa," he replied, "I've got one and my lungs are bigger than yours so even if you're excited we should be using about the same amount of air." He went on to let me know that we were going to go for a 100 foot dive. "That way you can always say you went to 100 feet on your first dive, an accomplishment that only advanced certified divers have made."

We had to time the swell surges to enter the water without hitting the rocks below, which looked harder than it actually was. As the swell approached the cliff, Bo signaled for me to go, and I entered the crystal clear water effortlessly and began to breathe from my regulator. Wow, this was a piece of cake. We began to descend rapidly, clearing our ears as we went. Bo kept smiling and giving me the thumbs up signal, and I would reply with the same sign. Everything was going great as we approached the 100-foot level. Then it all went horribly wrong. I was starting to have an incredibly difficult time trying to breathe.

Bo signaled to his depth gauge, showing me that we were at 100 feet. Having never been at this depth, I didn't know what it was supposed to feel like, but it was hard to imagine that the pressure alone was making it this hard to breathe. Soon the horror became quite clear. It felt like my eyeballs were popping out of my head when I realized there was not a molecule of oxygen to suck out of my tank. Dead empty, the tank was completely out of air and we were over 100 feet down.

My mind became very clear. I realized that if I dropped my tank and shot for the surface I would get bent for sure, so my only hope was that this master diver would notice that his friend was out of air. I trusted that before I drowned he would revive me one way or another.

I grabbed onto his wetsuit at his shoulders and began kicking for the surface. At first he didn't realize what was going on, but then it became very clear. I had to take a breath of something, so I took in the ocean water, and boy did it feel good. This was my first taste of the strange phenomenon that takes place before you are about to die. I was amazed how good it felt and even more amazed that no one ever told me you could breathe water. What a comforting feeling it was to realize you can breathe water.

What was really happening was that I was drowning, but in the moment it was very peaceful. About that time, Bo got the regulator in my mouth and brought me back to sound thinking. We buddy breathed until about 30 feet, and then slowly made it to the surface. His neglect almost killed me. His expertise saved my life. This would become the dangerous pattern of our relationship. Happy to be alive and wanting to trust him, I continued to listen as he revealed what else was up his sleeve, an adventure that would make this one look like child's play.

Stories… Truth Or Fiction? 1977-79

(Some of the names are changed to protect the innocent.)

On one of our fishing trips, Bo began recounting adventures from his days as a South African fighter pilot. He was a mesmerizing storyteller and spoke of being shot down by Zulus, who had been trained by the Cubans and Russians to fire heat-seeking missiles at any aircraft that flew over the interior of Africa. He captivatingly explained how South Africa had created the largest producing gold and diamond mines in the world. Several times a year, the owners of the diamond compounds would pay the South African Air Force to drop cement along the high tide marks to prevent the diamonds that had washed ashore from washing back out to sea. Bo said he had flown a few of those missions and explained that there were so many diamonds out there that these shiny rocks would not hold much value if it was not for the manipulated distribution schemes set up by the diamond companies.

Companies like De Beers marketed diamonds skillfully with slogans like "A Diamond is Forever" and created a social standard of how much one should spend on a diamond for his lover. If you did not spend your monthly salary times three on a diamond for her, you were not much of a guy. They injected a collective guilt trip upon the men of the world and sent the eyes and perceptions of women spinning madly for these flashy rocks that were now supposed to gauge how much you loved your woman.

The real story is that there is a surplus of diamonds but the elite distributors carefully control how many are released into the market at any one time. This assures a stable price, and the diamonds retain a high value. De Beers felt that if they could get diamonds regulated the same way gold was regulated, they could control the monetary system of the world; a lofty and devious goal.

He went on to tell me a story about the time he had to eject from his jet after he sucked up a heat-seeking missile. He initially camped by a river in search of food close to where his fighter went down, but soon he started making his way down the river and living off his survival food. This was where Bo spotted what he thought was an animal of some sort that had been carried away by the swiftly running river. He waded into the river to drag the carcass to shore, but as the carcass came closer, he realized that it was the body of a man.

Was this the native who shot him down?

Bo grabbed the native by the arm and pulled him to shore. He was blue, but the coldness of death had not overtaken him yet. Bo began to resuscitate him, and after a few minutes the native began to spit water and regained consciousness. This man was not aligned with those who shot him down, but was rather a worker in the Kimberley diamond mines and was in the process of smuggling diamonds. He was also the son of the commissioner of mines in Maseru, the capital of Lesotho. His name was Mpokoane, a name I could not even begin to pronounce. I do not know what his father's, the commissioner of mines, name was, but Bo called him Warren. The Kingdom of Lesotho is a landlocked nation, an enclave fully surrounded by the Republic of South Africa. The whites gave the native population land that had been totally mined and stripped of all gold and diamonds. They did still find a few here and there, but it was not valuable land. However, the people smuggled out the diamonds from the white South Africa's Kimberley Mines and ran for a few hundred miles back into the safety of their sovereign villages. Once safely back, the warrior gave the smuggled diamonds to his chief and then attempted to legalize them through the commissioner of mines. In order to do this, the native must have digger's papers. The commissioner of mines would authorize a native to look for raw diamonds in the riverbeds of Lesotho by giving him digger's papers. If the runner had not been granted digger's papers, he would have to go through his other tribal members who did.

A raw diamond is illegal anywhere inside the borders of South Africa. At this time in apartheid South Africa, the punishment for anyone caught in possession of a raw diamond was severe. If you were white and caught with raw diamonds, it was a mandatory 20-year sentence. If you were black, you were shot on the spot.

Bo had saved Mpokoane's life, and tribal culture required a reward. He tried to give Bo the diamonds he had hidden up his bum, but knowing the penalty, Bo wanted nothing to do with those raw diamonds. Mpokoane pleaded with him to take them, but Bo refused. "If you will not let me pay my debt to you, please come and visit me in Maseru and you will see I am who I say I am," Mpokoane requested, as the sound of helicopters in the distance meant a rescue team was on its way.

Bo was picked up and flown back to Cape Town, and he never mentioned a word of his meeting with the native. A year later, on holiday, Bo decided to visit Maseru, which is situated close to the South African border. He found his way to the commissioner of mines' compound and decided to check out Mpokoane's story.

The guards were apprehensive of letting Bo inside, but when he mentioned Mpokoane's name they sent in word, and soon a very large man emerged from the building. He greeted Bo and said that the commissioner would be glad to see him. When Bo entered the compound, he could not believe the display of opulent wealth, in drastic opposition to life outside its walls. Within a few minutes, Warren appeared, and he was even bigger than the man that greeted him. Warren's Zulu heritage was apparent.

Warren told Bo that he was indebted to him and wanted to reward him for saving his son's life. To refuse his gift would be an insult. He brought out a large tray of raw diamonds and began grading and rating each stone, adeptly documenting each flaw. Bo had never seen so many diamonds in his life. After Warren was done grading each stone, he poured the diamonds into a large envelope, lit a candle, and sealed it with his wax stamp and the seal from the Commissioner of Mines of Maseru. He handed the parcel to Bo and instructed him not to open it until he gave it to customs at his destination outside of South Africa. Let them open it and enjoy the shock in their eyes.

This was a fortune in diamonds, but he knew he couldn't accept them because it would certainly mean decades in jail. He promptly told Warren that he could not go back to South Africa with these. Warren just laughed and said that he was not going back to South Africa, at least not yet.

"I appoint you Assistant to the Commissioner of Mines of Maseru." The title would grant him diplomatic immunity in all black nations he passed through. "You will never set foot in white South Africa, and everything you do will be within the limits of the law," Warren reassured him. "Once in Germany or Belgium, you'll be able to collect the large profits you deserve for saving my son."

It sounded like too much to believe, but since he was on holiday for the next few weeks and nobody would miss him, he figured why not see if it would work. It wasn't long before he was issued his paperwork and escorted to the airfield. Mpokoane had his own little military escort see Bo onto a private aircraft, parcel and paperwork in hand. If everything went well, he would be in Europe in less than 24 hours. It was all very simple.

He landed in Zambia and was told he would be switching planes there and was passed along with quiet nods and subtle gestures from the underground African National Council. The well-greased wheel of their operation cleared Bo's paperwork and quickly had him on a jet to Belgium. It wasn't long before the plane touched down in Antwerp. With a nervous sweat upon his brow, Bo entered the customs line.

He was so nervous that he was going to end up in jail that he almost stayed in the transit line and never attempted to clear customs. When he finally handed the agents his passport and his papers from Warren, he was partly waiting for the cuffs to come out. The agent took one look at his paperwork and motioned for another inspector to come over. This was it, jail for sure.

The other agent took one look at the paperwork and said, "Please follow me." He was escorted into a private office and told that due to the amount of stones he was carrying it would be safer for him if they kept things discreet. The look of awe could not be hidden from the custom agent's face as he handed the parcel back to Bo.

"It is not often that we see a parcel of this size," the customs agent told Bo, "but since they're raw, I'm sure you're aware there will be no duty. However, if you leave the country with these stones you must declare them." Everything Warren had said was absolutely true.

As Bo exited the customs area of the airport, he saw a sign with his name on it. He introduced himself to the gentleman holding the sign and was led to a waiting limousine. It was a short drive to the office of a Mr. Shultz, a diamond appraiser and dear friend of Warren's. To say Shultz's office was palatial was an understatement; this was a man worth hundreds of millions of dollars.

Shultz introduced himself, sat down, and began grading the stones. His next comment verified that Warren was once again true to his word and the expectation of the diamonds' worth was accurate. Shultz casually asked Bo if he would accept $250,000 for the parcel. Bo couldn't believe what he was hearing. Seeing Bo's hesitation, he replied, "Cash? Or, perhaps you'd like me to set up a very confidential account for you in case we have future dealings."

With a lump in his throat the size of a golf ball, he muttered, "A confidential account would be best!" Within a few hours he was back at the airport staring at his deposit slip, still in shock over his good fortune. Then he booked a flight back to Cape Town, which proved to be a very big mistake.

When he arrived in Cape Town, his passport said he was in Maseru less than 72 hours before flying to Antwerp, then the diamond capital of the world, a travel itinerary that sent up red flags by the dozens. The customs agent in Cape Town immediately called in an agent from the IDB (Illegal Diamond Buyers), which is along the lines of the United States CIA. They went through his things but found nothing but his itinerary and a slip of paper with Warren's name on it.

Bo had sent all the documentation of his new account in Europe to his family in Denmark, so there was not enough evidence to hold him. He was released. According to Bo, his military career was also ending at that period of his life, so he returned to his fishing and wreck diving along the sleepy village of Sea Point. It was not long before Bo had purchased a beautiful cigarette racing boat, which he used to not only enjoy its open ocean speed but also as a state of the art treasure hunter and dive poacher's dream vessel. He would work under the cover of the darkest nights in search of the lobsters and abalones that crept and crawled through the real treasures of the hundreds of sunken ships that had gone to their watery graves full of gold, silver, and priceless artifacts. These ships, now swallowed by the deep blue, no longer elegant with their huge masts and billowing sails and now disguised by beautiful reef, lay home to many species of creatures, none more foreboding than the great white shark.

Bo would swim amongst these magnificent creatures that guarded the priceless treasures, remaining in the bowels of the sunken ships of the Skeleton Coast. Even to enter the domain of this aquatic monster whose sole purpose is feeding on everything and anything was an impressive feat in its own right. Bo earned every nickel he made sneaking off with what the great whites cared little about: the lobsters, abalones, and, when luck would have it, a doubloon, cannon, or gold coin. These sunken wrecks had to be searched for quietly and out of sight from the lurking eyes of other wreck divers, all looking for the treasure that could bring them a hero's notoriety and retire them for life. What lies under the sea is anyone's to go after, but the find is only yours if you remain on it and have the permits as salvage divers to make it legally yours.

Bo had better equipment than the local harbor patrol and the fish and game wardens, so even though they knew that someone was setting traps, there was nothing they could do about it. He would enter the water in the dark, with no moon and in the early mornings, filling his boat to capacity, and be out of the water by daybreak. He made deliveries like clockwork three times a week to the five-star restaurants that secretly dealt with him, always one step ahead of the fish and game officers. His police scanners and knowledge of the treacherous reefs in the area made him quite a legend.

Not only was he diving for lobsters and abalone, but he also kept his lifestyle in high gear by hiring himself out as a dive master and guide for those in search of the famous wrecks off the coast. On one of his capers, Bo led a group to a wreck that he had found with cannons dating back to the 1700s. They were feeling ambitious and decided to use dynamite to extract the cannons, but unfortunately for Bo and the salvage team that had hired him, they did not protect the explosives well enough on board the salvage vessel, and they blew their own boat up, leaving Bo and the crew in the water for several hours. This little caper, according to Bo, landed them all in jail, and Bo was incarcerated for several days. He even told me that Nelson Mandela was in the cell next to him at Robin's Island, where he spent the weekend in his wetsuit playing chess with Mandela.

He was finally released due to lack of further evidence, but the damage had been done. Bo was now listed on Interpol as a suspected poacher as well as diamond smuggler, so with the shit hitting the fan all around him, he decided to move to Hawaii.

Leaving the country was no easy trip. He was searched from head to toe and even escorted into the private room for a very painful look inside his cavities. He missed his flight and quickly booked the next available flight to the US; he never looked back. Forty-eight hours later, he was in sunny Hawaii. He thought he would be able to live comfortably on his quarter of a million dollars, but now, five years later, most of the money was gone. With the ocean not even coming close to providing him with enough money to pay his monthly expenses, he had devised a plan to return to Africa, and I was a big part of that plan.

So that was the real story explaining his presence in the islands, at least as it was told to me when we were out fishing, where he even pulled out a corroborating newspaper article that confirmed the explosion and the subsequent rescue. I was absolutely amazed at Bo's tale, and I had no reason to disbelieve him, especially since my *Hawaii Five-O* buddy Ric Marlow introduced him to me as the original Crocodile Dundee, and Irene, Ric's wife and Bo's childhood friend, had nothing but respect and care for him as well. Sometimes we just want to believe that these stories and the people who live them really do exist. I did, and was ready to go along for the ride.

Africa: Diamonds or Death

Apparently, Bo had been in communication with Warren, who was saying that plenty of fat cattle (large stones) were ripe for the picking. Still too hot on the international smugglers list, Bo could not carry the stones since he would definitely be interrogated, searched, and possibly incarcerated for even returning to South Africa. Messing with the diamond trade is very risky business. Another problem was that Bo could not take just anyone to this area of the world where a white man was a definite target and the natives would kill you for your shoes. He needed somebody who could handle himself. If I were interested, he would split everything with me fifty-fifty.

"So, I'm the sacrificial lamb," I responded, immediately skeptical. I was not wild about walking around with a big target on my back, but Bo said he had thought it all out. If I could fly my hang glider over the Zulu and Swahili Villages, the natives would think I was the spirit bird coming to take their souls to heaven. The natives were still very superstitious, and once they saw that I was not only the spirit bird but could shape shift into a man, I would not be harmed. Bo had been looking for someone like me to carry out his plan and claimed the rewards could set us up for life.

He continued to sell the mission, saying that an American would not have to clear customs in South Africa but could stay in the transit lounge until he reached his destination in America. A diamond does not have any value until it is cut, so we would not even have to pay any customs if we declared them raw. Bo said he needed an American that had balls and wouldn't get his throat slit as soon as he was left alone. He knew he needed me to pull this off, and he set the hook well and was reeling me in.

He said his family would invest $10,000 and if I could match it, we were set to make a killing. The year was 1978 and the South African rand was valued at 80 cents to the dollar, but his relatives would sell us rands at 50 cents to the dollar. With 40,000 rand, we could easily quadruple our money.

He was very convincing, and the excitement of the adventure began to build in my core. I contacted a few friends who eagerly jumped on board after I explained the plan and the possible payoff. We would spend the next 30 days training, because we had to be in the best physical condition of our lives if we were to survive this mission. Our rigorous regimen included martial arts and archery practice. Bo was a master archer, and since we could not travel with weapons such as guns, we would pack the bows, which would be our only protection. We purchased Bear breakdown bows and aluminum breakdown arrows that could all fit into a briefcase. Our silent killing weapons, just in case.

The only potential flaw in our plan was the bounty of unknowns. Nevertheless, we carried forward, purchased our tickets, got the necessary shots, and 30 days later set off for the diamonds. My cover story was that I was a stuntman and filmmaker coming to South Africa to do a hang gliding documentary. The title for the film, just as Bunker and I had planned: "Return Flight to the Land of the Endless Summer." With my stunt work flying hang gliders for *Hawaii Five-O*, we decided to use my slight notoriety for all that it was worth. I packed up my Eipper glider in the long solid cardboard tube that it had originally been shipped in from California to Hawaii. We hoped a glider would add legitimacy to the story that we were location scouting and looking to conduct test flights in the area before bringing an entire crew. I also packed several photos and some Sony beta-max tapes, including copies of my flying episodes for *Hawaii Five-O* along with photos of me with the stars of the show. We figured this would be enough to take the heat off of Bo. If I was there to fly the Twelve Apostles, Kilimanjaro, and Table

Mountain, Bo could play the role of my guide, a legitimate excuse for his return, and we began putting our plan into action.

The first leg of our journey in 1978 was to Chicago, where we would make sure our paperwork was in order and obtain our visas issued by the South African Consulate. Nick had recently opened up a restaurant there and invited us to stay with him. He even let us use his limo to get around and obtain our various visas. Nick was intrigued with the plan and said he would consider investing if this first mission worked, as he escorted us to the airport and wished us luck.

The next stop was Denmark to meet with Bo's parents and arrange the money exchange of dollars to South African rands. Bo's father contacted all his relatives in South Africa, saying that were eager to get their money out of their increasingly unstable country. They were more than willing to make use of our plan to exchange their rands for dollars. South African law only allowed for the removal of 10,000 rand twice a year for holidays. No other money could leave the country. The largest bill in distribution was a ten-rand note, so if you were trying to smuggle money out of the country you would need several easily discovered suitcases filled with paper notes. One hundred dollar U.S. bills were of greater value and also perfect for smuggling out cash.

We flew the 18 hours from Germany to Cape Town, by far the longest plane ride I had ever been on. But I can't complain, as I came damn near joining the mile high club when we got lucky with a couple of Swedish girls on our flight and had some fun in the bathroom. I was young and taking it all in as a grand adventure. Everything was laced with a tinge of excitement, but it got real in a hurry once we landed.

Two agents immediately spotted and approached us as we disembarked the plane. They flashed their badges and asked Bo to come with them; not a good start. I figured I could not make things any worse and decided to get involved. "Hey, he's my guide," I said. "We are here to do some location scouting for a film I'm doing." They asked to see my passport and dismissed me, firmly letting me know that this had nothing to do with me. Bo was simply a South African citizen who had not returned for over five years so they had some papers he needed to fill out. If everything checked out he could rejoin me shortly.

I was cleared through customs without delay and headed for the baggage claim. While waiting, I found a restroom and was surprised as several black men went rushing out nervously upon my entry. It seemed strange but I did not think more of it until taking a closer look at the sign outside. It read "NON WHITES." This was my introduction to Apartheid, South Africa's system of legal racial segregation. The year was 1978 and it felt horribly wrong.

Under the blazing African sun, I sat outside roasting with all my gear, waiting and waiting for Bo. Then a hearty man who looked to be about 60 pulled up in a Land Rover and yelled out, "Are you John?" I nodded. "Welcome to South Africa. I'm Bo's Uncle." He asked about Bo, and I filled him in on the officials who had detained him. "So he got the welcoming committee did he?" he offered nonchalantly. "Don't worry mate, Bo can handle them. Let's get your stuff loaded." We lashed the glider, still in the tube, to the top of the car and found a little restaurant for a beer and a bite to eat.

Bo finally emerged an hour later. "These boys have a long memory," he said. "It really pissed them off that they couldn't find anything." It turned out his dual citizenship, as he was born in Denmark, helped enable his return to the country. Then Bo turned to me and said, "I told you they wouldn't hassle you." He explained that they were not looking to bring any unneeded attention upon themselves as many in the international community raged against as their barbaric ways. The whole world was watching South Africa, and I started to realize that this place was like nowhere I had ever been before. A tension hung in the air, like a ticking bomb waiting to explode. A time of accountability was approaching for countries in violation of basic human rights, and white rule in South Africa now faced serious opposition.

We headed for the cliffs of Cape Town to Bo's uncle's cliffside estate. The place was magnificent, even decked out with two large cannons in the front yard that his uncle had found while diving around an old sunken shipwreck. He had restored them to their original splendor and even made them capable of firing. It was all regal and breathtaking. Beautiful was an understatement as we looked south to see Table Mountain majestic in the distance. Bo had contacted some of his climbing buddies to let them know he was bringing a Hawaiian stuntman to fly off this famous landmark of Cape Town, but little did I know that he was planning for us to climb its sheer cliffs in the process. Luckily for me, the weather did not cooperate the following day, and we settled for taking the tram to the top. Along the ride, Bo pointed out ant-like spots along the vertical face of the mountain, and as we came closer, those ants turned into climbers.

We met with the rest of Bo's family the next day, and they explained the various ways they had been cleverly smuggling money out of the country. Bo's father had a manufacturing plant that produced lamps and medical equipment like wheel chairs and such. They stuffed money into all these products, using any hollow opening that could be sealed either by welding or the firing procedure involved with the porcelain lamps. They saw the coming turmoil and wanted their money out any way they could find.

I took off my flack jacket that was stuffed with $20,000 and handed the money over to his uncle. They counted out 40,000 rand and packed it into a suitcase. I asked Bo if he thought we would be searched, but he felt we had a better than fifty-fifty chance that they would leave me alone, especially since going to Lesotho was only technically leaving the country. Since Bo had been gone, the only planes that were now allowed to fly into Lesotho were small commuters. Some private jets did get through, but it was very risky flying over the interior of South Africa. Besides the risk of being shot down by a hand-held missile, few private jets had the capacity to make the long journey without stopping somewhere for fuel.

CHAPTER SEVEN

If You Can Dream And Not Make Dreams Your Master

We left the following day for Maseru, Lesotho, and, as predicted, no one even looked inside my bags. So far, so good. The Maseru airport was a dusty little airfield in the middle of seemingly nowhere but was crowded with black Africans. A Humvee pulled up and skidded to a stop in front of us, and then one of the largest human beings I have ever seen climbed out. It was Warren.

The Legend Of Laquaba

"Ah Singgagna, you made it," Warren said, embracing Bo in a big hug. "And I see you brought Laquaba with you." Singgagna was Bo's African name, meaning the frog, and Laquaba was the bird spirit that flew the souls of warriors to the heavens. Laquaba became my name here after Bo told them quite a tale about who would be carrying the stones.

Warren immediately asked me when I was going to fly. I gingerly explained to this large man anxious to see my magic that it would not be this trip but the next time when I could be camera ready and shoot the movie I was writing. He did not seem to process my excuse and repeated, "Singgagna has told me all about you, and he says that you can fly like the birds. Can you fly here, now?" I could see he was operating with some primitive concepts, so it would be best to play along. I was in his country and was supposed to be the reincarnation of a legendary spirit; so not wanting to let him down I said I needed a cliff or mountain to fly off.

Warren wanted to see me fly so much that he had the excited anticipation of a small child. "There is a small mountain by the Swahili village, he could fly there," he continued.

"That is where I want him to fly," Bo chimed in. "I want those villagers to know that this is Laquaba and hopefully they will leave his shoes intact and his body for that matter as well."

I felt like I was at the end of the world, a healthy apprehension that filled my mind as we climbed into the Humvee and headed for Warren's compound. We arrived to an enthusiastic greeting from Warren's son, Mpokoane, who was obviously overjoyed to see Bo and hugged him tightly. Bo introduced me as the Bird Man, but Mpokoane already knew me as Laquaba.

"Can you fly to the heavens like the great Laquaba?" he asked right off, and I could only respond with the truth, as I knew it.

"I can fly like the birds. Only angels can fly to the heavens; they have special wings." I pulled out a series of photos of my flying at Makapuu. The childlike innocence of Warren and his people instantly struck me, but I never forgot Bo's warning that in the blink of an eye they could become tigers, devouring you without a second thought.

Warren, who had ventured off as we spoke with his son, now reappeared and asked if we were ready to do business. "The money is right here," I said, pointing to the suitcase.

"Several runners have contacted me anticipating your arrival, and I have informed them that you will be staying at the Queen Victoria Hotel. They will be contacting you there soon," Warren delivered this message in his solemn business tone. He said that he would get started on the paperwork, but then shifted back just as quickly to a jovial nature and declared, "Let's eat, you must be starved." Two young women brought us out a feast of wildebeests and ostrich, yet I still could not believe that I was in the deep heart of Africa.

Bo told them that tomorrow he was going to take me to the mountain above the Swahili village, and we would check the wind to see if I could fly. They all agreed that if I could fly over the village it would insure my safety for the duration of my stay; nobody would dare mess with the spirit of Laquaba. Mpokoane wanted me to land right in the center of the Swahili village because he planned to drive ahead and predict my coming.

"The Swahili are so superstitious. I'll bet they will give me their stones when they see you fly," Mpokoane excitedly said. "You really can fly can't you?" I assured him I could, but only if the conditions were right. Bo just laughed at it all and told Mpokoane that before I became the great messenger from the gods we would need a ride to the Queen Victoria Hotel.

Mpokoane brought the Humvee around and we took off for our humble accommodations. Along the way, we sped by a beautiful hotel and casino, and Bo explained that Maseru had become a mini Las Vegas for South Africans. To see this palatial casino hotel plopped here in the middle of nowhere inspired a double take.

"Is this where we are going to stay?" I asked.

"Not this trip," he answered.

Up the road was a rundown looking building with a rusty sign: Queen Victoria Hotel.

"This is where we are staying," Bo offered coolly.

"Why do we have to stay here?" I asked. "We can surely afford the casino." He quickly assured me that we were safer here at the Queen Victoria. The place was a dump, but it was to be our home for the next few days so I would have to get used to it. A huge black woman greeted us as we unloaded. Bo had stayed there before, and the woman, Goula, instantly recognized him and displayed a memorable three-tooth smile.

"Ah Endadie, you are back," she said. "And who is your handsome friend?" Bo introduced me as the Bird Man and mentioned that Warren had already christened me with an African name, Laquaba. "Is he really Laquaba?" she perked up.

"Warren thinks so," returned Bo.

"Well, he must be Laquaba then," she said, and then with a shy smile she whispered to me, "I'm not ready to go just yet."

She assured us that she had saved a special room for us, as we followed her. I could not believe how absolutely filthy the place was; a tent probably would have been a better idea. When she tried to wipe the beds off, it only propelled a great cloud of dust into the air. "Believe me, it's safe here."

Bo tried to appease my obvious disgust. He then began removing all the bedding and shook his sheets vigorously.

"What in the world are you doing," I asked.

"There is a little bug that lives in this area of the world, and if it bites you, you can die instantly," he calmly replied, still whipping his bedding about. Great, I thought, of all the ferocious things in Africa that can kill you, I'll probably die of a tiny bug bite. The safest place to be seemed like it might be up in the air in my hang glider.

"Why are we staying in a place where the bugs can kill you?" I asked. "This is Africa," Bo said, "and the tribal problems are always lying beneath the surface." He explained that you couldn't put various tribal groups together, including the Swahili's, without provoking a fight to the death. A few weeks of calm will go by, but eventually the drums of the opposing tribes will start on one end of town, and then the Swahili drums will start in response. Then one day the streets fill with stick-wielding men running about and beating the crap out of each other. Then the military comes in and fires a few warning shots, and they all run away. This goes on for a spell, building up to a riot, and the first place the mob goes is that casino. It had already been attacked several times. "You do not want to be at the wrong place at the wrong time when the natives get restless," he concluded.

That night at the Queen Victoria, the runners began to arrive, but the stones were small. I was expecting much larger diamonds, but since I knew nothing about this business, I left it all up to Bo and trusted the best was yet to come.

The following morning, we were up at the crack of dawn. The magnificence of an African sunrise was unforgettable; looking out over the plains it was as if you could see forever. Not much pollution here—in this neck of the woods, you could almost make out the curvature of the earth. A few minutes later, Mpokoane pulled up, honking his horn wildly.

"It's show time Laquaba," Bo yelled.

When we finally reached the hill overlooking the Swahili village, the wind had picked up, and totally out of the wrong direction. There was no way to fly off this hill. I asked Mpokoane if the wind was always out of this direction, and he confirmed that it was. All this way and our plan for protection would not work. Our last hope was that the wind would calm down or shift directions. It never did, and I never flew. We were left with our own resources of intuition and observation to keep us safe.

We drove down to the village, and Mpokoane introduced us to the chief and told him of the African names his father had given us, Singgagna and Laquaba. Mpokoane proceeded to warn them that if anyone tried to hurt or steal from us during our visit they would be subject to punishment by him and his father. He told them we were also very dangerous men and had special powers. The villagers gathered around us and jabbered at us in Swahili when I took out my Polaroid camera and took a picture of one of them. The flash shocked him, and he jumped back. With a magical wave of the hand and some rambling gibberish, I presented the rapidly appearing image to the chief. He stared and stared. Even Mpokoane looked on in awe, saying, "You have stolen his soul!"

"No, I only borrowed it," I said. I turned the camera toward the villagers again and they all jumped back. A few cried, "No Endadie, do not steal our souls."

"Tell the others Singgagna and Laquaba mean you no harm," I was really playing it up now. "We are your friends sent from the Great Spirit." I spent the next four days checking the weather, but it was not going to cooperate. However, so much for hang gliding, my camera did the trick. I was sure glad I brought my Polaroid.

A few days later, we received a call from Warren telling us that the parcel was ready. We headed over to his compound, and he greeted us warmly once again. "I heard you made quite an impression on the Swahili," he said to me.

"I guess they have never seen a Polaroid camera," I joked.

"The Swahili are very superstitious. You must be careful with them," he returned. He then told us how our parcel had been documented and sealed and warned me not to open it until I got to my final destination. He ordered his guards to accompany us to the airport. A good thing, as it was quite evident that we were being followed as we pulled out of the compound.

"We have company," I said. Bo looked behind at the car following.

"Looks like we have a send-off committee," he said with a laugh. "Guess it wasn't such a secret. When we land, they'll come for me. They can't touch you. No matter what they say, don't clear customs. Book the next flight to the U.S. and surround yourself with people at all times," he turned serious. "You'll be a harder target that way."

"What do you mean target?"

"You have their stones. They want them back. But they can't touch you if you don't clear customs."

Three agents approached us as soon as we landed in Cape Town. They went straight for Bo, demanded his passport, and asked that he follow them. Everything was going as planned. I went over to the TWA desk and asked about the next flight to New York. There was not a flight until the following morning, but I booked the flight and asked for the transit lounge.

Two of the agents that had escorted away Bo approached me as I waited in the lounge. They were very courteous and addressed me by my name. "Mr. Thorp, how has your filming gone?"

"Very well, thanks."

"To show our appreciation for your film's promotion of South Africa we have set up a complimentary suite at our finest hotel for you. Would you please follow me?"

"No thanks. I will wait right here."

"Why would you want to wait here when we're offering you a beautiful suite?"

"I don't like the way you treat people around here. You treat the blacks like they're animals," I said boldly. "I'd rather sleep on the floor." They tried to tell me that I just did not understand the full complexity of the situation in South Africa, and they scoffed at the idea that the Kaffirs, their derogatory term for black South Africans, were anything but a hair above a wild animal.

I asked them where they had my guide, and they only returned my questions with questions of their own.

"How long have you known this man?"

"I hired him as my guide, other than that I don't know a thing about him."

They again asked why I did not want the hotel room they were offering, and I said that I was not going to take a chance on missing my flight and repeated that I would stay right here.

"You should be very careful, Mr. Thorp."

"That is just what I'm doing."

The Big Payoff

Bo was still nowhere to be found the following morning, but when they called out my flight, I went straight for the gate. The two agents we had talked to the day before were waiting for me at check-in.

I spotted my hang glider being loaded on the oversized cargo carrier and noticed that the cardboard packaging had been duct taped together. "So who cut into my glider?" I asked. "That cardboard tube is what protects the wings, and you will be responsible for it." The agents signaled for the handlers to bring my glider over to me. It looked as if they had just cut the cardboard to see that it really was a glider inside, and when I looked at the leading edges and the stoppers at the ends of the aluminum, they looked as if they had not been touched. All this suspicion and no one had even looked inside of the glider tubes. Ideas of future hiding places began to dance in my mind.

"Your guide is not who he says he is," they began. "He has quite a history here in South Africa. We are aware of your meeting with Warren, and you should be warned that he is under investigation. This is serious business and we are concerned for your safety."

"Excuse me, but I have to catch a plane," I said sliding past them, hearing the final boarding call. I was shaking to the core while handing over my trembling ticket and passport to the desk clerk, but soon let out the biggest sigh of relief upon hearing, "You may board the aircraft now Mr. Thorp." The glider and bags were loaded onto the plane without delay. We were safe for now, and, more importantly, I had a few diamonds wrapped around my waist with all the documentation, including the wax stamp from Warren that confirmed that the stones I was carrying came out of the Maseru Lesotho riverbeds and mines.

When I landed in New York, my first call was to my old buddy Johnny Kuhl. Johnny was a highly decorated New York cop that I had met in Honolulu when he was handling security for a songwriter and performer. He told me if I was ever in New York to give him a call. There was no better time than now. First, I had customs to get through.

I handed my passport to the customs agent, and it only took a few seconds for my name to come up on Interpol.

"Do you have anything to declare?" he asked.

"Only this," I replied and lifted up my shirt to unzip my money belt that held the parcel of diamonds and emeralds. Two more customs agents joined us now at the podium, and the first agent said, "He is declaring this."

"You'll find everything in order," I said coolly. "Documented and sealed by the Commissioner of Mines in Maseru, Lesotho."

The three agents could not help but broadcast their amazement as they inspected the parcel. They looked on in disbelief, but could say nothing more than, "Everything is in order. A raw diamond has no value until cut. The same goes for these emeralds that he is carrying. There is no duty Mr. Thorp. We must warn you, though, that if you try to take these stones out of the country, you must declare them."

I assured them I would and offered a cheery, "Have a great day." We had pulled it off. Everything went just as Bo had said it would. The only thing left was to sell the stones.

Johnny met me at the baggage claim and seemed glad to see me. "So what brings you to town?" he asked. I said I would tell him all about it on the ride to his place. Whenever we passed a cop, they would nod or smile. He seemed to know everyone and I could not feel safer in anyone else's company. He had quite a reputation for being a tough but fair cop. He was sure surprised at the site of the diamonds.

"You're one lucky son of a bitch," he said. "I'll bet you really pissed them off. They shoot people for this type of smuggling and don't think twice about it." Johnny had a big safe in his apartment, and I knew my parcel was safe in there with his wide assortment of guns. "Let's go get a drink," he offered. We went to one of his favorite watering holes, where a few turned into many. Johnny had to pick me up off the floor by the end of the night. It had finally caught up to me just how close I had come to spending a very long time in a South African jail, or worse, much worse.

I caught the next flight to LA that morning and then back to Hawaii. Kim was at the airport waiting for me and let me know right off that Bo had been released and was going to make it back in a few days. I held her tight and told her how much I loved her. Bo called that night and said that he had contacted his guy in Germany and that we had a solid connection to sell the stones.

Our investors could not believe their eyes when we rolled out the parcel. They picked through the stones and chose a few for themselves. Everyone was happy and relieved that it had gone so well. I had decided that was enough excitement for quite a while and that this would be my last trip.

Much to our disappointment, the wholesale diamond buyers were critical of the stones. They said the color was off and the clarity was not the greatest. The only thing to our benefit was the size of the stones. They would cut nicely but would not yield the kind of profit Bo had told me they would. We were able to cover the expenses of the trip and pay the rent for a few months, but that was about it. The investors made about 30% on their money, but this was certainly not the mother load as I was led to believe and for which I put my neck on the line.

Bo's explanation was that they did not know what they were talking about and that we should have had them cut ourselves. He promised we would have made a lot more money that way. "Next time I will find a cutter and that way our profits will be much greater," he continued. Hindsight is twenty-twenty I thought to myself.

A few weeks later, we got a call from the wholesale diamond buyers and they were pleased with the way the stones turned out but wanted to know if we could get colored stones as well. Bo quickly assured them we could but told them to give us some samples so we could match up the exact color they were looking for. He called me and said that the wholesalers wanted to sponsor our next trip. Going back to Africa was not an appealing idea. We had gotten lucky at many points the first time through, and then to barely make a profit really took the wind out of my sail. It just seemed like a lot of risk and very little reward, but after some encouragement from Bo, I started to come around. He promised bigger profits this time, and he reminded me of how much fun we had and said that we could find a place to fly this time, surf, dive, and really have a nice vacation on someone else's dime. "It is all about the adventure," he pleaded.

He finally talked me into it. Bo contacted Warren to warn him we would be coming and to have him keep an eye out for good stones. Warren informed Bo that Russia, afflicted with severe financial hardships, was overloading the diamond market with their stones. This massive dumping of stones was causing the price of diamonds to plummet. He said this was probably the last chance to secure a parcel that could set one up for life. De Beers was buying everything they could get their hands on, stolen or not. The only way they could stop the prices from falling was to buy up the excess inventory and pull them off the market. Any black African even suspected of running diamonds was either missing or turning up murdered. Mpokoane, Warren's son, was among the missing, and Warren was deeply troubled.

It sounded like turbulent times in Maseru, but a few nights later Bo called and our trip was all set. "You in?" he asked. Unable to resist the idea of the big score, two weeks later I was with him on a flight to Cape Town. I looked out the oval window as the plane pulled up to the gate and saw the same welcoming committee that had greeted us the first time. I pointed out the agents on the tarmac and Bo said, "It's nice to see we're loved." We walked down the stairs, and as soon as they spotted us, they headed in our direction. "Here come the bloody Nazis," I chimed in.

"Mr. Bo, will you please come with us?" they said, not wasting any time. I smiled and asked them, "Remember us? We are here to do our movie."

"We know who you are and why you're here," they replied. "And it's not to make a movie."

They had nothing on us since we were not carrying any money this time. We felt it was safer to have the money wired directly to Maseru when we had the parcel in hand. I was more than accommodating as they searched me thoroughly. We each had about $5,000 in cash, not enough for them to do anything with, and they released us about five hours later. I kept thinking that this was more hassle than it was worth, but the possibility that it could set us up for life kept me going forward with the plan.

"If you two as much as sneeze in the wrong direction, you're out of here. Now beat it!" they sternly warned.

Only a couple of months had passed, but I could tell things had changed around the airport in 1979. The "WHITES ONLY" sign was gone outside the bathroom, but the blacks were still using their filthy designated bathrooms. Nothing had really changed about their segregation other than the signs.

The Cape was spectacular. Bo pointed out the Twelve Apostles mountain peaks and the cliffs along the coast that went on for miles. I noticed right off that the wind was blowing right up the face. This was the place to fly. Unfortunately, I never did have the opportunity to fly in Africa, but on this trip, I would end up happy just to make it out alive.

Another Trap For Fools

We headed for Durban the following day, flying along the Indian Ocean coastline. Bo had set up meetings with a group of jewelers who had a line on emeralds, rubies, and sapphires. Disappointingly, these colored stones were very small and already cut, which meant they would have to be declared. But Bo convinced me this was a good deal and that everybody would be happy. Paying a couple of thousand rand for this parcel felt like a bad start, a feeling that probably should have been heeded.

Determined to make the most of our visit this time, we checked into a nice hotel on the beach and went straight for the surf. The waves were small but most distressing were the dangerous currents and sharks signs posted everywhere. We rented a couple of boards and paddled out into what felt like bath water. I was actually surfing in South Africa, fulfilling a long held dream generated from watching Bruce Brown's classic surf flick Endless Summer. The reality was not as romantic as my dream. The water was an ugly brown and really did look sharky. We caught a few waves and started paddling in when I felt a sudden tug on my leg. It sent me off, yelping wildly. Then Bo emerged from out of the water behind me, once again laughing hysterically at his own antics. He was certainly amused easily, and I was already getting tired of his kind of fun.

A quick plane ride and we were back in Cape Town the next day. Bo's brother met us at the airport with more disconcerting news. Our friends in the IDB paid him a visit looking for us and made it clear that we would be arrested if we even tried to get on a plane to Maseru. Bo looked at me and said, "So we will drive. It will only take us a couple of days to get there, and they will never know that we were there."

Back on the road again, we were passing through a game reserve when Bo abruptly pulled off the road. Springbok, or deer, as we call them in the States, wandered about everywhere. "Hey Laquaba," Bo started. "See how close you can get to those springbok, and I'll film you." He handed me an orange, which apparently they went crazy for. I got out of the car and slowly started walking toward the gentle animals. Every time I looked back at Bo, he would look up from the camera and signal me to go further. I had a strange feeling that I was being watched. The next time I looked back at Bo I was startled to see he had his bow out, fully drawn and pointed in my direction. Then out of the corner of my eye, I caught a glimpse of a large brown flash, gone before I could turn and focus.

"It was a lion," Bo said, breaking into hysterics again. "But don't worry, you're too skinny Laquaba. Mr. Lion wants the springbok, not you."

"You are out of your mind," I yelled. "Quit trying to get me killed." I felt like nothing more than entertainment for a madman.

Upon another gorgeous sunrise, we arrived at the Lesotho border, where you had to get out of the vehicle, fill out paperwork, and personally hand it to the guard with your passport for inspection. Just as we started to pull away, I let out a scream of, "Oh shit, my passport." I had left my money belt with my passport at the stand where I had filled out the visa slip. I jumped out of the still rolling car and flew back to the podium. As everything slipped into slow motion, I leapt over about ten villagers already reaching for the money just in time to snatch the belt out of one of their hands, saying, "I'll take that." My heart was doing a couple thousand RPMs. Not a smooth start at all.

The guards at the border barely paid us any mind as we handed over our paperwork. I recognized one of them from Warren's compound and overheard him saying to another guard, "They are Laquaba and Singgagna, very dangerous." I asked Bo if he heard what the guard had said. He nodded and said, "I think they remember us, our reputations precede us!"

It was instantly apparent that we were arriving into a very different Maseru than we had left behind. The place looked like a war zone. The Queen Victoria had a big hole blasted through the wall of the lobby, and a rickety sign stated the obvious, "Closed." We would definitely stay at the nice casino now. As we pulled into the once posh estate, we had to pass through a new razor wire lined fence surrounding the grounds. It looked more like a prison now than a hotel.

Once inside, everything appeared to be operating normally, and I was actually quite amazed at the beauty of the interior. We checked in and were shown to our room. Now this was more like it. The room was large and overlooked an Olympic size swimming pool. "Ah, a pond for Singgagna the frog," Bo commented.

We wasted little time in venturing over to Warren's compound, anxious to see what he had in store for us. I was absolutely shocked at the drastic changes since we had left only a few months ago. Everything was dilapidated and riddled with bullet holes. Mpokoane, recently returned from a runner mission, attempted to explain what had happened. Everyone was scared to bring stones into the village, since most of the runners who did business with his father had already been hunted down and shot. A policy of zero tolerance was in effect. It was not going to be as easy this time.

"The men who have your parcel are Angolan tribesman, men of honor," Mpokoane continued. "Their parcel has many big stones. I have seen it, over 5,000 carats."

"We don't have the money for 5,000 carats," I said to Bo.

"My father wants part of the parcel," Mopkoane chimed in. "We will be partners. How much can you put in?"

We explained that we had about 50,000 rand ready to be wired if the parcel was good, but our money guys were already feeling apprehensive since our first parcel was of subpar color and clarity.

"These are Angolan stones and the parcel is beautiful, not like your last parcel," Mpokoane returned a little too quickly.

"So when can we see them," I said, already skeptical and thinking, here we go again.

"They do not want to be seen with us, so we must meet them at the location," said Mpokoane. "It is approximately 100 kilometers from here, far away from the eyes of the IDB. My father and I have made a plan. I will travel in the night and meet these men and make the deal. They know me and trust me. When can you get the money?"

"It can be wired immediately," said Bo.

The money arrived the next day, and we delivered it all to Warren, who looked tired. "Ah, Bo," he said, "Things have been rough ever since you left." He went on to describe how the IDB had tried to trap him several times. Men came in and claimed to be working with us. They brought a lot of money and went around the authority of the chiefs, having the runners bring the stones directly to them. They created a great deal of mistrust. How they smuggled the stones out, he had no idea. They had not returned, but they had purchased over 100,000 carats.

"The tribal chiefs think you are involved and want nothing to do with you," Warren continued. "This big parcel from Angola may be our way out. The amount of money they want is nothing for a parcel of that size. We just got word that the parcel is ready. If Mpokoane does not leave immediately, they will return to Angola, since they already fear for their lives. He must leave tonight."

Sensing another trap, I did not have a good feeling about any of it, but Bo was fully confident in the security of our money since Warren was not only involved but also putting up the lion's share of the money. Mpokoane left that night and said he would return within a week. Bo and I returned to the hotel, and, with nothing else to do, we made ourselves comfortable by the pool. A collection of very attractive South African women lined the poolside, and we were very thankful for a diversion from our anxious concerns with the diamond trade.

A week went by and then two without a word or sign from Mpokoane, and even Warren was becoming quite worried. We were all restless, watching the hours tick by each day. We set up cardboard boxes as targets to practice our archery, and the villagers lined up every morning to watch and let out great cheers when the arrows found their mark. Our morning workouts also included our katas, kicking and punching the heavy bag. With fit bodies and worried minds, we waited and waited for Mpokoane's return. We went to Warren's compound every afternoon, but all Warren could say was we must be patient.

He also warned us about leaving the hotel at night, since the chiefs were throwing all the blame of the recent problems in our direction. Bo asked Warren to set up a meeting with the chiefs so that we could speak with them and clear our name, prove we were honorable men and that we had nothing against them. "Please ask them to meet with us so they can hear the truth," Bo requested. Warren would do his best but could not guarantee anything. But later that evening he left a message that two chiefs had agreed and we could meet them at dark. Shortly after sunset, a knock came at our hotel room door, and two large chiefs entered our room.

"All white men are messengers of the devil," were the first words out of their mouths. "If you leave our country now, we will spare your lives." They got up to leave, but we pleaded with them to hear what we had to say.

"We are honorable men, and we were not part of the deception," Bo tried. "We want to help you rid this country of these evil men. I have never lied to you. We have come to fight the evil that surrounds you."

"We are going to kill all the whites!" insisted the chiefs, unmoved. "You must leave now!"

"Not until we get the diamonds we've paid for," I said. "We have a deal with Warren, and Mpokoane should be back soon with our parcel. Then we will leave."

"Our warriors plan to kill you in the night," one of them threatened, talking directly to me. "The men that said they work for you, they will not return. If they do, they will never leave alive. We will kill them in the night and take what they have. Then they will come for you."

"They will die if they try," I answered quickly as I reached down and pulled my bow from the side of the bed and fired a single arrow at the door. A lucky but perfect shot, head high and dead center, that sent a clear message to the chiefs. Bo looked at me, his eyebrows raised, and then added, "If they come for us, you better pray for them."

"I, Laquaba, will take their souls," I declared, hoping they had heard of my earlier soul stealing Polaroid camera exploits. It must have been the shots of tequila at the pool that gave me the balls to go up against these threatening primitive chiefs. I had to chuckle as the two large men squeezed past the arrow as they exited the room.

"You've learned well Laquaba," Bo said. "What a shot."

Another week went by, and then another. Almost five weeks had gone by without a sign from Mpokoane. I was not very optimistic about our chances at this point and started to worry how we were going to explain to our guys that their money was gone and there was nothing to show for it except the few colored stones purchased earlier. I was sure we had gotten burned. Our money was running out and so was my patience.

An apparent miracle arrived at our hotel room door a few days later when another runner Bo had worked with in the past made it through and presented some amazingly beautiful stones. The runner said the complete parcel was over 1,000 carats with each stone in the five to six carat range, the type of parcel we had been looking for from the beginning. The only problem was that Mpokoane still had all our money. Bo told the runner to meet us at Warren's office in two hours and to bring his digger papers with him.

We called Warren and told him about the runner, Gato, and the parcel. Warren was skeptical, saying, "He is a thief."

"I don't care what he is if he has the parcel he says he does," argued Bo. "Your son has had all of our money for over a month now. If you will help us secure this parcel we will save face with our investors and even have enough to come back to complete the deal when Mpokoane returns."

"I will take a look at the parcel," Warren conceded, "but I won't guarantee anything."

At this point I did not trust anybody, feeling like we got ripped off and Warren was part of it. I was thoroughly fed up with the diamond business, but figured I would carry this out to see what could be salvaged from the trip. We waited and waited for Gato to show up at the compound, and just before we were to give up on him, he arrived.

My heart leapt from my chest when he rolled out the parcel on Warren's desk. This was an incredible parcel, the stones exactly as he had described. These diamonds had to be worth a fortune. However, my jubilation was short lived as Warren's face quickly turned to anger and he shouted, "Get these stones off my table. This is a trap."

"What do you mean a trap?" I questioned.

"These are police stones. I have seen this parcel before," said Warren.

"How do you know," I persisted.

He picked up one of the stones and thrust it into my face, bellowing now, "Look!" He pulled out his loop and under the loop you could plainly see "SAP" scratched into the stone, South African Police. "Every stone has it, and you can bet this man has no digger papers."

Bo grabbed Gato by the throat and lifted him off the ground, yelling, "Where are your papers?"

"At my village," he said.

"You little shit," Bo screamed. "Warren, I had no idea. Is there anything we can do?"

"Get these stones off my table," he demanded.

"What if we get his digger papers? Will you legalize the stones?" Bo would not give up.

"If you can get his papers, I will do this for you, but you must not touch these stones yet. Do not take possession until we have them sealed in a parcel. Now get out of here before the agents show up."

"Can we use a vehicle to go to his village?" Bo continued to plot.

"Take Musha, he will drive you. You've got to be quick; we are caught in the middle of a trap."

Trembling Trigger Fingers

My heart was in my stomach after going from complete joy to "oh, shit." Now we were planning on ripping off the cops, and I knew that this trip had gone from bad to a lot worse. Bo continued to hold Gato by the neck as we dragged him into Warren's truck. We drove for a tense hour before arriving at his tiny village. Bo tore Gato out of the truck and took him directly to his hut, and I followed close behind.

Gato's wife's eyes revealed seizing terror as Bo screamed at her to get his papers. Frozen in fear, she hesitated for a minute, and then Bo spoke to her in Swahili and handed her 500 rand, which she took with a visibly shaking hand. She lifted a mud brick out of the wall to retrieve the hidden papers. "Here Endadie," she said. Bo stuffed them into Gato's pocket. We dragged Gato back to the truck and sat him between us. "Let's get out of here, fast," Bo yelled, and Musha threw the truck in gear and roared off.

I saw it coming in the distance but could not quite believe it. Out of a huge approaching dust cloud emerged ten to fifteen military jeeps with machine guns mounted and aimed at us. They were setting up to block us, and Musha started to slow down. Bo desperately yelled out, "Hit it! Don't stop!"

Musha stopped, and the police force of Maseru instantly surrounded our truck. A man came to the side of the vehicle and stuck his nine-millimeter semi-automatic pistol to the side of my head. The barrel trembled and bumped nervously against my temple.

"Take it easy," I said, trying to calm this obviously frightened cop. "That thing could go off."

Then Bo started yelling, "Take that gun out of his head before I shove it up your ass."

Slowly rolling my eyes over to Bo, I said, "Hey, the gun is at MY head." They demanded we get out of the vehicle, and as we did, they grabbed Gato and began leading him to another vehicle. Bo, unfazed, continued to berate them, yelling, "He is with us. You can't take him." They just kept shouting for us to get on the ground.

As we laid face down in the dirt, I kept waiting to hear the sound signaling the end of my young life, the explosion of an executioner's bullet. I looked over at Bo as he continued to grumble, "He is an American and we have done nothing wrong." This was the crisis situation we had trained for, what I trusted Bo could lead us through, and I kept expecting that at any minute the great soldier would kick the legs out from under the leader, grab his gun, and shoot the others. That moment never came.

They radioed back and forth, checking our papers thoroughly. If they found the digger papers on Bo, we were dead for sure, and I watched in terror as they reached into his pockets. They came up empty handed. They kept our faces in the dirt for an hour before the head cop came back and said that we could go but had only 24 hours to get out of Maseru.

We went back to Warren's compound and told him everything that went down, but he already knew, having been detained as well. He was very relieved that we had taken his advice and did not take possession of the parcel, another sure signing of our death warrant.

This was enough for me. I considered myself lucky to be alive, and within hours we were on our way to Cape Town, where I caught the next plane back to New York. Bo remained behind in an attempt to salvage the trip and see if any of his other connections could come up with some diamonds. I was through with the diamond business.

Bo did not return for another six weeks, but the story he told upon arrival made things even more bizarre. He said that Mpokoane had returned with the parcel a few days after I left, so he drove back to Maseru to pick it up. Warren arranged for him to fly with the entire parcel to a Mr. Shultz in Germany, oddly the same exact trip that had landed him in trouble the first time and warranted my entire presence. Bo then said Shultz examined the parcel and agreed to transfer the funds into his account like before, but not for a few days. Bo left the office with the parcel stuffed into his boot. When he got to the street, two men converged upon him from each side, and as they grabbed him, he felt the jab of a needle. Apparently injected with heroin, he started to black out and they threw him into a van and took off. Just before he drifted off into drug induced sleep, he felt them pulling off his boots and knew that they had found our stones.

According to Bo, he was thrown into a pile of snow in a dark alley infamous for drug activity. There was a small bag of heroin and a few thousand dollars planted in his pocket. When the police found him the next morning, he was barely alive, suffering from hypothermia, but he miraculously survived. He was arrested and hospitalized, and a week later was released. How he talked his way out of that, he never did say. Bo could really tell a story, and, unfortunately, I believed them for too long.

Why did I believe in him? Here was a man who was so brilliant in so many ways, why would he have to lie? He was very convincing, right down to the stones in my hand, but the truth as he told it only existed in his own head. Sure, I had seen the potential to make money in our diamond trade. I had watched this guy do amazing things and never saw a sign of fear in his eyes, no matter what mess we had gotten ourselves into. I considered him my best friend and the brother I never had, but over the years more discrepancies in Bo's history and character would eventually be aired. I'm not even sure if this supposedly decorated military pilot had ever held a pilot's license in his life.

Yet, it was a hell of an adventure, and if experience is the finest teacher, I had a world-class faculty. I had failed to trust myself over the assurances of a shiny story and a dazzling storyteller, a lesson I would never forget. We went our separate ways and I was quickly back to soaring the friendlier skies of Hawaii. It was not long before *Hawaii Five-O* had another script for me.

CHAPTER EIGHT

If You Can Think And Not Make Thoughts Your Aim

A Lie Can Cost You Your Life!

If I have been saying "me" or "I" in reference to any stunts, forgive me. In the stunt business it is all about the people that surround you, because to make any stunt work, it takes a coordinated team effort. Every moment of viewing pleasure one sees at home on their television or in a movie theater runs between thousands to millions of dollars per minute.

When the directors yell action, they must have full confidence that each unit is prepared and ready to perform, because in the end, wasted time is wasted money. As I mentioned earlier, after pulling off a stunt on the first take, the set was ecstatic, with the actors, extras, and especially the producers thanking me and congratulating me on pulling off an efficient stunt. However, any praise needed to be directed toward what the team had accomplished. As the captain of our team, I accepted the praise, but back in the trailer I would reward my team equally or more than I had been rewarded. Beyond the applause and recognition, there was no better feeling than the pride of knowing we gave them everything they wanted and then some, often in one take.

One of the keys to a well-functioning stunt team or even an efficient set is honest communication. Anything hidden is eventually revealed, and the results can be costly. One experience, which could have cost a human life, comes to mind from the beginning of the next season, season nine, of *Hawaii Five-O*. The episode, "Heads You're Dead," called for the kidnapping of a yacht crew to facilitate a drug deal. They cast me as one of the kidnapped crewmen who were to be thrown overboard and then tossed a leaky raft.

The show was shot about a mile or two offshore, and the weather conditions were absolutely miserable, even warranting small craft advisories. Almost everyone was seasick, and one of the crewmen actually had appendicitis out there and had to be rushed in to the hospital.   My group, the yacht crew, consisted of the boat owner, who was given the small part of the captain, the female detective who was undercover, and an anonymous crew member played by a young actor, and me.

When the scene called for us to be thrown overboard, the new actor seemed very nervous, as well as being extremely seasick, and he actually started digging his fingers into me before they tossed him over. Well, they flung him off the boat, and sure enough, the man could not swim. To prevent a drowning, I had to immediately dive in after him. He had deliberately told casting that he was a good swimmer, but his lie was obvious now for all to see.

The next shot was of the kidnappers throwing us the leaky life raft. We all began swimming for it except, of course, our new actor, who was just flapping his arms behind as we left him and headed for the raft. The next take, he was the first in the boat. I put a flotation band around him, beneath his shirt so he could stay up. People would do or say anything to be on *Hawaii Five-O*, including lying and then almost drowning in those lies. He cost us time and safety, he lost respect and trust; and since he was throwing up most of the time, I even got one of his only lines added on top of my own.

"I heard you helped out with that actor," Jack later told me on the Coast Guard Cutter used to rescue the yacht in the shoot. "Thanks John, I knew you would pitch in if things got rough and you certainly saved his butt. This was a really tough show to shoot. Thanks, you did a good job!"

After that wild day out at sea, they asked me to stunt double for several actors that were uncomfortable in different situations. Going above and beyond was bringing in positive attention, and the casting director for the show soon began acting as my agent, getting me gigs when other productions came into the area. She was proud of me and would brag about the local talent of the islands. I was often the first local hired. She knew the people who looked out for the overall good of the crew and the shoot. There is no room for egos or selfishness on a set and pitching in beyond your designated duty is what gets you noticed and called back.

Death Defying For Hbo

You could hear a pin drop after I relayed the tragic news, silencing the room with the shock of it all, but it was the next question that caught me completely off guard.

"Do you have anyone to replace him?" asked HBO's producer. Was he really asking me this? I immediately said that we could not even think about that at the moment and excused myself before saying something that I may have been sorry for later. On my drive back to the house, the tears came and went as the nightmare slowly shifted to reality, but it was also impossible to let go of the line producer's words, still burning my ears. An emptiness gutted my core. I was sadly experiencing the brutally cold nature of the industry, a sickening realization that some people really do not care, and a lesson that I will never forget.

It all started in 1978 when I formed one of the first aerobatic formation hang gliding teams in the world. Except for inverted flight, we completely simulated the formations and maneuvers of the legendary Blue Angels. In addition, we created our own unique aerial dog fighting competition. We would attach 50 foot long crepe paper streamers to our control bars, and the task was to chase down the other pilots and pull them off. It was a very exciting competition for the participants, as well as for the tourists below. One wrong move meant the possibility of a collision or a forced landing, so you really had to know Makapuu's cliff like the back of your hand, where there was lift and where there were big sinkholes. We would even chase each other down to the telephone wires not more than 50 feet above the road. Each of us five pilots would put in 20 bucks, and the last man with streamers would take all, but the winner was responsible for the beers after we landed. It was all for fun.

Someone must have seen us performing and the news traveled fast, because it was not long before HBO contacted me about filming an aerial display for their new specialty sports program. Their show was in the same mold as ABC's successful *Wide World of Sports*, which a year earlier had featured me in a hang gliding piece done by sports programming pioneer Andy Sidaris, who became a good friend and promised to bring more stunt work my way.

HBO was looking for the extreme, and they saw us as the perfect fit for their new show entitled *Death Defiers*. It was later renamed *Thrill Sports*, but we were grouped with other innovators truly chasing the edge, speed skiers and base jumpers. The ski segment featured record holder Steve McKinney barreling down the shockingly steep slopes of Storm Peak at speeds over 120 mph. Carl and Jeanine Banish would be featured in the next segment on base jumping, highlighting their jumps from fixed objects (cliffs, bridges, or buildings) with their late throw of the chute and short glide down. The show would end with our hang gliding segment, which was to include formation and aerobatic flying as well as a dog fighting competition.

I would be the technical advisor and stunt coordinator and would also negotiate our deal with the HBO producers, who had flown in from their New York office.

My select team included Duff King, David Darling, Steve Rahefield, and Ed Ceasar. I had the HBO producers drive out to Makapuu, and after they witnessed the aerial stunts firsthand, they immediately wanted us all onboard. My normal rate was $1,000 per flight, and I requested that rate for everybody on the team. At first they balked at our price, but I informed them that once up, we could stay up as long as they wanted or needed. The standard fee became $1,000 per landing. If they wanted us to go up again it was another $1,000. This protected us from running up and down that hill all day because they missed a shot. With a couple of takeoffs per day, that was not bad money, especially when we were getting paid to do what we loved doing anyway.

With gusting winds over 40 mph and rain squalls, the weather did not cooperate for the first day of shooting, so I held a team meeting to make sure our priority was safety first. We all agreed that we would not attempt anything that we would not do without the influence of the cameras or, more importantly, the money. Nobody was about to get hurt or possibly killed on a shoot under my control. Also, we had decided to choreograph and stage the dogfight just as any stunt was scripted. No exceptions, we wanted to pull this off without a hitch.

A week went by with no change, the wind only got stronger and the forecast was not good. The strong winds were creating genuinely death defying flying conditions, but we had another pilot meeting and decided that we had to try and give them something. The only possibility would be at sunrise the following day.

The wind was still gusting the following morning, between 35 and 45 mph, but the wind direction was better, coming straight in. We decided that Ed and I would attempt it first. Ed was probably the best at high-speed wind conditions and would be first off. We had walkie-talkies on each pilot and with all the ground crew. Everything was set. I climbed down and tied myself in, and Steve brought the nose of Ed's glider over and handed it to me. We all knew we were attempting something on the edge of our sport, which amplified our focus. Conversation was kept to a minimum, except for Duff, who had the wind meter and was calling out the speed.

"Forty-five and holding, 47, 45, okay now 40 and holding," Duff was screaming over the howl.

With 40 being about as good as we could get, Ed yelled at me to lift the nose and asked, "How does it feel?"

"Stronger than shit," I said.

"Just hang on to me brother," said Ed.

"Still holding at 40," Duff shouted at us.

"Up, up," Ed said, looking me straight in the eye and then shouting, "Go!"

I did not even have to duck. Ed went straight up a thousand feet in what seemed like a second. He just kept climbing and climbing, and the cameraman said he was nothing more than a dot and had to get lower. I radioed to Ed that he needed to get lower, and all we got in response was a laugh as he offered, "Yeah right!" They had gotten one spectacular takeoff but that would be it. I was up next and asked Ed how it was.

"If the takeoff doesn't kill you, you'll be fine."

I got my glider ready, and the wind was holding steady at 42 mph, a little stronger than Ed's takeoff, but this looked like my only window. My wife, Kim, looked at me as I taped on the big radio and asked, "Are you sure about this?"

"No," I replied, "but Ed made it, and my glider is even smaller and should have a little better penetration. This is what it's all about, honey."

We all knew safety was first, but the thrill was hard to deny. I hooked in and motioned "ready" to Steve. He walked my glider over to Duff as I struggled to keep the glider from taking off prematurely.

The wind speed was bouncing around from 45 to 42, and I told Duff to lift the nose. Although already knowing the answer, I looked him straight in the eye and asked him how it felt. It was stronger than anyone had ever flown before. When I heard, "42 and holding," I told Duff to lift it up higher. Then came the amazing power of the wind as it caught my glider, and there was no choice but to tell Duff, "Go!"

It felt like being shot out of a cannon pointing straight up. I was going straight up, and then a little backwards, and even after pulling the bar all the way in the glider was still rocketing upward. Finally, it began to back off, and I cranked a turn to the left. By the time I looked back at the launch spot my glider was already a mile down range and the crew was nothing more than black specks.

Ed and I eventually paired up and radioed down to the other guys to let them know we did not think it was a good idea for them to attempt the takeoff. Steve was getting his glider ready. Clearly, there was no keeping him out of the air. As a top glider designer with the mind and balls of a true test pilot, he was eager to test his craft in the most adverse conditions possible. Steve's launch was the same; straight up, backwards, and in a hurry. The three of us teamed up at about 4,000 feet, laughing at the craziness of what we had just done. "What a rush," we screamed at each other. We did not do it for the money, but for the edge, testing our limits with faith in our experience and abilities.

The wind velocity continued to increase and both Duff and Dave decided to pack it up after our constant urging of "Don't do it!" We then directed the film crew to the gap at Makapuu. By flying about a mile out to sea we were able to lose altitude, but every time we even tried to get close to the cliff, up we would go, disappearing into the clouds again. At least they got the spectacular takeoffs, and in the high wind, the landings would amaze them too. All we had to do was get over the landing area and we could use our sail to slowly parachute straight down. No one had ever seen anything like it.

The weather forecast called for lighter winds the following day, and sure enough, it was down in the 30 mph range. All five of us got into the air and successfully performed the formation flying, but the dog fighting competition would have to be saved for an even lighter wind day. With the weather still fighting us, we took a few days off to re-evaluate what we had shot and rethink our plan. One of the executives at HBO mentioned that since we were having trouble shooting from the ground, why not mount cameras on the gliders? We had never mounted a heavy movie camera on a hang glider, and now we were being asked to be cameramen as well as stunt pilots. I started to realize that these guys had very little understanding or appreciation for the difficulty of what we had just done for them. We were making it look too easy. We all knew one wrong move could mean a swift death.

After some consideration, I came around to the mounted camera idea. We were supposed to be the best and this was our chance to show the world our amazing sport. But it was true; we were not getting the shots we needed to showcase what we were accomplishing. Even though the cameras were not in our contract, we all agreed that we were flying for the sport and for us. We looked at each other and said, "Let's do it."

We would have to counter the weight of the cameras, since hanging them off the keel would require an equal amount of weight on the nose. A slight discomfort with the idea crept in as we started designing. Once again, we were attempting something no one else had ever tried before, but that night we had another meeting and everyone agreed it would look spectacular. Steve was confident the gliders could handle the weight, so we called the producers and told them it was a go. We would have to specially build the mounts for our gliders, which would take a day or two and give us a much-needed break.

The following day Steve finished a new aerobatic glider he had designed specifically for the purpose of pulling off a complete aerial loop, supposedly impossible in a hang glider. Steve believed that removing the top wires could allow enough stress on the glider to get all the way around, and that day we all went out to the cliff to see Steve test fly this groundbreaking high performance glider. Before the entire team, after doing several steep wingovers, Steve did the impossible, completing a full loop. We all hooped and hollered and doused him with a bottle of champagne as he came in for his landing. It dawned on me what an honor it was to be amongst this group of men. The bond of respect we had for each other does not happen too often. I loved them all and left the cliff that day feeling on top of the world.

I had a meeting scheduled with the line producers for later that afternoon, and I could not wait to tell them about the surprise we had for them. While I was driving into Honolulu for the meeting, Steve was heading back for the cliff. He wanted to show his fiancée, Blyth, their astounding new accomplishment. She had designed and sewn the sail of this glider constructed to do the impossible. Blyth was an excellent seamstress, as well as one of the few female pilots that flew the cliffs of Makapuu. Each sail she created was a unique masterpiece, and combining her talents with Steve created an impressive glider design team. As I arrived at my meeting, Steve was jumping off the cliff for Blyth.

Just before telling the HBO producers about the added part to our dog fighting scenes, I was pulled away by an urgent call. It was not possible to immediately accept or believe what I was being told. Steve was dead. He had pulled off the first loop effortlessly, but, unfortunately, he went for two in a row, the second one smashing him into the launch pad directly in front of Blyth, and killing him instantly. The chilling reality of death was slammed back into my face. We had lost, no longer defying death at all. Death had clearly won once again; the fragility of life was embarrassingly exposed. I came back to the table fighting the tears that could not be denied.

"We have a problem," I said. "Steve just hit the cliff. He was killed instantly."

I was greeted by nothing but silence and blank faces. That is when I was shocked to my core when one of the HBO producers asked if I had someone to replace him. It was obvious that their concerns were not about us. They cared only about the show.

How dare he ask me, seconds after I had just lost a dear friend, who I had in mind to replace him? A man had just died, yes, doing something extreme and which he loved doing, but these producers seemed incapable of any empathy, seemingly detached from what it means to be human. Had it been beaten out of them by the business? Was it never there in first place? Something was seriously wrong here, and I had to remove myself from these heartless automatons as quickly as possible.

Steve's funeral was three days later. Gary Wilson, a commercial jet pilot and stunt pilot, took Steve's ashes up in his Pitts Special and scattered them over the launch platform and the Ko'olaus Mountains. It was Steve's wish, as well as mine, to have his remains scattered over the cliff and the ocean below. Tommy Hauptman, our legendary local helicopter pilot, flew over and dropped flowers at the landing zone. It was a touching tribute as we all stood arm in arm saying our final good-byes to one of the best glider designers in the world. Tomorrow we would fly for Steve.

The next day the conditions were once again strong, but the wind was right on. An eerie silence pervaded over everyone as we set up our gliders. Once we had the weights balanced and the cameras mounted it was show time. The four of us had our preflight meeting and said a prayer for Steve. Once again, we honestly asked ourselves if we were flying for HBO or for ourselves. We all agreed that we were flying for ourselves, for Steve actually, and we dedicated this flight to him.

Ed was the first to take off, and when I readied myself upon the launch pad, my glider felt very awkward with all the camera weight. Nevertheless, my takeoff was picture perfect, feeling divinely guided. A single Mauna E'wa bird rose with me, hanging tightly off my right wing.

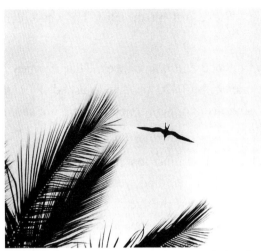
Our constant companion after Steve's death, the lone Mauna E'wa bird

"Hey Steve, is that you?" I yelled and the bird acknowledged my question by following me wherever I went. Duff and Dave joined us in the air and were equally amazed how this bird stayed with us through all our maneuvers. We all felt this was Steve letting us know he had made the transition and was fine on the other side. We felt it surely to be a sign, especially since Steve had named his new glider the Mauna E'wa. With his spirit flying with us, guiding us, and protecting us, we were emboldened to carry out the rest of the shoot.

The filming went perfectly as we performed the dog fighting competition before a beautiful Hawaiian sunset backdrop. When we landed, one of the producers met us at the platform, once again stunning me with what he had to say. "Where was the fifth pilot?" he asked.

"He is dead," I answered back sternly.

"Well, we contracted for five pilots," he said. "Don't you have someone that could fly the same glider that Steve flew the first day of filming? We just need to match that shot."

I could not believe that they were more concerned with matching up a shot than with honoring our fallen brother. We could not use just any pilot, with the hazards of the conditions and flying in a formation. There was only one pilot that had flown Steve's glider design, but he lived in Alaska. I told him about Tom Veer, and he said to go ahead and check his availability. Thinking about the circumstances under which I contacted Tom still brings back that empty feeling in my stomach. He had heard about Steve and agreed to fly over and double for him. I informed the producer that we had a double for him, but they would have to pay for his airfare and hotel accommodations and pay him the same rate as everyone else. Tom arrived the next day and took Steve's place in the shoot. The rest of the filming went off without a hitch.

We made sure the HBO show was dedicated to Steve, and the final caption of our segment highlighted the stark risks involved in our new sport: "Steve Rahefield died while doing what he loved, flying hang gliders." The irony of this special, originally entitled *Death Defiers*, is that all but one of the featured performers in each of the segments was killed doing what they loved. Carl Banish died base-jumping, and speed skier Steve McKinney also died tragically, hit by a drunk driver while he slept in his car. In addition, not only did we lose Steve Rahefield during our filming, but we also lost Duff King, who passed during an attempt to fly off the cliffs of Molokai on another high wind day. They will all be missed greatly. They were all the best at what they did, and three died doing what made them feel alive. The cameras, the movies, and the television programs may share the thrill of their daring actions with the viewing public, but they will never completely capture the experiences these men had in claiming their unique place in space and time.

Bullets and Babes "B" Movies

Staying true to his word, Andy Sidaris contacted me a few months after the HBO shoot. Looking to go beyond his sports television role, Andy was branching out into film and requested my gliding and stunt services for a movie he was writing, directing, and producing called *Savanos Seven*, later shortened to *Seven*. He was highly respected for his work as the first director of ABC's *Wide World of Sports* (a position he continued for 25 years) and for his Emmy Award winning direction of the 1969 summer Olympic Games, as well as for his work on ABC's Monday Night Football. However, perhaps foreshadowed by the

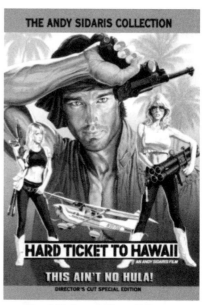

Hard Ticket to Hawaii Poster
One of Andy Sidaris' first films

creation of what he called the "honey shot," close-ups of cheerleaders and pretty girls in the stands at sporting events, Andy had a bawdy flare and would let it run wild in his Bullets, Bombs, and Babes series of B-movies, also known as his Triple B series, produced between 1985 and 1998, and almost entirely shot in Hawaii.

In 1978, Andy was just beginning to hone the craft of the tits and ass (T&A) action flick, and he had not forgotten the flying I had done for him earlier. Crazy enough, he brought me on to double for a black actor named Christopher Joy. The world of stunts today is a little different than it was then. Guys could double for girls and so forth. Now it is strictly gender for gender and ethnicity for ethnicity. Fortunately for my finances, they could not find any black hang glider pilots then, and they did not hesitate to dress me up in an Afro wig, complete with black face and body paint. With Christopher's help, we had a ball as I learned to mimic every one of his motions, and from a distance you really could not tell who was who.

The stunt called for me to take out a mafia boss by flying over him in my glider while he was golfing, and dropping a hand grenade on him. Once again, it would take some creative artistry to make this outlandish stunt look real. The air above the golf course made for an impossible place to fly, but when I warned Andy about this, he said that he would provide a helicopter for me to get the same over-the-shoulder POV shot that I had told him about from my first *Hawaii Five-O* shoot. When I went to meet with the helicopter pilot, he immediately flew off the handle, enraged that we were trying to tell him what to do with his machine. Despite our past evidence and reasoning, he flat out refused, saying it would throw off his CG (center of gravity). I was astounded by his ignorance and stubborn reaction to our request, and Andy was furious. The stunt was scheduled for the following day, and we had to get that shot. I knew somebody who just might be able to save the day.

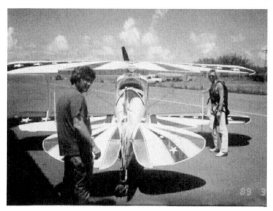

Pitts special: Tommy Hauptman and I getting ready to go up and break a few blood vessels in our eyes

I wasted no time in calling my good friend and helicopter pilot virtuoso Tommy Hauptman. Tommy's specialty was lifting. He had a contract with Hawaiian Electric, lifting and setting electrical line poles, and I often helped him for some extra money, hooking up the loads under his Hughes 500D. We had established a solid friendship based on trust. Indeed, I trusted his flying abilities beyond those of any other pilot, even enough to share the same airspace with him while in my glider.

Tommy knew exactly where his prop wash was at all times. The turbulence from a chopper can knock a hang glider clear out of the air, but Tommy would sit not more than 20 yards from me, a big smile on his face, knowing that his prop wash was sufficiently down and away from the clean air that sustained my flight. We would chase each other through the sky, Tommy with hundreds of jet-propelled horsepower and only the wind to power me, just a couple of carefree kids playing hide and seek in the clouds 2,000 feet above Waimanalo.

The following morning, we awoke to the roar of Tommy's chopper landing on the front lawn of the hotel. I ran out to meet him, and he signaled for me to jump in. Off we went to do some location scouting. The stunts would be saved, and Tommy and I were going to be the heroes. Every morning we would buzz the hotel at sunrise to wake everyone up, the crazy stunt guys at it again. The hotel warned its guests that a movie was being shot on the premises, and they apologized up front for the early morning disturbances. It is absolutely amazing what you can get away with while shooting a movie.

The filming went off without a hitch, and everyone was blown away by Tommy's abilities. And once again, we did every stunt in "one take." Tommy and I really had saved the day, and Andy never forgot me, as I would have plenty

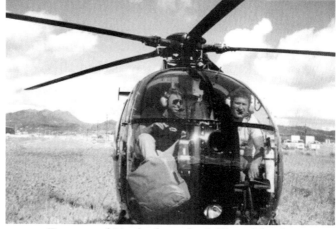

Tommy and I in the four wheel drive of the sky, the "Hughes 500 D"

more fun running about his sets with the gun-toting Playboy and Penthouse playmates starring in Andy's future T&A flicks.

Life was good and never ceasing to amaze me at every corner. It got even better when a few days after the shoot I got a call from Tommy, who told me to meet him at the schoolyard close to my house. He came flying in and landed on the baseball diamond, where I jumped in. He asked me if I felt like landing on top of a waterfall. Sure enough, we flew off and he landed us on the top of a waterfall that was well over 100 feet down from the top of the cliff. He backed that Hughes 500D into the trees, actually trimming the tops, using his rotor like a weed whacker, and he said to me, "I bet no one has ever drank from these waters." I was able to hire the best pilot in the world and he took me to places that I had never dreamed one could reach, proving trust and loyalty can achieve the impossible and unexpected.

Teaching A Foxx To Surf

The next job appeared just a few weeks later when NBC's hit production *Sanford and Son* rolled into town to launch its sixth and final season with a location-filmed jaunt to Hawaii. I was asked to read for the part of the surfing instructor and got a role featured with both of the show's stars, the volatile and legendary icon Redd Foxx and Demond Wilson, who played Sanford's son, Lamont. My part, as the surfing instructor in this episode entitled "The Hawaiian Connection," was to teach a drunken Redd Foxx how to surf. Now they really had me in my element, on the beach.

The shoot was a blast, and although I had heard all the infamous tales of Redd's battles with the show's creator Norman Lear, everyone appeared to be enjoying the filming in Hawaii, and all were in high spirits, some higher than others. During the wrap party, I sat directly across from Redd at dinner. He had taken a liking to me over the course of the shoot, and after dinner, Redd motioned for me to meet him in the bathroom for a little dessert. At this period in time, the late '70s, cocaine was prevalent and generally accepted. There were often times when producers would actually assign someone from the set to supply the actors with the white marching powder, seemingly everybody's drug of choice. Cocaine was definitely Redd Foxx's drug of choice.

I gave Redd a few minutes and then excused myself and followed him to the restroom. Redd's feet were visible below the stall doors, and a foul odor was permeating the room. I turned to leave due to the stench, thinking I should leave the star to his business, and Redd gruffly called out, "John, is that you?" The stall door opened and there stood Redd holding a spoonful of cocaine.

"Here," he said. "Try this."

Of course, I reluctantly obliged, not wanting to insult the star. With a sniff of the marching powder, Redd let out a whooping holler.

"How does nigger shit smell?" he yelled between eruptions of wheezing laughter.

CHAPTER NINE

If You Can Meet With Triumph And Disaster
And Treat Those Two Imposters Just The Same

The next gig that came my way was ABC's *The Six Million Dollar Man*. Once again, it was a trusted *Hawaii Five-O* connection, Margaret Doversola, who contacted me to read for another interesting part. The episode centered on a spaceship that crashed, releasing a bunch of robed mutant wanderers about the island. These mutants had contracted a rare disease that slowly turned them into monsters, which was the make-up artist's dream or nightmare, depending on how you look at it, transforming beautiful people into grotesque monstrosities in a matter of hours.

I played one of the aliens that was turned into one of the "uglies." The hours and hours of make-up were bad enough, but what really got my goat was an actual goat. I was given the part of a mutant goat herder, so I had my own little billy-goat co-star with me at all times. When offered a role with animals, make sure you receive hazard pay. That goat proceeded to butt me all day long, trying to ram that pointed horn of his up my butt every time I turned my back on him. The 17-hour production days are one thing, but when you have to fight off an ornery little creature determined to sodomize you, it really amplifies the tedium and aggravation of those epic days on set.

Six Million Dollar Joint

At the lunch break, I went to seek some relief, and a group of us snuck off for a little of the wacky tabacky to calm the nerves and get through the day. We were thoroughly enjoying ourselves when we heard a familiar voice.

"Hey, it really smells good over here."

We all jumped and turned around and were more than a little surprised to see that we were busted by none other than the Six Million Dollar Man himself, the show's star Lee Majors. He had followed us off the set with a healthy suspicion of what we were up to, but he quickly put our fears at ease when he reached out for the joint and joined our circle. You will have to ask him if he inhaled or not. After that startling encounter, Lee and I became fast friends.

I was still working the door at Nick's Fishmarket, and Lee came in often to join me for dinner on the nights he was not filming. We confided in each other over those meals at Nick's, sparking a friendship that has continued for years. It was actually during the filming of our episode that Lee received word that his beautiful wife Farrah Fawcett wanted to separate, which eventually led to their divorce. He was still very much in love with her and was shattered. To add insult to injury, Farrah had fallen in love with Lee's best friend, Ryan O'Neil.

Lee continued to lament to me how he had even pushed them together, asking Ryan to accompany Farrah to a few events while he was shooting on location. When Lee confronted Ryan and asked him to back off, Ryan regretted that he could not; he had fallen completely in love with Farrah and said that she was in love with him too. With friends like that, who needs, well, you know the rest. Farrah and Ryan stayed together until her untimely death due to rectal cancer in July 2009.

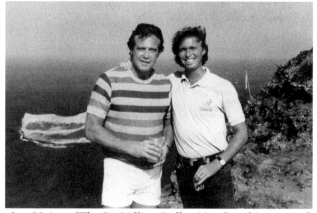

Lee Majors, "The Six Million Dollar Man," and I on top of the Makapuu launch platform

Stunts Unlimited

Recalling a similar lesson my Pop Warner football coach ingrained in me decades earlier, I found that the life of the stuntman was one of sacrificing your body to glorify your soul. As a stuntman, you enter promptly when called and pull off the stunt on the first take, most often because the complexity of the stunt could only afford one take. And then, ideally, you walk away without a scratch. If you do get banged up, you do not tell a soul; you return to your trailer and patch yourself up. You're paid to take the fall and if you screw it up it's your fault. You take your injuries and wear them with pride, never taking an extra dime from the production company for your pain.

The stuntman's relationship with the rest of the production is a unique one, and it takes a certain type of person with a certain type of attitude to thrive in the industry. A few young stunt performers embodied that special something more than anyone else and came together to put a lasting imprint upon the stunt world. In late 1970, Hal Needham, Ronnie Rondell, and Glen Wilder set up an elite organization called Stunts Unlimited. After they brought in long-established stuntman Dick Ziker, they only invited another ten members, including Hollywood A-lister's like Bobby Bass, Buddy Jo Hooker, and members of the Epper family, including mother Jeannie. A few limited others who showed a determined talent would later be accepted after an intense private and studied screening process, but the group was nearly impossible to join.

The Stunts Unlimited performers quickly established a reputation for being the best and complaining the least. They literally took over the stages at Universal, Warner Brothers, and Paramount, sometimes roller skating from set to set and doing the biggest stunts without getting a scratch. If you wanted to guarantee the best shot, it was well known that you needed Stunts Unlimited.

They quickly became an elite fraternity, and the common sentiment amongst the group was that if you were not a part of Stunts Unlimited, you were a second-rate stunt person. This angered many of the original organizations, like Stuntman's Association, and the competition was on. Those excluded from both organizations began to form their own organizations, like International Stunt Association and the Hawaii Stunt Association. When a job was landed by one of these organizations, they would only hire within their group. The key to all jobs was the stunt coordinator. If the stunt coordinator was aligned with your organization, you had a guaranteed in.

Dick Ziker and I met through a mutual friend, Dusty Gaines, at Nick's Fishmarket. Dick had also been an early aviator in the hang gliding world. Dusty quickly filled Dick in on my hang gliding accomplishments, and a few beers later we became great friends. All it took was a trip to the top of Makapuu to introduce Dick to this world-class hang gliding spot. The wind was stronger than any place Dick had experienced, and when I said it was perfect he agreed to launch me. A straight up take-off and a little fancy flying ended with a perfect landing and an earned respect from Dick Ziker. He literally gave me the shirt off his back and a hat and t-shirt that said Member of Stunts Unlimited. Although I never became a member, I wore the shirt, belt, and hat with great honor.

As tough as it was to be independent, I was never a member of any stunt organization except my own, which I founded in 1979 and named Stunts Hawaii. As an organization, we refused to kiss anybody's ass and held on to our integrity to build a solid reputation. Later, when Andy Sidaris once again held true to his promise and brought me on to his next sexy-girls-with-guns flick, he made me stunt coordinator, which meant my entire Stunts Hawaii team was on the job. Although most of Andy's work was

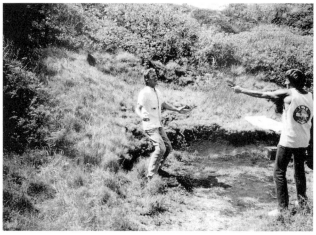

playfully tongue-in-cheek, he was a skillful filmmaker who worked on shoestring budgets. This film, *Hard Ticket to Hawaii*, really kicked off his Triple B collection and starred Dona Speir and other

Getting shot by one of my stunt performers

Playmates. Andy used these beauties as the dangling carrots, enticing me to give him a super buddy deal on my stunt coordinating fees.

"Come on John, give me a deal. Remember, who wouldn't want to be on a deserted island like Molokai with seven stunning Playmates?" Andy would say, knowing my weakness all too well. Reduced fees or not, we still had more than a good time shooting, with our stars running about half naked for most of the filming. And the stunts

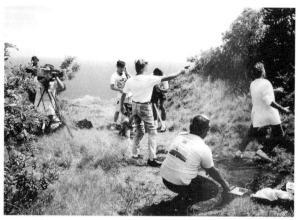

Behind the scenes: how to simulate a shooting sequence

were wildly outlandish. Blowing an actor out of a building and dropping bombs from a motorized hang glider was great fun. Also, who do you think the leading ladies love to be with off the set? The stunt guys, of course.

All joking aside, it was a great pleasure to bring in local Hawaiian stunt talent and take the stunt coordinator and second unit director seat. Stunts Hawaii is still in operation today, but is on hiatus, taking a break, as it is known in the industry.

Never Listen To The Director

Not long after my work with *The Six Million Dollar Man*, Dick Ziker, now the president of Stunts Unlimited, showed up on the island and offered me a stunt role on an episode of *Vega$*, the ABC detective drama starring Robert Urich. I did not hesitate to accept. I was ecstatic to work with a legend like Dick Ziker, and also excited that I would be doubling for Lorne Greene, known to many as Ben Cartwright of *Bonanza*. Pernell Roberts, who played Ben's son Adam Cartwright, was also going to be on the show, and they were both given parts as villains, roles they happily welcomed after years of playing America's good guys of the West.

Lorne had become very hard of hearing, which made things difficult because as his stunt double I had to communicate to him where I had ended up at the end of a cut. I practically had to scream at him so he knew where he was supposed to be for his close-ups. It was awkward to be yelling at one of my childhood heroes, and later it made for an interesting moment during one of our most difficult stunts.

The big scene of the show called for Lorne's murderous character to race a boat away from a pursuing helicopter. Dan Tana, played by Urich, was going to stop him by dropping down from a helicopter to light the boat on fire and then be lifted away just seconds before the boat blew up. My part was to dive from a flying bridge, approximately 30 feet in the air, as the boat exploded. The stunt was tricky, and Dick decided he better be the one to double for Robert Urich.

Done up in my wardrobe of a gray wig and a white silk suit, we sped out into the turbulent ocean, rough that day with six to eight foot swells. The timing had to be perfect for Dick to drop onto the boat, set it ablaze, and then be carried off in the helicopter, clinging to the skid and flying away to safety as the boat exploded in the background.

Dick and I were in radio contact, but with all the noise of the boat, the helicopter engines, and the whipping blades above, the walkie-talkies were useless. For some reason, the director was on board with me, out of sight from the cameras in the boat's cabin. He was determined to be in charge of this stunt and kept telling me to take his signal to jump. He had me completely confused when he frantically started yelling for me to dive off as Dick hit the deck. It felt off to dive without the boat being on fire yet, and I paused, but the director kept on yelling at me.

"Go! Go! Go!" he yelled.

So I went. I felt the wind catch me as I dove, and I just barely cleared the deck and hit the water at about 35 mph. Diving from a speeding boat that was also 30 feet in the air and awkwardly hitting the water felt like my body was being ripped in half. When I came to the surface the rescue boat was already right there, and I let out a sigh of relief to have survived a really tough stunt.

Dick came speeding over in another boat, pissed off. Not only was it dangerous for him to be jumping from the helicopter in those rough seas, but he was looking out for me, knowing better than anyone how close the blades were coming to my head. It could have been feet but it sure felt like inches.

"What the fuck were you thinking about?" he screamed at me. "Why did you jump? I hadn't even lit the boat on fire."

I tried to explain that I was taking orders from the director, who was very adamant that it was time for me to jump.

"Fuck the director," he said. "You listen to me. It's your ass that's going to get killed, not his."

I would have to do it all over again. After I talked with Dick, the director came over to me, shrugged his shoulders, and said, "Sorry, I thought you were supposed to jump." I learned a big lesson that day from Dick on chain of command. Directors direct everyone on a set, except for the stunt performers, who always take their final cues from the stunt coordinator. I was caught dead in the middle of their conflicting demands that day, but it would never happen again.

Well, we had to do it again and now my wardrobe was ruined, which meant I would have to wear Lorne's clothes since there were only two sets. It was an entertaining scene, me taking off Lorne's clothes as I yelled at him, trying to explain why we needed his clothes. He was so hard of hearing he did not have a clue what was going on. He had the funniest look on his face as I pulled away. It was more than a little weird to see old Ben Cartwright wrapped in a blanket, standing confused in his underwear.

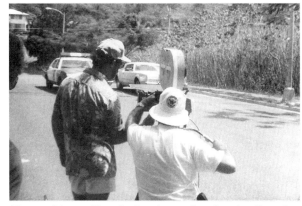

Me crashing a Lincoln Continental under the direction of Ronnie Rondell on the set of "Hawaiian Heat"

Dick and I repeated the stunt once again, and this time I even gave it a few seconds extra, making sure the boat was really smoking before I dove from the flying bridge and landed with a thud into the churning Pacific. This time it was golden. Dick came around and pulled me from the water.

"Now that looked good," Dick said.

As satisfying as it has been to run my own organization and participate in this exciting profession, in no way do I aim to place myself next to the Dick Zikers, Ronnie Rondell, Joe Hooker, the Eppers, and many others in the storied halls of stunt history. In comparison to their legendary careers, my foray into the stunt world has been a twinkle, but it has been a bright one, as I feel blessed and honored to have been hired by these giants and to have worked alongside the truly elite in the stunt business.

The Birth Of *Magnum P.I.*

I arrived at Nick's that night after a wild day of shooting for *Vega$* and was immediately directed to Lorne Greene's table. He had asked the guys at the front door to tell me to stop by, so I went over to say hello and was pleasantly surprised to find several familiar faces. There was my good buddy Ric Marlow and, sure enough, my new friend and Hollywood producer Glen Larson, who somehow knew just about everybody. Since Lorne had already filled them in on my hazardous exploits of the day, they gave me a little round of applause and invited me to join them at their table for dinner.

I had been introduced to Glen through Nick's when he became a regular customer around 1978. He always took care of me generously at the door, and in return his glass of Robert Mondavi Cabernet was always full and just the way he liked it. He knew that I was "in the business" so he treated me as a member of the family, a family he obviously held a powerful position within. He usually came in with the movers, shakers, and A-list stars, and word was that Glen could sell a television series with 10 episodes to a network without even doing a pilot. With creator, executive producer, or screenwriter credits for shows including *Battlestar Galactica*, *BJ and the Bear*, *The Hardy Boys Mysteries*, and even *The Six Million Dollar Man*, Glen's reputation was already established, but his biggest successes were still to come, including *The Rockford Files* with James Garner and a little show in Hawaii that would soon capture the attention of the nation.

Many times Glen came in with only his wife and family. One day, after discovering that surfing was one of my specialties, he and his wife asked me to take their son Chris to the beach since he was just learning to surf. Honored that they trusted their son in my hands, the next few days I watched over him in the surf off of Waikiki. One night when I brought Chris home Glen invited me to stay for dinner. It turned out to be a star-studded affair with Dolly Parton, Norm Compton, Paul Williams, Don Ho, and my friends Dick and Jennie Jensen. I was flattered to be welcomed to the table, and they all treated me as an equal, or at least someone who was a bit of an exciting mystery. Glen asked if I would take them up to the top of the cliff so they could watch me fly, and, with the wind in full cooperation the following morning, I performed a beautiful flight in front of one of television's biggest producers.

I had already pulled off an intense stunt with none other than Dick Ziker (twice). I was sharing several hundred dollar bottles of wine with my childhood heroes Ben and Adam Cartwright. I was dining with good friends in a restaurant I practically had the run of. I could not imagine how things could get much better—and then Glen started talking about creating a series featuring a James Bond type who flew hang gliders and lived on the North Shore of Oahu. He asked about the consistency of the wind conditions, and I enthusiastically reassured him that 90% of the time I could pull it off.

"If I was to write a script, would you be interested in being the technical advisor?" Glen asked me directly.

One of Hollywood's top producers was asking me to collaborate with him on a television series. Now I was really feeling like I had the world by the tail.

Glen followed through and began penning the initial screenplays for our new television series. He would often call at strange hours to ask technical questions about what was possible to do while flying a hang glider. It was all happening, and he told me that the series was going to be called *Magnum P.I.* For the show's starring role of Thomas Magnum he had in mind a relatively unknown actor who was currently starring in a cigarette commercial by the name of Tom Selleck.

I would be the stunt coordinator for all the hang gliding and would be in a position to work as a stunt double and even get some bit-part acting roles. The series would not begin for a few months, but Glen confirmed that it was definitely a go. With time to spare, I decided to take a break and head for the mainland to visit my good friend John Allen. John had become one of the finest entertainment attorneys and had recently negotiated the largest contract for a television actor with NBC and his client Robert Conrad on their series *Baa Baa Black Sheep*. I could use John's expertise to negotiate my own contract with Glen and CBS.

Upon arriving in California, I got word that another one of our hang gliding community was killed at Makapuu. I was sobered by the reality that another friend's ashes would be sprinkled over those cliffs. Two other guys in California had recently been killed as well. One even landed in the high tension wires above the Pacific Coast Highway in Malibu, unfortunately making for some gruesome front-page news. Hang gliding remained a very unforgiving sport.

I arrived at John's house, which sat at the top of Mulholland Drive, and was greeted by Voltan, the 150 pound Doberman pinscher, not growling but welcoming me with wagging excitement. I had actually delivered Voltan from my Red Doberman, Pele, when I was breeding Dobermans in Hawaii. Each potential parent for my pups was scrutinized like an adoption agency. If the yard was not perfect or they revealed anger issues, their application was denied. I kept the runt of the litter and named her Amber and the pick of the litter and named him Kahn. John lived in a mansion that had a five-acre fenced yard, and he loved animals; I had enthusiastically helped Voltan become John's new best friend.

John emerged from his house and yelled at me to make myself at home; he was with somebody at the moment. That somebody turned out to be actor Larry Manetti. John was representing Larry, a co-star on *Baa Baa Black Sheep*, which did not look like it was going to be picked up for a third season.

Larry had heard about the new series to be filmed in Hawaii and had recently auditioned for the part of Rick, one of Magnum's sidekicks. I told him about my involvement with the show and how excited I was that CBS had bought ten episodes, and especially that Tom Selleck was going to open the series in a hang glider scene. Larry confirmed that the series had been picked up, but thought the story lines must have changed. He did not recall anything about hang gliding.

With a sick feeling growing in my stomach I called Glen and listened to him explain how CBS would only approve the show if the hang gliding was scrapped. They were scared away by the recent bad press and told Glen they were not about to have people dying on their sets. Glen had already hired me as the technical director, but with this monumental change, there would not be anything for me to technically direct. I would be used as a utility stunt performer, as needed. Glen told me to look at the good news: the show was on. He assured me that he had several other projects coming up and he would find something big for me.

Glen had teamed up with a major writer and producer of commercials, Don Bellisario, to rework Magnum into a private investigator who worked with a pair of Vietnam buddies reunited in Hawaii. The show first aired in 1980 and was immediately a towering success. I worked on the initial episodes and was always greeted warmly on set. *Hawaii Five-O* had just stopped production, and *Magnum P.I.* slid right into its place, using many of its locations, props, and, especially, personnel. My loyal connection Margaret Doversola, who was assistant casting director for *Hawaii Five-O*, upgraded to casting director for *Magnum P.I.* She gave me every opportunity to audition for guest acting roles. Even with the changes I was

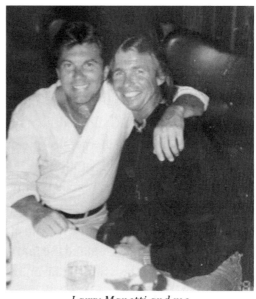

Larry Manetti and me

in a great position to be used often for both stunts and small roles. *Magnum P.I.* was clearly Hawaii's production juggernaut, and I was thrilled to be on the inside.

Magnum Betrayal

When you dream big it is often necessary to reconcile your ambitions with reality. By doing so, I had come to terms with my father and also with the true nature of my flimsy marriage. In the entertainment business, however, reality often comes looking for you when you least expect it, like a sweeping ax ready to cut you down.

Being a regular on the set of *Magnum P.I.* made me privy to the inside scoop of a blockbuster prime time show dominating American television. Don was apparently pissed off and complaining about sharing royalties with Glen on the creation credits of the show. Don never really gave me the time of day, knowing full well that I was a friend of Glen's. Glen confided in me that he had given Don his big break, pulling him out of the commercial world, and felt that Don still owed him, owed him big. One day while visiting Margaret in the production office, I overheard Don unabashedly ranting about how he deserved all the credit for the success of the show. It was obvious that Don did not feel he owed anything to Glen.

A few weeks later, I received a call from J.C., Glen's personal assistant, who said that Glen was flying in on his private jet and that he was anxious to talk with me about new projects in the works. I was invited to join him and Dirk Benedict, the star of *Battlestar Galactica*, for a University of Hawaii and BYU football game at Aloha Stadium, BYU being Glen's alma mater. He and J.C. arrived in his limo to pick me up. All was light and enjoyable at the game before he excused himself from J.C. and Dirk and asked me to join him in a private VIP booth. Once we were alone, I quickly learned the actual purpose of my invitation. He knew I was on the set on a daily basis and asked me point blank if Don was badmouthing him in front of the crew and saying that he deserved all the credit for the show and its wild success. He assured me that our conversation was confidential, even reminding me that he was the one who had written me into the show and Don was the one who had written me out of it. I was nothing more than honest and confirmed that Don was indeed upset. Glen thanked me profusely and said again that this would go no further than that room.

BYU won by a landslide, and the four of us had a fabulous dinner at Nick's afterwards. Several hundred-dollar bottles of wine later I was starting to get that warm fuzzy feeling again, like the night we had spawned the idea for *Magnum P.I.* He promised that I would be considered for stunt doubling and acting roles in anything he produced and went on to mention a series he had in mind about stuntmen and how he would love to have me involved. Unfortunately, it was going to be shot in the mainland, but I if I wanted to leave Hawaii, he was positive he could find a place for me. I felt like one of Glen's trusted friends, like he was inviting me into his inner circle. He did not even try to hide how cozy he and his assistant J.C. were becoming. As I returned home in the limo I was seemingly back on top.

My sweet dreams were interrupted by a ringing telephone. It was Larry Manetti yelling at me, "What the fuck did you tell Larson? There are attorneys everywhere and your buddy Glen has been spouting off all morning that you are his spy on the set." My stomach churned as the reality sunk in. Glen Larson had completely betrayed me, taking me from the top of the world to the bottom in a matter of hours.

I was seriously worried. Hawaii is a very small place where everyone in the business knows everyone else. I knew I was only as good as my last stunt, and now I was seen as a traitor on the only hit show in Honolulu. It was going to be nearly impossible to get any more work after this. I tried to talk to Don but he refused to see me. Margaret could only do so much and regretted that my only mistake was telling the truth. If I had one major flaw on set it was that I was too honest; the television and movie industry is not an honest business. So much for this crazy world, I was thinking as I left, disgusted. They buy you and sell you like a cheap bottle of wine or, in this case, a several hundred dollar one, it now seemed.

CHAPTER TEN

If You Can Bear To Hear The Truth You've Spoken Twisted By Knaves To Make A Trap For Fools

It took several years for my dad and me to start speaking again. After he started seeing me on television and heard from my sister that I was practically running a restaurant, he decided he better come see what kind of life his "son the bum" was making for himself out there on the islands. Time definitely heals, and he decided it was time to forgive me.

A few weeks after we spoke on the phone, my dad and stepmother, Judy, touched down in Hawaii, and I went to pick them up in Nick's stretch limo. Both my father and Judy, who he had met at his church bowling league, could not believe the car. Arriving at the million-dollar estate I was renting, my beautiful wife Kim and our three Dobermans greeted us as we pulled into the private drive. I gave them the grand tour of the home and the couple acres behind that opened up to a breathtaking view of the windward side of Oahu. I possessed everything my father could possibly envision for the successful modern man, and I must admit I was pleased to show it off just a bit.

The surprises I had in store for my father were just beginning, the next stop being Makapuu cliffs. I was anxious to show my father the freedom I had found in hang gliding and determined to show him that I had ventured off all those years ago in order to teach myself to fly. Setting up my glider, I waited for another pilot to come by who could assist me in a wire launch, but no one showed up. Kim had launched me before, but we had just lost another good friend off the cliff, making her nervous about launching me.

She did not feel good about the wind conditions either and asked me not to fly.

The wind was absolutely howling, but the direction was starting to come around. Setting up the glider meant that I was committed to the flight, which only came after judging the situation. Breaking it down would mean an error in my assessment. I trusted my intuition in leaving home for Hawaii all those years ago and was not going to stop trusting it now. I was meant to fly that day and knew who was destined to help me.

I turned to my dad and asked if he would launch me. He looked over the edge of the sheer cliff at the thirteen hundred foot drop.

"Son, are you sure about this?"

"The direction is good. I just need you to hold the nose down until I say I'm ready. All you have to do is lift it slightly and off I'll go."

I pointed to the launch box rope, which we had added after a couple of launchers got kicked and nearly fell right off the cliff (apologies to a battered launch man were almost always a case of beer), and I showed my father how to tie in. He was getting more nervous by the second. As I took the rope from him and showed him the correct way to tie it around his body, it really did feel like a right of passage, the passing of the torch as the father becomes the student and the son becomes the teacher. I carried the glider to the edge of the cliff and went through my mental checklist like all pilots do.

My dad confirmed that he was ready but was obviously getting shakier by the second. His nervousness eventually infected me too. Everyone was tense, especially our on-looking wives. Kim assisted me in carrying the glider over to my father, handing the nose to him as I hooked myself in. He was shaking so badly that I seriously considered backing off and taking us home. We were all psyched out, but I felt we should carry out the flight and directed him to lift the glider over his head. When his head came under the glider, his eyes were full of terror. I yelled over the howling wind for him to pay close attention.

"Remember Dad, pull that wire the wrong way and you just killed your son."

That got his attention, a little harsh, but it jolted him into the moment and his shaking subsided. I could tell he was with me now, his concentration sharp. I began shouting for him to lift the nose higher and higher. When I noticed he was starting to tremble again, I brought him back one more time.

"Dad, if you don't pay attention, remember what can happen. Now, believe me, I do not want to die!"

I had returned my fate into the hands of the rock of my life. "All right, let 'er go!" I said. I stepped off and rose a hundred feet in seconds. As I soared away in the smooth trade wind air I turned back and flew past my dad, spinning around backwards in my swing seat, and yelled, "Thanks Dad, I'll see you on the beach."

Flying past him as he stood at the edge of the cliff, I could see a gleam in his eye, and I instantly recognized that glimmer as the most important breakthrough in my life. The chip on my shoulder plummeted thirteen hundred feet down as I flew higher and higher, knowing that my father respected me and that I had earned it.

To make a perfect landing on the beach that day in front of my father was the taste of honey much sweeter than wine. My father promptly informed the people on the beach gathering around my landed glider that it was he

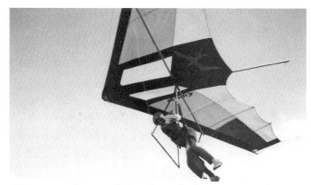

Moments after my father launched me in my 16' eipper

who had launched me. What a day! It was the launch of a new relationship for us, and surely my mother was glowing with happiness at the site of her husband and son reunited in love and admiration.

After I soared in front of my dad, we sat on the beach watching the sun go down, feeling the healing strands of time as he told stories of the past. Gaining his full attention, I began leading him toward the memories of his early days to set up my next surprise. I casually mentioned that I still had the picture of him in his little piper cub airplane. A twinkle in his eyes returned that I had not seen since the days as a kid sitting in his lap while he told stories from his youth as a daredevil pilot. It only took a little baiting on my part and he broke into my favorite story of how he had taken up my grandmother for the ride of her life.

I sat content, feeling like we had come full circle, listening to him again tell the story of how deathly afraid my grandmother was to fly. He had coaxed her to come to the airfield to see the new plane that he had just purchased with a friend, a new piper cub. He had only recently passed his flight exam but felt he was already a very qualified pilot. She was absolutely against the idea of going up for a ride, but he finally convinced his mother to sit inside and see how it felt. He strapped her in, demonstrating for her how safe everything was, and then decided it was time for her to lose her fear of flying. He reached across and closed the door. Before she knew it, they were already in the air. He had also just recently finished aerobatic training, and he took the plane and my grandmother through their paces. For the rest of her life, she would always mention how amazingly smooth every flight was after that first one.

He was shining now with the memory firmly returned. This was the perfect time to tell him what was in store for him next.

"Well Dad, I have another surprise for you. I just bought a third partnership in a Piper Cherokee 150. I got my private pilot's license six months ago."

"You're kidding me," he let out, laughing now with apparent joy. "Let's go flying!"

The following day, my dad, my stepmother, Kim, and I were down at the airport first thing in the morning getting my plane ready for a flight to Kauai. My father was watching me closely during the pre-flight checklists. His face went from concerned scrutiny to proud appreciation as he watched his son thoroughly inspect the plane, but his jaw dropped when I pulled out my swim fins and stuck them behind the pilot's seat.

"What, none for the rest of us?" he asked.

I explained that in case we had to ditch I could stick them into the doors to prevent them from jamming. I was covering every flaw, never forgetting what a fellow stuntman had told me: "Find the flaw, the flaw will kill you." Flying a plane is serious business, especially when the lives of others are in your hands. I do not care how good you are, things can happen. It is never wise to treat casually the climbing into a single engine aircraft to fly over 100 miles across the Pacific.

I finished loading our things and asked my dad to come in and sit next to me since Kim was insisting he take her front seat. As we began taxiing out I had my father take the yoke (stick or steering wheel) and ride the pedals with me. Moreover, I gave him the throttle as I radioed the tower that we were ready for takeoff. I motioned for my father to push the throttles all the way forward. He reached full throttle, and we began to rocket down the runway. I kept my hands off the yoke that day in my little Piper and looked my father dead in the eye.

"She's all yours, Dad!"

"But I haven't..." he began.

"Either fly or die," I said teasingly, holding my hands up by my shoulders. He took the yoke, gently pulled her off the ground, and away we went.

"You crazy son of a son of mine," he said, now smiling with me. He flew us all the way to Kauai and only relinquished the controls to me at about 50 feet off the deck. I did not want to take the stick, but he said, "We have others to think about, not just you and I." I took over and brought us in with a perfect landing on Kauai. My father's decision reminded me of an old piece of aviator wisdom: "There are old pilots and there are bold pilots, but there are no old, bold pilots." We had beers together that night and talked about the flight over and over as only a father and son could do. My father and I now shared the same arena, and the two of us were actually having a conversation as friends. These were truly some of the finest days of my life.

A Very Bad Idea!

The next day we decided to fly over to Nii'hau. I invited my two good buddies John Black and Pono Ouye to accompany my dad and me. Once again, my dad and I shared the controls, flying the 20 miles west of Kauai to reach this private and mysterious island. We flew around the backside of Kauai along the Na'pili coast. Not more than a quarter mile out to sea, we noticed a Navy ship lying dead in the water. I took control and, acting like a kamikaze pilot, dive-bombed the big ole Navy boat. We buzzed them at probably only 100 feet above the deck, just a friendly gesture of entertainment.

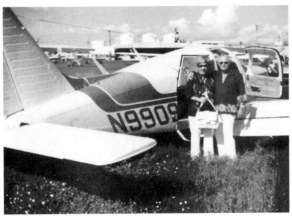

Big Al (my dad) and Judy (my stepmother) next to my Piper Cherokee 097

Feeling like a plane full of adventure seekers, we circumvented the island and realized that there was not much to look at other than a muddy lake, so we headed back toward the west side of Kauai at about 50 feet off the deck. When you are that close to the water you really feel the 110 mph you are traveling. As we got closer to the west side of the island, I noticed a few more Navy vessels, so I veered off to the north to avoid the Barking Sands missile-testing site. At least I thought I had avoided it.

Well, timing is everything, and it turned out to be a bad time to buzz a Navy boat and to fly this close to Barking Sands. I was flying a normally acceptable distance from the site, but since they happened to be testing that day and because I had already violated their airspace around the Navy boat, it was not long before we had company. The next thing I knew I had an F-15 flying on each side of me, flying slower than I ever imagined was possible. As I flew low across the ocean toward the testing area, they had dispatched the two fighter jets to either escort us out of there or shoot us down.

Busy giving them the Shaka sign and waving, I only got a couple pissed off looks in return and then a big thumbs down. I rounded the northeast side of the island and radioed the tower at Lihue; we then realized we were in big trouble.

"Cherokee 097 please be advised that you have violated military airspace," the tower responded. "You will proceed directly at 220 degrees on a long final to Lihue. All other traffic has been vectored out of the area until your aircraft has been searched. Please proceed to the west end of the airport and wait for further instructions."

They let us move on promptly, but it took me almost a year and several apologetic letters to the FAA and the Navy before I was finally taken off probation for that little stunt. So much for kamikaze runs on the Navy.

We decided to fly back to Oahu the next day, but when we went to start the plane, it would not turn over. In the course of all the excitement the radio was left on and now my battery was completely dead. Not about to leave my plane on Kauai, I called my buddy to bring down his car battery to help jump-start the plane. There we stood, my dad, stepmother, Kim, and I (my flippers in hand), jump starting my airplane like a Dodge pick-up.

They could all fly back commercially, and I would get the plane back to Oahu alone. No use in continuing to push our luck after almost getting blasted out of the sky by the Navy the day before. Despite my insistence that it was the safe and smart thing for them to do, my father put his arm around me and said, "I will fly her home with you son. Hell, I know that the battery is only needed to start the plane. The magneto is what keeps it going."

Sure enough, she fired right up with the jump-start and the magneto checked out fine. My dad started to climb in, and then Kim yelled, "Well, you're not going without me." And Judy said, "I'm going too."

It was a quiet flight, with all eyes on the control panel and ears on alert for any changes in engine pitch. We took a collective breath of fresh air when Oahu came into sight and the power plant at Waianae was under us.

A smooth landing back in Honolulu ended another adventure. My father would tell the story repeatedly for years to come. What a wonderful man he was. Not only had he seen me fly, but his new confidence in my abilities set me soaring even higher.

Unforgettable Days

So many days go by and are forgotten. Day after day they just drift by with no lasting memory. I have been blessed with many days that I will never forget; none more unforgettable than the day my father said he would help me fly my plane home from Kauai. I had finally earned my father's respect, and after that day I began seeing my life in a new light. Constantly challenging myself and my limitations had indeed manifested my dream of flying and taken me beyond any life I could have imagined. But I had also filled my days with an insatiable quest for the next ecstatic moment, the next good time, the next adventure.

When I said goodbye to my father, it was once again the twinkle in his eye that revealed what I had been missing. It was not the adventure itself, the thrill of the narrow escape, but rather who was standing by you at the end of that adventure that left a lasting imprint. Life now appeared shockingly too short. I needed to be spending each fleeting day with the people I loved and trusted. Unfortunately, in some cases this was a lesson too late.

The other person who helped me fly back that day from Kauai, who unhesitatingly leapt aboard the plane to brave the journey home by my side, was my adoring wife Kim. She gave and gave, but I did not see her and her love. I never lied to Kim about my wandering eye, and to be honest I never really considered myself married. Few people even knew that I was married. My job at Nick's Fishmarket put me in the perfect place to attract women, and I seized many of those opportunities. I always drew my lines of how far I would go and was always cautious of any sexual act that could lead to impregnating a woman, but it was all for the vanishing pleasure of the moment. None of my one-night stands came close to the love I had found with Kim.

Sadly, when I finally opened my eyes and started falling truly in love with her, she was already falling out of love with me. My wicked, wicked ways and the lack of honor I had shown for my wife was ultimately too much to overcome. It was too late. Our marriage ended. Regaining my father and losing my wife made it abruptly clear that life is simply too short to not show the people you love and respect how important they are when they are still with you.

The Treasure Of The Sierra Madre

As long as I was open and willing, new opportunities and adventures had never ceased to come my way. Sure enough, just weeks later I got a unique job offer from Dennis McKenna, formerly known as Jupiter. He was working on a documentary of the indigenous Tarahumara people of Mexico's immense Barranca del Cobre (Copper Canyon). His wife, Dulcy, was close to giving birth, so he needed someone to cover for him and go down to the Sierra Tarahumara region in the northwestern state of Chihuahua. He wanted me to supervise the production and handle the Nagra field recording sound system. I had never been a sound operator or a producer but decided it was time to expand my horizons in the motion picture industry.

I met Dennis in California, and he began my education on the Tarahumara, or Raramuri, as they call themselves. The name Tarahumara was what the first Spanish called these Native American people. They continued to live in caves, under cliffs, and in small wood and stone cabins in remote areas, carrying on a simple life undisturbed by modern technologies. They are an incredibly hardy, quiet, and considerate people, but they are not to be taken lightly. According to legend, the Tarahumara are the last protectors of the treasure of Sierra Madre, the hidden gold mines of the Incas and Aztecs. Dennis went on to inform me that ten years earlier a group of explorers went in search of the gold and were later found beheaded.

They are also well known for their running abilities, both out of tradition and necessity, since it is their only mode of transportation and many of the small communities are very far apart. Dennis said that they solved many of their internal disputes by running ultra long races, some lasting several days. Raramuri means "runners" in their native language, which they have kept alive along with their unique culture.

It sounded like a first-rate adventure. I asked what helicopter company was flying us into the canyon, and Dennis explained that we would not have the luxury of helicopters. We were going to the middle of the Mexican poppy fields, and the growers would shoot down any chopper that came close. So we would have to trek it in. Our guide would be one of the top Mexican authorities working with the DEA, Oscar Chin Vega, who was heading up Operation Condor, which focused on eradicating the country's poppy production. Oscar was also a good friend to the Tarahumara and was in the practice of bringing them coffee, beans, and tobacco during droughts or crop failures. Regarding him highly, the Tarahumara were going to make Oscar a tribal governor and we were to film that ceremony. We would also be filming their large Semana Santa festival, Easter week, which is a unique mixture of both Christian and Tarahumara beliefs and celebrations. We had plenty to cover and only a slight idea of what to expect.

The adventure began by flying into a little dirt field on a high plateau seemingly on another planet. It was clear this was not your ordinary voyage when after squeezing between high cliffs and landing on a narrow strip of dirt we were met by people in loincloths. This group of primitive service workers carried the $100,000 worth of equipment off into the jungle on their backs as we slowly followed behind on mules. With Oscar in the lead with his double .45 pistols crisscrossed about his chest, we could have been following Poncho Villa himself. Several hours later, we began to hear the resonating beat of distant drums that would unceasingly provide the soundtrack for the next ten days. It felt as if we were stepping further back in time with each step, deeper into the remote lands of these hermetic people.

We camped that first night by a riverbed, as the continuous drumming grew louder and louder. The drums were used to scare off evil spirits, and since the Tarahumara often perceived the white man as evil, it seemed that they were attempting to drum away our intrusion. Around three in the morning we were startled awake by the drums, now right on top of us, and the sounds of rustling in the bushes around our camp. On the other side of the stream appeared a group of about 20 Tarahumara in their full native dress. They began throwing rocks into the river and yelling at us. Oscar told us to remain calm and not to move. He said they were checking to see if we were evil. This rock throwing went on for over half an hour before they began doing a formational dance in counterclockwise circles, and then suddenly disappeared back into the darkness.

As the sun came up we continued our journey and soon arrived at an old church built for the Tarahumara by the missionaries in the early 1800s. This is where the hundreds of Tarahumara would gather for the annual celebration of Semana Santa, the only time these isolated tribes would gather together, and we were going to have the opportunity to capture the amazing event. Oscar knew a family that lived nearby, and they invited us to stay and rest as they prepared for the ceremony. They were a close family, and you could see in their eyes as well as their actions that they really loved and cared for each other. One of their sons had been killed in a mining accident, and his widowed wife and child were in the care of his parents.

The patriarch, a sturdy man in his forties, had carved a plow from a large fallen branch and cultivated his land with this primitive tool pulled by an ox. Strapped to his plow and oxen, the man tilled the earth that sloped at no less than a 45-degree angle. When he finished, he unhooked himself, revealing deep gashes from the straps, which he ignored, and anxiously wanted to show us the toys he made for his children and grandchildren. He was also very proud of what looked like a violin, which he also crafted with his handmade tools. He played a few notes, and I was amazed at how wonderful it sounded. He had created the instrument as a gift for a friend and it would be played at the coming celebration. He even demonstrated for me how to make a brush out of a pinecone.

I was amazed by their resourcefulness. They provided for everything they may need, but, most importantly, I was moved by the happiness they derived from their simplicity and their genuine respect and love for each other. I felt privileged to spend this time with them.

We spent the night with this family and awoke to nibbling bites at our ears by little pigs. We packed up our things and headed back for the church, the center point of Semana Santa. Just before we reached the church, we came upon a group of people preparing the sacred clay in the riverbed. The water was crystal clear and the children were having a fantastic time playing in it. It was not long before I could no longer help but join in their fun. I stripped down to my shorts and climbed the highest rock to dive from, making quite a splash with the children. Our only communication was our laughter, through which our mutual joy was well understood.

I had brought along my trusty magic box, the Kodak Polaroid camera, and began taking instant pictures for the children. It was a big hit among both young and old, until I ran out of film and lost my magic. It actually got a little hairy when an elderly man, who had already started in on the ceremonial Tesguino drink, started demanding a new picture, following me around and belligerently insisting that I perform my trick.

Tesguino is made from fermented corn and makes for a very potent type of alcoholic beverage. The women make this drink with a blinding kick exclusively for this celebration, and it hits like White Lightning, rendering you staggering drunk. It occasionally inspires hallucinations. It was one powerful concoction, and these Tarahumara had been drinking it for days when we arrived at the church. One of the chiefs filled a gourd full and offered it to me. I started to say, "Thank you, but no thank you," when Oscar informed me of the huge insult I was about to commit, so I drank the foulest tasting liquid to ever cross my lips. Fighting the urge to throw it up as it when down, I smiled my thank you and handed the gourd back to the chief, who smiled back with a wonderful toothless grin, refilled the gourd, and handed it back to me. Soon I didn't know if I was about to shit or go blind, and when no one was looking, I staggered off into the bushes and threw up.

We filmed the rising full moon as the ceremonies began. They were rich with tradition and mixed cultural inspirations. The Tarahumara carried out the festival, and we kept the camera rolling. The dramatic conclusion to the event was a live dramatization of the protectors of Christo at battle with the enemies of Christo. The enemies, covered with the white sacred clay, looked ghostly, and they seemed to have consumed much more Tesguino than the protectors of Christo. The fight began in an orderly manner, two men squaring off, an enemy and a protector wrestling sumo style. No punches or blows were allowed, but whoever was thrown to the ground was then mounted and humped for a few moments, a quite homoerotic triumphant ritual. The winner would then square off with the next combatant. These mini-battles were going on all around us, a semi-controlled sumo riot.

I guess the losers did not enjoy getting humped all that much, and things got ugly when a few crazily drunken men began throwing punches. All broke out into a perpetual cycle of chaos; the drunker they were the more likely they would get their ass kicked and then promptly humped. We could not believe the footage we were getting. We were thrilled until the violence eventually became directed toward us. Both the drunken protectors and enemies ganged up on us, pushing and shoving our film crew. We wasted little time shutting down the lights and heading for our campsite, but a group started to follow us until the revered Oscar stepped in and the excitement ended. We all decided this would be the final night. We had the shot and tomorrow we would head home.

I knew that Dennis would love some of the ceremonial masks and mock weapons, and I had my eye on one of the ceremonial drums as well. I was hesitant to ask, but Oscar negotiated the sale with one of the chiefs, and I became the proud owner of these fantastic artifacts that I cherished and held with the highest regard. While I was busy packing my new prizes on my pack mule, a very drunken man suddenly accosted me in an attempt to take back the drum and mask. Once again Oscar stepped in and settled things down. He explained that all the crafts and instruments created for the ceremonial purpose of driving away evil spirits were traditionally burned at a closing ritual of the festival. I felt horrible that I was not made aware of this tradition earlier, but Oscar and the liberal chief felt that no one would miss a few souvenirs, especially since the majority of the men were passed out anyway. My masks, the gourd, and my drum hang on my living room wall to this day.

As we rode out of town, we left behind a sea of dead drunk, painted men lying about the ground and church. Whether this was ceremonial or not, I was saddened by the sight of these otherwise considerate and noble people reduced to this sufferable state at the hands of drugs and alcohol. We had great footage of these amazing people and their grand annual celebration,

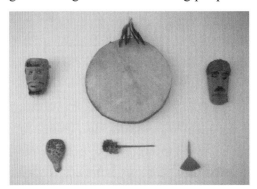

but perhaps most touching were the quiet scenes and the images of the biting straps of their sacrifice encountered in their homes. After their wild voyage to the thrilling edge of euphoria and madness, the Tarahumara would pick themselves up and return to the integrity of their family lives. With just one more precarious takeoff in our little

The ceremonial Mask and Drums of the Tarahumara Indians

single engine airplane, we too would be on our own way home, and I could not help but think of my father and the home that I had left in search of the edge so many years before. I couldn't hide my smile as the plane lifted into the air.

The Courageous Genius Of Dar Robinson

Shortly after the documentary on the Tarahumaras, I was back in Los Angeles working with Dennis on a new company we were forming and Dennis was financing called Production Machine. We offered the first truly computerized financial production system, complete with state-of-the-art computers that kept tabs on the entire production. We could give a producer a financial update at any moment during the shoot, showing if they were running over or under budget and what was causing the shortages or surpluses. This was unheard of technology in these days. Usually it was weeks or even months before you found out where you stood with the budget of a major feature film, which allowed for the common disappearance of sizeable chunks of money that were simply written off as production costs. Our machine worked a little too well, and those unscrupulous producers and production managers, who had grown used to lining their own pockets, did their best to keep Production Machine away from their shoots.

Dennis and I were also working on a new project with Barry Mahon, an Ace WWII fighter pilot, hero, and dear friend of Hollywood legend Errol Flynn. Barry had traveled the world with Flynn and was involved in over 80 films. I had just come from a production meeting at our offices in Hollywood, where we were working on getting the rights to a comic book character that was famous in the '50s. It was going to be a great opportunity for me to stunt coordinate as well as co-produce this TV series about a comic book superhero who was also a fighter pilot. It sounded like an action-packed show—plenty of stunts and plenty of work. We would need the most talented stuntmen and women to pull it off.

I was feeling really good about the meeting that day with Barry, so I stopped in at the Baja Cantina to have a couple of drinks and check out the ladies before heading home. I was thinking I might keep my luck going and score a little darling to take up to the house, originally owned by Eleanor Roosevelt, located at the top of Latigo Canyon, that I was sharing with Dennis and Dulcy McKenna. They were out of town so I had the mansion to myself. I pulled up a stool at the bar and ordered my usual, tequila and a beer. The bartender recognized me, and we started talking about the new series and about all the wild stunts we were planning. That was when he asked me if I knew of Dar Robinson. I had heard of him. His reputation was well established in the stunt world, but I had never met him. After excusing himself to the back room, he came back with a man who would quickly become my best friend and most trusted mentor in the stunt business.

Dar was well known for falling out of a window in a Burt Reynolds movie, *Sharky's Machine*. Dar, doubling for the villain, Henry Silva, fell from 22 floors up. He not only set a record by falling 220 feet, but he went out of the window backwards, which had never been attempted before. He was also well noted for taking over the show *That's Incredible* when the network switched to stunt performers after the independent dare devils kept getting badly injured or killed. Dar turned *That's Incredible* into a showcase of the stunt world, pulling some of the greatest stunts the world had ever seen, and was one of those who always seemed to walk away without a scratch. He never did break a bone in his body doing a stunt.

It was easy to see what a nice guy Dar was from the very beginning. Lacking a showbiz ego, he was just one of those great guys. We began comparing notes on who we both knew in the industry, and it turned out that we had several mutual friends who were either actors or stunt people. I told him about the series we were working on and asked if he would be interested in helping out. He said he would love to be involved, so we set up a meeting for Dar and Barry the following day. As they say, the rest was pretty much history.

Dar had made his inroads into the stunt business in a similar fashion as me: with his talent. He was an expert in gymnastics, and even set world records on trampolines. My stunt specialties were hang gliding, horses, cars, snow skiing, water skiing, and surfing, but high falls were something on my list of things to master. He really wanted me to teach him to fly hang gliders, and the deal was that if I would teach him to fly, he would teach me to fall. Dar took me under his wing and began instructing me on falling from buildings into airbags, motorcycle stunts, everything from fight stunts to fire falls; he knew it all. Dar really finished off my education as a stunt professional with our private training sessions over at his friend Bob Gerkes's place. Bob's backyard was fully equipped with a full circus trapeze, high wires, and trampolines. If you signed a release, Bob would let you go wild on his equipment. He even had air rams that could pitch you up to 15 to 20 feet into the air to hopefully land on the designated airbag. It was a stuntman's heaven.

Teaching Dar To Fly

Dar had held up his end of the deal. So it was my turn now. I had mastered falling; it was time for Dar to fly.

CHAPTER ELEVEN

Or Watch The Things You Gave Your Life To, Broken, And Stoop And Build'em Up With Worn Out Tools

I invited Dar to Hawaii and took him to my favorite training spot in Maui, an area facing into the trade winds just below Haleakala Volcano. With the help of my buddy Sam Nottage, who volunteered his gliders and expertise, we hooked Dar into a large glider and gave him the basic instructions of how to shift his weight into the turns. Dar was an expert skydiver, but hang gliding and skydiving are two very different sports. The good news was that he was not afraid of speed or heights, and Dar's confidence and proven abilities in the stunt world made me feel more than okay about sending him off.

His first two flights were very short, but he landed on his feet both times. I instructed Dar to let the wind fill his sail and go up with the rising air and not to pull in so fast, which was limiting his distance. This was not about falling, as in skydiving; this was about learning how to fly. I held the nose of the glider and waited until I felt the wind pick up. I told Dar to really run this time and not to pull in but to push out. With the next wind cycle, I looked him directly in the eye and told him, "Run hard." I let go of the glider wires and Dar ran off at full speed. He pushed out as instructed, and this time he went straight up. A quick learner, he responded perfectly as the glider began to stall. He pulled in, picked up speed, and was off again. I ran below him and saw that as he attempted a turn he pulled in and began picking up too much speed. He sent himself into a down-wind dive. I yelled at him to turn into the wind instead of going with it as he was doing, but the wind had him good and was taking him straight toward the earth. He heard me yelling and tried to correct but overcorrected, which created a stall over a bush-filled gully. Now he really was plummeting while both Sam and I yelled at him to push out. But our screams fell on deaf ears as Dar plowed through the bushes and came to an incredibly abrupt stop.

I ran down to where he had landed, and did not see any movement. I was immediately worried that Dar was badly injured or worse. It was a rough looking crash, and I thought, "Oh no, I just killed the best stuntman alive." But my heart soon lifted as the glider started to move. He slowly emerged from the gully with the broken and twisted glider wrapped all around him. He wore a big grin on his face.

"Wow, let's do that again," he said. We would have to get another glider. That was enough for the first day, and I said we should head to the beach and check out the ladies. On our ride down from Haleakala, Dar was full of questions about what went wrong and how to correct his mistakes, realizing there was a lot more to hang gliding than he thought.

The following day the weather did not cooperate for training, so we headed back to Oahu. I welcomed the opportunity to show Dar the best and most dangerous hang gliding spot in the world, the cliffs of Makapuu. Dar was impressed with the view. Since it was just the two of us, he agreed to launch me. Obviously, he did not have a problem hanging off the launch platform and gave me a perfect launch. I rose a thousand feet straight up and put on a show. Buzzing overhead, I did all the craziest aerobatics possible. Dar took my truck and drove down to the beach to pick me up after a perfect landing. All he could say was, "Wow." Now he understood all the weight shifts I had been talking about during his flight. I was showing off a bit but was proud to have earned the respect of a man many still believe to be the most talented stuntman the world has ever seen.

Dar's Gift Of Inspiration

I was now both trained and inspired by the work of Dar, and my stunt career opened up as I became more versatile. With the huge success of *Magnum P.I.*, Hawaii became the place for everyone to try to sell a series. Several came and went. In 1984, I became involved with one of these fleeting but ambitious projects, *Hawaiian Heat*, starring Robert Gentry. Ronnie Rondell of Stunts Unlimited stunt coordinated 11 episodes before the show was cancelled. Ronnie used a host of local Hawaii stuntmen, including me, in almost every episode. Knowing you are only as good as your last stunt, I successfully pulled off every single stunt in one take. With the likes of Dar and Ronnie, I was truly in the company of elite stuntmen, and they helped take me to the top of my game.

The World's Greatest Stuntman

Of the many stunts Dar performed for the television show *That's Incredible*, a few truly amazing ones stand out. He jumped off the CN Tower in Toronto with a hidden parachute, drove his Bradley GT over the edge of the Grand Canyon only to parachute to safety as the car exploded on the rock-lined bottom, and pulled off the first air-to-air transfer ever performed.

The astonishing transfer was from one plane to another. Dar jumped out of one airplane at the same time the pilot of another airplane put his biplane into a dive. The biplane released a small parachute from the tail that slowed his aircraft down to 120 mph, matching the airspeed of Dar's free fall. They fell together for over a mile as Dar maneuvered himself closer and closer to the other aircraft, and then at the last minute climbed onto the wing of the biplane, which was still diving straight down. The pilot detached the parachute, pulled out of the dive, and safely landed with Dar perched on his wing tip.

Determined to push the envelope of the stunt world, Dar decided to return to the CN Tower for another free fall, without a parachute. He would use a rapid decelerator mechanism that involved attaching a wire to his leg to slow his fall and eventually stop him before he slammed into the ground. Dar would later tell me that everything in preparation for this stunt went wrong.

Ky Michaelson developed a big brake drum contraption that would allow Dar to free-fall for half the distance down the tower before Ky would gradually apply the brakes. They had the apparatus set up on top of the tower, and attached the 185 pound dummy to the harness suspended from the wires attached to the big break drum. They let the dummy go and the free fall began, but when Ky went to apply the brakes a malfunction occurred. The wire cable began smoking and then the drum began to melt, causing the wire to break. Dar's dummy double splattered into hundreds of pieces on the ground below. Everyone looked at each other and said, "Oh Shit!" But they were not about to give up the stunt. Ky was immediately on a plane back to Michigan to get the parts to repair the decelerator. By the time he returned, the weather had gone to shit. The wind and rain became so strong that the stunt was postponed.

Dar had recently started dating Kathy Lee Crosby, the female host of *That's Incredible*, and it was evident that she really cared for Dar and was concerned for his safety. She did not want him to attempt this stunt, especially after the chilling result of the equipment malfunction. Kathy's concern and the nasty weather were really making this a tough one for Dar. When the wind backed off for a few hours, they got a second chance to test the decelerator. They attached the dummy, but just before starting the free fall, the wind picked up and slammed the dummy into the side of the building.

Each stunt had a specifically allocated budget, and due to the malfunction and weather delays Dar had spent most of his money and had very little to show for it. The high wind conditions continued and Dar's resources dwindled. The shrinking budget and poor weather really began to worry everyone involved, and for the first time ever I could hear glimpses of apprehension in Dar's voice as he described the stunt to the local media. The overall weather forecast was still dim, but it looked as if the wind might die down the next morning. Dar had a sleepless night, knowing it was now or never.

That gloomy morning, he gathered his team on the top of the building, led them in prayer, and then looked each member of his team in the eye and said, "Well, they say if you're going to die from a high fall you are normally dead before you hit the ground." He tried to make light of the dark possibility. "If the wire breaks and I hit the ground, roll me over and you will find sand in my eyes because they will be wide open as I fight for my life the whole way until I hit the ground."

He told all present that he loved them and then began his stuntman's chant: "Oh what a jerk I am." When repeated quickly it was supposed to sound like a sacred Hindu chant. He yelled the chant all the way to the edge and as he pushed off the lip of the tower to begin his free fall. Happily, it went perfectly, and the biggest sighs of relief came from the team who helped him pull it off. There was not a dry eye among them as Kathy Lee hugged Dar at the base of the tower.

Just a few weeks later, Dar was at Knott's Berry Farm where he broke another world record by jumping out of a helicopter 311 feet above the ground. A light meter recorded Dar's airspeed. When he crossed the beam, he was traveling at an amazing 86 mph. Stunt after stunt, I witnessed Dar take things one step further. And he was just warming up.

In Search Of The Flaw

Dar invited me one day to go to Houston, Texas, where he was going to be performing in a thrill show headlined by a car jumper by the name of Spanky Spangler. Dar was going to jump from the top of the Houston Astrodome with a wire around his leg using an updated rapid decelerator. "A piece of cake," he said.

He was taking the gig to build up funding for a wild stunt he was crafting that nobody had ever seen before or even dreamed was possible. He believed he could free fall from a mile up without a parachute and land on an airbag, but the airbag would need to be the size of a football field and over five stories high. He started monitoring his airspeed while in free fall and felt that with the help of a specially designed suit he could slow his descent to a little over 100 mph. He was dead serious about pulling this off and started looking for the suit that could slow him down, just like Rocky the squirrel. The planning and calculating that went into every one of Dar's stunts was always impressive.

I quickly accepted his offer and was on my way to Houston, eager to help the greatest stuntman in the world with his latest spectacle. Nick Nicholas, of Nick's Fishmarket, had just opened a restaurant in Houston. When I let him know I was coming he offered us the use of his limos and insisted we use his restaurant for the after show party. Life could not get any better.

We arrived at the Houston Astrodome and met with Dar's right-hand man, Kenny Bates. Kenny was testing the rapid decelerator from lower levels and working his way up. I helped Dar develop a harness similar to my hang gliding harness to help distribute some of the strain from the fall. This harness supported your whole body and could be hidden under your clothes, preventing an overload on your ankle joint and the gruesome possibility of ripping it out of the socket.

Dar's wardrobe would cover the wire and the harness, making it look as if there was nothing to stop him from slamming into the arena floor. For the test runs, he set up an airbag directly underneath the platform that would be raised up to take us to the top of the Astrodome. We climbed onto the platform that was attached to a pulley suspended from the top of the dome. The other end of the rope was attached to a truck by the exit. When the truck backed out of the exit, we would be raised to the top. Dar asked me if I would like to try the stunt out, and I jumped at the chance. I would have the added safety of having the airbag underneath, and since I was about 30 pounds lighter than Dar it would be a good test. "You can be the test dummy," Dar chuckled. Gary Benz, Dar's manager and good friend, also had just arrived and was with us at the top of the dome. Gary weighed the same as Dar, so after I tried the decelerator, Gary would give it a try as well.

We spent hours walking around on the beams above the dome. Dar insisted we cover the whole rooftop, looking for the possible flaw. "John, you have to look for the flaw because there is always a flaw somewhere," he instructed. "Just remember, the flaw is what can and will kill you. Always looking for it has kept me alive." This was priceless advice. We looked and looked, and once he was confident that he had covered every possibility, he allowed us to perform the stunt. The fall was incredible, and, best of all, I barely felt the tug on my leg. The harness worked.

The night we did the stunt they had me up in the rafters with a dummy we had constructed and loaded with watermelons. The announcer described the death-defying stunt, how the great Dar Robinson was about to make a fall like no other from the top of the Astrodome without a bag to break his fall. The floodlights filled the arena ceiling, revealing a figure suspended from the platform. The announcer asked if everything was all right up there. There was no reply. He repeated the question again, and then asked for the lights to be brought up, as if something was not right. The spotlight went to the rafters, and then there was another long pause before the announcer asked, "Is there a problem?" The audience gasped as a figure fell from above. I had let the dummy loose, and it plummeted to the arena floor, splattering the 20 watermelons inside the dummy, covering the front row in red juice and pieces of watermelon. The screams turned into a giant collective sigh of relief as the spotlight went to Dar while balancing on a board rising to the top of the Astrodome. The drum roll, the fall, it all went perfectly.

We capped off the show with a celebrity automobile destruction derby. It fittingly came down to only Dar and Spanky Spangler battling it out in the end. Dar, who had preserved the front end of his car by attacking everyone in reverse, knocked out Spanky Spangler by blowing his radiator. Afterwards, we had a police escort to Nick's Fishmarket, with Dar in one limo and me in the other, jumping from car rooftop to car rooftop as we paraded down the streets of Houston. We owned the city that night. The stunt performers gave the people a little more than they had paid for.

We had a great dinner at Nick's and returned to the hotel with a woman on each arm. Everything is a little fuzzy after that, but I was told the next morning that I was wandering around the lobby in my boxers looking for my dates. In the company of Dar it felt like we could pull off anything, except knocking out my crazy hang over. My head was killing me.

Straight To The Heart

Dar was a romantic. He led with his heart and wore it courageously on his sleeve. He loved to be in love and always seemed to be in love with some of the most beautiful women in the world. Moreover, they were in love with him. One day he called me, in Hawaii, after he had broken up with an incredibly beautiful actress. He was shattered that she just couldn't handle being in love with someone who would risk his life for money. She did not understand that the risk was minimal for a well-trained and diligent stunt performer. We are showmen and actors playing up the risk and drama of the stunt, which makes everyone believe that we were content to toss our lives away. In reality, it is always just another day at the office. We do not want to die and do not plan on dying.

I told him the best thing for a broken heart is another heart. I happened to have a good female friend who had recently broken up with her husband. She was a knockout, but she was a little crazy. She actually had stabbed her ex-husband and faced jail time if he pressed charges. Fortunately, he dropped all the charges and she was a free woman. Ironically, she had been crowned Mrs. Hawaii and had then dumped her husband. She was half Japanese and had an exotic look, just the style Dar loved. I told Dar about her, that she was going to be in L.A. and I would set them up. I warned him right away that this gal was hot and fiery. Whatever you do, I warned him, do not fall in love with her. Have a good time, make uncommitted love, but whatever you do, remember she is dangerous, both physically and emotionally. She will tell you everything you want to hear, but you must not fall into her trap.

Dar assured me he was not looking to get in another relationship for a long while. A few weeks later, with his little head doing all the talking, he informed me he was in love. No matter what I said, he could not be talked out of this new "love of his life." What had I done to my friend? I just wanted him to get laid and forget about his heartbreak, not fall in love all over again, especially with someone gorgeous but dangerous. I warned him about her violent side and that she had a drug history. Not that she was any different from me or anyone else in the Candyland of drugs in the early '80s. Dar had been one of the few that had never done any drugs. He was as clean as it gets. In fact, the first time he ever smoked a joint was with me.

I introduced this pure and clean human being to his first joint. He was not feeling so great after his first hang gliding session, so I offered him a little antidote. Some good old Maui Wowie. He told me he had never done drugs, and I assured him that pot was not a drug, but a sacred herb. After smoking this sacred herb with me, we got into a very deep conversation. Unfortunately, that conversation was interrupted by a beautiful female friend of mine who happened to be walking down the beach and had spotted me in the beachfront bar. As I talked with her, Dar got up and wandered off.

An hour or so latter I realized that Dar was still missing. We went in search of the world's greatest stuntman and found a familiar looking pair of tennis shoes sticking out of a row of bushes. Attached to those tennis shoes was none other than the world's greatest stuntman passed out in the bushes. Dar was an innocent and honest man, and that is why this new relationship bothered me greatly and it was all my doing.

Dar returned to L.A. and was pleasantly surprised to find her still in town. He called me to let me know that she was definitely interested in him. I warned him once again to be careful. He assured me that he was being very careful and was non-committal. I reminded him that she loved the drug of choice at the time and to be very careful of the mood swings that accompany people who use that drug. He assured me that she was clean and that he had never been happier. I explained to him that I had run into her and knew that she was not as clean as he thought she was. I actually went to the extent of recording her with my girlfriend at the time, who was just about as mean and manipulative. They were beautiful, but they were after one thing, the party, money and a good time. To this day I am not proud of the following event. In my heart of hearts I was only trying to protect my friend and undo a hook-up that I should have never made.

I sent my girlfriend into the bathroom with a voice-activated recorder to get the two of them doing the powder I will refer to as the "Devil's Dandruff" on tape. When my girlfriend returned to the table, I excused myself and listened to the recording. We had entrapped her into saying many things that would crush my friend. I had the proof I needed to spare my friend. Or so I thought.

I told Dar that he was being lied to and that I had recorded her with my girlfriend. Dar was extremely angry with me for doing that, and it seriously threatened our friendship. He came by my house the next day demanding that if I did have a recording he wanted to listen to it. He said he had taken her to her doctor and her doctor told Dar that she was clean and drug free.

I am sure the doctor was a good friend of hers and would say anything to cover for her. It sickened me that this woman had divided our alliance. A few weeks later, she was pregnant with his child, and a few months after that he made her his wife.

Word got out that they were battling all the time. Dar's manager, Gary Benz, and I had remained good friends, so Gary would keep me apprised of the situation. He said that she would show up unannounced on the set while he was working and create problems, damaging his career, because no one wanted to deal with his wife. Dar actually was fired from a show due to her behavior on the set. He had never been fired from a show. I never should have set him up with her. I have blamed myself to this day for performing that introduction. But love is blind and I was now witnessing the truth of that statement.

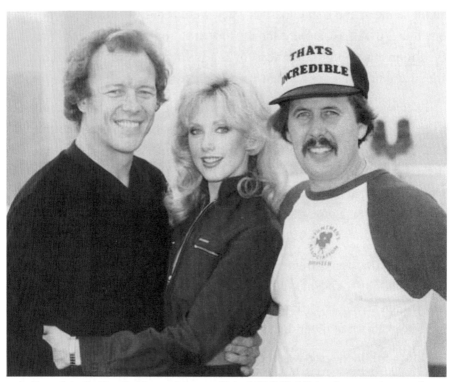

From L to R: Dar Robinson, Morgan Fairchild & Ky Michaelson on the set of
"Thats Incredible"

CHAPTER TWELVE

If You Can Make One Heap Of
All Your Winnings
And Risk It On One Turn Of Pitch And Toss

I know you are all wondering what stunt it was that caused this terrible accident. Well it was no stunt at all. The first three letters are the same—- S T U—but unfortunately the ending is P I D. Stupid.

It was the biggest breakdown literally and physically. It became one of the biggest breakthroughs and changed my life forever. I can only express this as a miracle. The following is the true story of how it all happened. Let me forewarn you once again this is not a pretty story and one that I'm certainly not proud of. But as they say the Lord works in Mysterious ways.

I awoke relieved, happy to have escaped from a bad dream. Then, slowly focusing, my eyes made out the intravenous drip bag seemingly floating above my head, and I began to decipher that I was in a hospital room. My bad dream was no dream at all, but a nightmarish reality. I instantly suffered from the onset of excruciating pain and the flashing recall of the events that landed me here. My life had drastically changed.

The day before, January 6, 1986, I had awoken to another beautiful Sunday morning in Hawaii. I lay in bed with my girlfriend, thinking how lucky I was to live in paradise, to have a job I loved, and to have the freedom to fly at will. After a light breakfast, I went for my daily swim and a run on the beach with my two Doberman Pinschers. As far as I was concerned, I was blessed beyond imagination.

We were to attend a dinner party at my girlfriend's parent's house that afternoon and running ahead of schedule, we had time for a quick trip to the mall for her to exchange a Christmas gift. She assured me it would be a quick stop, but knowing what a quick stop at the mall can mean I had her drop me off at a friend's sports bar so I could watch the NFL playoffs.

I arrived at Foxy's Sports Bar at 2:30 and was happy to see a few of my buddies from Nick's. Foxy, the owner and bartender, greeted me warmly with a Corona and a shot of Jose Cuervo Gold tequila. "First one is on me," he said. Life was indeed good. I threw it down, took a swig of my beer, and found my shot glass refilled. I enjoyed the game, had a few pretzels, finished the second shot, and tried to settle my tab, knowing I was off to an early dinner party so I had better back off on the drinks. My money was refused again since one of my buddies, Dusty Gaines, had paid for the last one. This kind of generosity could mean trouble.

At 3:30 there was still no sign of my girlfriend so I ordered another beer. At 4:00, still no sign, so when Foxy offered me another shot I could justify it. Another hour went down and so did the shots, with plenty of beer, of course, to chase them. When she finally showed up at 5:45, I was feeling no pain. Naturally, we argued about how long she had been at the mall and about how much I had to drink. Funny how quick I was to blame everyone else for my drinking problem then.

Feeling too inebriated for a dinner with her parents, I said she should take me home or I could get a ride with one of my friends. She agreed to take me home, I waved a cheerful goodbye to my buddies, and off we went. Curiously, the freeway entrance flew by, and I asked her where she was going. "To my mother's," she said.

"Honey," I pleaded, "I'm in no shape to go see your family."

"You're fine and you're going with me," she said, refusing to let me off the hook.

I was a far cry from fine, and in my drunken mind I started scheming my exit strategy. She would have to slow down to make the right turn onto Black Point Road and I was calculating at what speed I could attempt a tuck and roll out of the car to escape the embarrassment of showing up plastered at her family's home.

Six Foot Six, 250 Pounds, And Bullet-Proof

As she slowed to make the turn, I reached for the door handle. But just before exploiting my stuntman training to avoid social disgrace, two joggers ran out in front of us and she screeched to a halt. I was out of the car before she even knew what happened, and now she was begging me to get back in. I refused and she continued to yell at me when a man in a Volkswagen convertible, waiting while facing her car, began honking and screaming for her to move. She was blocking the majority of the entrance to Black Point Road. She answered his vocal barrage and even threw in some bawdy sign language for good measure. Climbing out of his car, he headed toward her. He easily outweighed me by a hundred pounds, but I stepped in front of his advance and yelled, "Hey, calm down!"

He replied with a left hook that caught me along the temple. My instinctual survival mode kicked in. I sent a punch directly into his nose, breaking his glasses and stunning him enough to momentarily stop his advance. After regrouping for a few seconds, he lunged forward in attack once again. My training in martial arts paid off as I delivered a solid kick to his mid-section, doubling him over gasping for breath. I turned to my girlfriend and told her to get back into the car, and out of the corner of my eye saw him charging again, head down, blinded by the blood in his eyes. Despite meeting him squarely with a knee to his forehead, his momentum still carried us over, and I heard a horrible crunch as we both hit the ground. His head hit the curb, and with his full body weight on top of me, I landed on my back with my ankle by my head. This could not be good.

My assailant was unconscious and my right leg was bent in a scarily unnatural angle. My body was in shock, the adrenalin flowing and temporarily sparing me the overwhelming pain to come, and I asked the joggers if they had seen what had happened. They agreed that he attacked me first and was now a bloody mess. While they went to call for an ambulance, I looked at the gruesome position of my leg and figured that either my knee was dislocated or my leg was severely broken. My attacker soon regained consciousness and rolled off me, and I calmly told him that I thought he had dislocated my knee. When someone started yelling to get the police the big guy dragged his busted body to his car and took off.

No matter how hard I tried to justify the violence—I was protecting my girlfriend, he threw the first punch and I was defending myself—none of it mattered. When you resort to violence, everyone is a loser. And I had lost the most of all. Time after time, year after year, I had walked away from treacherous flights and high-level stunts without a scratch, had ventured through the African bush and Mexican jungle unscathed, and had surfed mountainous waves with only a bruised ego, and now as a result of a senseless incident of drunken road rage my body was shattered. My body and possibly even my future were taken down by a petty vice.

A crowd gathered around me and it was only a few minutes before the police and ambulance arrived. The pain setting in, I begged the paramedics for relief, for one more shot. The tequila shot got me into this mess, and, ironically, another shot, an injection, would end it. Everything went warm and fuzzy, and the next thing I knew I was waking from what I could only hope to be a horrid dream.

When I was fully sobered to the reality of the previous day, the doctors delivered the news that my life would indeed never be the same. My leg was broken into 56 pieces, the tibia plateau shattered like an eggshell. Talk about pain; I did not know what hurt worse, my hip or my knee. They had put me back together with three pins, twelve screws, and two plates worth of hardware and a bone graft from my hip to glue it all together.

When the doctor asked me if I wanted the good news or the bad news, I asked for the bad news first. He said that my career as a stuntman was over and that I would probably never surf, ski, or fly a hang glider again. In just 24 hours, I went from having it all to having nothing. Everything that I valued, that defined my existence, was gone.

The good news, well there really was no good news except that my Screen Actor's Guild insurance would pay for the knee replacement I was going to need. The doctor explained that he had put everything back together but did not think I would ever bend my leg again. I had one chance and that was a total knee replacement. I asked how long the artificial knee joint would last, and he could not give me a definite answer: 10, 15, maybe 20 years. I was 35 years old, and I thought of how I would have to go through this all over again before I was even 55. "Why me?" I asked myself, as well as God.

As I listened to doctors tell me that I would never again do the things that I valued, I felt my life was not only changed but that it was over. I was stricken with a horrible feeling deep in the pit of my stomach, so deep it touched my core, my soul. The sweat poured from my body as I felt an emotion that I could have never comprehended before. It was a desire to commit suicide, to end it all.

"Why me?" I continued to wail, and then it was as clear as could be. I was suddenly humbled, aware that something was bigger than me, bigger than what I was doing. God, the divine, whatever power resides above and all around, had my complete attention. With a split-second snap of my leg, I was now awakened to the truth that I had hidden from for years. I had been living only for myself, at all times glorifying the sacred "I."

My mind flashed back on all the partying, all the drugs and alcohol I had consumed in the past years, and I was not so astonished anymore at how this could happen. I had made the choice to disrespect the gift that was my body. Feeling invincible, I had starved my body of all the nutrients that it needs to survive. This was a drastic intervention from the highest source, and I knew I could either wallow in misery or I could turn this negative moment around and extract from it a blessing.

I thought of my mother and how she suffered gracefully with her debilitating cancer, her faith unwavering. When I had asked her why God was angry with us and why she had to die, she assured me that God's plan was of love and forgiveness. She said we only died because men had made the choice to live apart from God, to seek to become gods themselves. In faith, in a return to the source, we would carry on past what we could possibly imagine both here on earth and beyond. My mother's vehicle, her path to God, was her Christian faith, but I had learned and accepted that many devout vehicles lead us back to the giving "One." Faith was the key.

The foundations of her teaching comforted me now, and I began to wonder how these doctors could tell someone that they would never walk again or that they only had months to live. Doctors had given my mother only months to live, yet she lived year after year for over eight years, holding on to instill her impenetrable faith in her family. I knew I would honor her struggle by accepting the power of such faith, and it was that faith that pushed me forward to believe that no matter what the doctors might say, I could be healed.

I checked myself out of the hospital fearing they would operate if I slept. My good friend Leonard Gion seemingly came out of the woodwork and offered me a safe haven to rest, away from everyone. The little cottage he provided for me sat right beneath Makapuu. Like a bird with a broken wing, I had no choice but to wait faithfully for what would come next.

Five Foot Ten, 150 Pounds, And Made Of Glass

No matter how many sermons, lectures, instructions, or words of wisdom you hear, experience is the teacher, the only true teacher. Having fallen, my faith was being tested to its limits. A new challenge was before me, a challenge to heal myself, to prove the doctors wrong. The mission was to come back to the life and career I loved. In the back of my mind were the stories of elite athletes who suffered catastrophic injuries but returned the following season after amazing recoveries. What were they doing that helped them recover from injuries that would have crippled most others for life? What did they have access to?

Refusing to accept the limited reality that the doctors were offering in Hawaii, I decided to call my old friend Lee Majors. He agreed that a knee replacement would automatically make me a liability in the stunt world and no production company would come near my $60,000 knee. A slip or fall on set and they could find themselves paying me for life. "Getting older is a bitch," Lee lamented. "There are 100 younger, faster guys ready to take your job, and they do not have a $60,000 knee."

My only hope was to try something alternative. He recommended a clinic in California where he and elite professional athletes were being treated electrically with space age instruments. "We have the technology, we can rebuild you," he joked.

Lee could not remember the exact name of the electric therapy instrument but thought it was called the Acu-Jack or something like that. It sounded very familiar, and amazingly enough, it turned out that I had briefly come across the technology three years earlier.

Good old Jupiter, Dennis McKenna, was offered a space at a medical clinic in Huntington Beach while he was promoting our oil filtration system. When I visited Dennis he had pointed out two small devices, the Electro Acuscope and Myopulse, in the progressive small clinic called Prevention Medical. The doctor there, Dr. Duvendack, MD, swore by the results of these machines. But I was healthy then and never gave them a second thought. I was surely thinking about them now; I just couldn't remember what they were called.

I packed my bags and took off for California in search of what I was still calling the Acu-Jack. In my search came a very troubling discovery about the state of our healthcare services.

As I entered the elite clinic recommended by Lee, they herded me off to a large couch with about ten other people. They were all doing various exercises, what I now call getting the lotions, potions, and range of motions. Squeeze this, push on that were the frequent commands from the non-emotional drones clearly set on processing us in and out as efficiently as possible.

There was a single therapist and an assistant for ten injured people. With six podiums and six padded benches, they could treat sixty people an hour. It was a mill. The head physical terrorist, I mean therapist, gave orders to her assistant while referring to us by our injuries. "The knee" gets the ice, "the shoulder" gets the heat, or "the ankle" needs fresh towels. I kept asking for the Electro Acu-something, but they looked at me like I was from another planet and tried to tell me Lee must have been talking about an ultra sound.

I could not help but notice the traffic of large men going past into a private room, and when I inquired who they were, the therapist said, "Oh, that's the Raiders and Rams football players. We treat them privately so they don't get hounded for autographs."

"I bet that is where you have the Acu-Jack thing," I responded. I received a sarcastic look and the same answer, "We don't have any new electrical healing device."

I left the clinic feeling like another cow milked for the last drop of my insurance dollars. When the insurance reaches its cap and you're still not any better, the healthcare system casts you aside like a steer marked for slaughter. There is no money in cure, just money in treatment. No one cares whether you get better or not, but what everyone does care about is getting paid. I had no doubt that it was all about the money.

That night I met up with Lee. He assured me that they had the electro stimulation device and that he would make a call to the top guys and get me a treatment. The following day I entered what could have been an entirely different clinic. The transformation was astonishing. I was greeted right away by a doctor: "Well hello Mr. Thorp. You must be the friend of Lee Majors. Would you please come with me?" You will never guess where. Yep, that private room I was eyeing from the cattle couches the day before.

The doctor immediately confirmed that they had the Electro-Acuscope and Myopulse, but in a syrupy sweet tone he said, "To be perfectly honest with you Mr. Thorp, we think these instruments are more hype and placebo than anything else." He continued to explain that the only reason they even had them was because the professional athletes requested their teams to purchase them after finding treatment had significantly quickened recuperation times. He stressed that there was just not enough clinical documentation to support any of their claims to offer it to the public.

"If you wish to try them, be my guest. But there are a few guidelines you must follow," he offered. "Rule one: cash only, $200 per day. Rule two: You don't mention this treatment to any of the other patients."

I found that peculiar, but he immediately reasoned once again that there was just not enough clinical documentation to support the claims. He thought it was great that the athletes thought it was helping them, but... "I know, not enough clinical documentation," I chimed in.

The real reason that more people were not treated with the Acuscope and Myopulse was purely economics. Why have one therapist providing individual treatment to "a nobody" for an hour when they could generate $200 per patient while seeing ten cases in that same hour? Plus, they were being fully reimbursed by the insurance companies.

I promised to keep quiet, and I got treated. I was off all pain medication five days later. Continuing regular treatment with both the Electro-Acuscope and Myopulse for six months, I was half-way home, walking, not perfectly, but walking on my own now. Unfortunately, my progress had come at a price of $30,000, and my money had run out. I was broke and still broken.

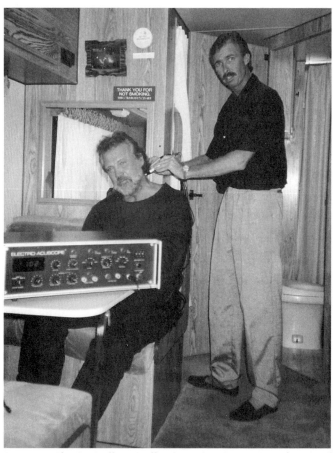

*Treating The Six Million Dollar Man, Lee Majors, on the set of
"Raven" television series filmed in Hawaii.*

CHAPTER THIRTEEN

And Lose, And Start Again At Your Beginnings And Never Breathe A Word About Your Loss

Did you ever wonder if we are all being diagnosed with electrical devices like EEGs, EKGs, and EMGs, then why are we not being treated electrically as well? If you have a heart attack how do they bring you back? With electricity! Remember the Frankenstein movies and the big jolting shock from above to generate life? It turns out that it does not take a big jolt of electricity to infuse health, just a very small current known as micro-current. Millionths if not trillionths of an amp are capable of taking a cell from a degenerative state to a regenerative state in a matter of seconds.

If not for a couple of my dear friends, Dennis McKenna and Lee Majors, I would never have heard about the miracles that were happening on a daily basis with the space age instruments. If this was good enough for the pros it seemingly should have been an automatic draw for all patients, but it was deemed too time consuming and therefore economically inefficient. I saw this as a horrible injustice, an injustice so great that it became my passion.

To complete my healing and learn more about these instruments charging me back to life, I tracked down the sales representative for the Acuscope and Myopulse. I found a man with a "used car salesman" attitude. Interestingly enough, he said he needed someone to treat horses, since he knew nothing about them. He also needed celebrity endorsements to help with the marketing. Thanks to my stunt career, my love of horses and wanting to be a veterinarian as a kid, I knew horses and I knew celebrities.

Underpants And Horse Stalls

After two days of training, I was officially certified to use the Acuscope and Myopulse. The distributor made a few phone calls and spoke to a veterinarian who was willing to try the devices on a few injured horses that were not responding to traditional therapy. "Send your guy in," said the vet. "If he is successful we will purchase the instruments."

The distributor hung up the phone and looked over at me with that telling salesman grin. "Well it's all set," he said. "There is just one thing. Have you got any collateral? These instruments are worth over $16,000, but it won't take long for you to pay them off with the deal I just set up for you. You'll get paid fifty bucks a horse, and you ought to be able to do ten horses a day." If he was right, it really would not take me long to pay off these instruments. Most importantly, I would be free to heal my leg.

I offered the pink slip to my car and a sunken treasure coin collection I had smuggled out of Africa to the salesman as my collateral. His eyes almost fell out of his head when he saw the dates on my coins. "These will do just fine," he replied. "I'll keep them right here in my safe." I proudly walked out of the office with the Acuscope under one arm and the Myopulse under the other, barely missing the weight of the coins.

I met with the vet the very next day at the equestrian center in Burbank, where he took me to the first horse and struggled to explain the horse's injuries: "He just won't stay sound." He felt the injury was possibly in the horse's shoulder, so I immediately went to work on that region. After about an hour and a half, the vet returned to assess the treatment. After trotting the horse out and around, he returned to say, "You sure did a great job on the right front. Too bad you wrecked him in the rear." There was no mistake; the horse was now noticeably lame in the rear hindquarter.

After I worked for another few hours on the rear hindquarter, the vet returned to repeat the same evaluations and the horse now showed lameness in other areas. I treated that damn horse wherever he revealed pain for over ten hours. The sun had long set when the vet trotted the horse out for the final time and returned with a big smile: "Well, you did it! He is sound!"

Great, but it took over ten hours to earn $50. How was I ever going to pay off these instruments?

I looked at my $50 and started thinking about how the salesman and the instructor of the two-day class that I sat through to get my certification referred to the treatments as acupuncture without needles. If one could find a way to systemically treat the entire horse first, all the little problems could be eliminated and the treatment time significantly cut down.

In search of horse anatomy books, I went straight for the library and found my holy grail, a book on equine acupuncture. I sat up through the night studying all the integral points on the body of a horse.

No Placebo With A Horse

I returned to the equestrian center early the next morning with my new guide under my arm and attacked my first horse of the day, treating all the master acupuncture points. Within 30 minutes, the horse was sound. They brought the next horse, and again I went after the master points. This time it took a little longer, but within an hour, this horse was sound too. Although the treatment on some horses took a little longer and on some a little shorter, I was rolling them in and out and gaining confidence with each treatment. In addition, the best part was that in-between each horse there was time to use the devices to treat my own leg. At sunset, over nine horses had been treated and my knee was feeling better and better.

Soon my reputation began to grow and even the owners of the horses started coming to see how I was healing their animals. It was not long before folks were standing in their underwear in a horse stall and watching their pain miraculously disappear. I thought for sure that any day now someone would come to throw me in jail; this was just too good to be true. However, it never happened, and the horses, the owners, and I were left alone to heal.

Just when everything was looking up, I was in for another rude awakening. I had the instruments paid off from treating the horses, had acquired a human clientele, and was recovering quite rapidly, maybe a little too rapidly. I started to feel six-foot-six, two hundred and fifty pounds, and bulletproof again, but, unfortunately, I was served a firm reminder that I was five ten, one hundred and fifty pounds, and made of glass with just a couple of plates and a handful of screws holding me together.

I slowly slipped back into my old ways. A few drinks became several drinks, and I was soon out in the bar scene again in full force.

It was June 13, which happened to be a Friday, my lucky day. It was just a little over seven months since my accident, and my buddy, David Backstrom, and I were invited to a bikini fashion show featuring another new girlfriend and a girl we were going to introduce to David. They arranged for VIP seats for David and I at the bar, right next to the roped-off section reserved for the models. Focusing my big Nikon camera and trying to position myself over the crowd, I balanced myself on the upper rung of a barstool. I felt someone bump my stool and looked around to find a long-haired scruffy dude standing next to me in the section reserved for the girls. "Hey, watch out," I warned him, "and you're in the models area." I could see the bartender coming over to help remove this intruder, but looked away when David let me know my gal was on her way out. I was refocusing my camera when my stool suddenly rocked forward, my boot slipped down between the rungs as I fell forward, and I came face to face with the floor. The scruffy dude had kicked the bar stool right out from under me.

Not a single broken bone in my entire stunt career, and now in less than a year I had broken my tibia, fibula, and femur twice, both times in alcohol-fueled incidents. You would have thought I would have gotten the message the first time to take a time out.

Once again, an ambulance sped me away to the hospital, and the doctors there had the same advice as before. Total knee replacement was my only hope to walk again. No way. My only hope would be to get out of this hospital as fast as possible; I had found the cure and it was not inside these walls. David would bust me out of the liability-leery hospital and return me to my miracle machines.

As we had planned, David came to visit me the next morning and brought my old brace that I had saved from my first series of breaks. He told the hospital staff that he was going to wheel me out to get a little fresh air, but once we were outside, he pulled my car around and off we went as if we had just pulled off a well-planned robbery. We sped away, David laughing and I part laughing, part crying in pain with every bump as we banged out of the parking lot.

We pulled up to the house I was raised in and surprised my dad. Had I not broken my leg once again I would not have returned to my home for one last visit with my father. I told him about the Acuscope and how it had helped me and hundreds of others. He said, "Well bring that thing in here. I've had a stiff neck for weeks and I couldn't go bowling."

Since I could not walk David went out to the car and brought the Acuscope in. I treated my dad for well over an hour and he said, "It still feels the same!" All the people I had helped, including myself, and here was my father saying it didn't do a thing for him. Maybe it *was* just placebo.

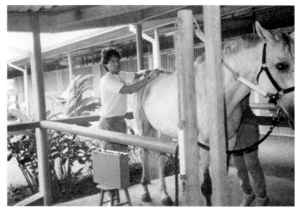

Barry Hilton offered me his home to recuperate, so I set up the instruments in his spare room and began treating myself all over again. If I was going to get well and stay well,

David Backstrom, my get away driver from the hospital, treating a horse using the Electro Acuscope & Myopulse

I knew the drinking had to go. This time for good, as I did not know how many chances I would be granted.

The following morning I got a call from my father, who was very excited. "Whatever you did to my neck, the pain is totally gone. You healed me, son, with that Acuscope thing. I know it was that machine because I have tried everything and I did nothing except let you treat me with that thing and my pain is gone. I'm going bowling! It's a miracle." Once again my heart felt that warm glow all over. My father believed in me.

Hot Springs Of Healing

Good old Dennis McKenna got word that I was busy healing myself again and came to me with an interesting proposition. He was set to invest in a rundown hot springs up in Big Bear, California, and he asked if I would like to go in as a partner with him and his wife, Dulcy. Dennis recounted the history of the hot springs, how they were once the healing grounds of the Serrano Indians, who would come to lay in the mud baths to treat their injuries. Having realized the importance of a spiritual recovery, this could be the perfect place for me to heal my spirit.

"John, I will bet you anything that if you join up with us we can create a wellness center out of these hot springs," said Dennis. It all sounded wonderful, but I was still worried about getting thrown in jail for practicing medicine without a license. He quickly assured me that he would contact a retired chiropractor that he knew in Big Bear who would probably like to work with us.

A few weeks later, we closed the deal on Pan Hot Springs and renamed it Eagle Valley Mineral Hot Springs and Spa. My clientele followed me up there, and the chiropractor, Dr. Bill Chaney, decided to come out of retirement to work with us. He moved his mobile home over and parked it right next to the hot springs. Dr. Chaney's wife was familiar with insurance billing, so she handled that part, Dr. Chaney did a few adjustments, and I handled therapy using the miracle machines, "the Electro Acuscope and Myopulse."

It wasn't long before we were featured in the local newspaper and Eagle Valley Mineral Hot Springs became the place of wellness in the Big Bear Valley.

Soon we were generating thousands of dollars per month, of which every penny was rolled over into remodeling the place and just barely covering the mortgage. But the money didn't matter; getting myself and others well did! The fresh mountain air, clean living, and the mineral waters were doing wonders on my body and soul.

Dennis pushed me to swim every day, and one morning I awoke to find a beautiful new bicycle. Dennis had bought me a state-of-the-art road bike and said, "You should be our example of healing, so let's go for a ride. Hell, if this stuff really works you should be able to run a triathlon a year from the date of the injury."

I could barely provide the full range of motion to pedal the bike, but after sitting in the hot mineral water and really pulling on my leg, centimeter-by-centimeter, my leg began to bend. When riding the bike became easy, it was time for me to start running. Although it was more like shuffling than running at first, my leg eventually started lifting higher and higher.

My Father's Final Words

I awoke to the sound of my phone ringing by my bed. It was my father. He had recently been diagnosed with an ulcerated esophagus. He told me that none of his physicians were around but this thing had really been bothering him. He told me the last time they took a look while he was in the hospital for his cardiomyopathy check-up, they stuck a scope down his throat and it damned near killed him with pain. He told me he was going to go to the emergency room and find out what the hell was the matter with his esophagus, which burned every time he ate anything. He further explained that this time he was going to ask them to give him some Valium or something else to alleviate the pain.

Two hours later the hospital called me and said that they did not think he would make it through the night.

At first they said they thought he was having a reaction to the Valium they gave him, and then they said they realized he was having a stroke. "Hell, he walked in on two feet this morning. What the heck did you do to him!" I asked. We are doing everything we can for your father was all they could say.

I jumped in my car and raced to the hospital, meeting my sister and stepmother there. They directed us to his intensive care room, and what I found shocked me. He was unconscious and his weight had dropped dramatically. I watched a vibrant sixty-nine year old man go to looking like he was 90 in just a few months. The doctors believed that he had a major stroke but they were prepared to do all the codes on him if he stopped breathing or went into cardiac arrest. I looked the doctor straight in the eye and said I think you have done enough. If my father goes, it is his time to go. I also felt that my dad was ready to go. My father had smoked all of his life and in the last ten years began drinking pretty heavily due to his marriage breaking down. The only thing that gave him joy was walking Voltan, the Doberman that I had given to my dear friend John Allen. When John could no longer care for Voltan he had given the dog to my father. My father loved that dog from the moment he laid eyes on it. I was glad that Voltan had given my dad so much pleasure in his final days, but it was my father's time and I accepted that.

If I hadn't believed that there is divinity the next event would assure me that there is. The minister who had been by my mother's bedside when she passed just happened to be in town and showed up at my father's bedside. I held my father's hand and told him that he was free to go. Everyone was watching the vitals, and I had told the doctors there would be no "Code Blue." I looked into the minister's eyes and instead of the tears he shed for my mother he had a knowing gleam in his eyes. I told my father to go to mom, that she was waiting. I visualized them in their cute little clothes and their cool shoes in the picture at the beginning of this book, and I saw my mother reaching for my father's hand. I said once again "Go to her, Dad," then I watched the monitor utter its last few beeps, and then flat line. He was with her. His death was a beautiful death. My father was with my mother once again and I knew he was happy for the first time in a long time.

We let his body rest for three days and then we buried him next to his beloved Eva.

Three weeks later, I got a call from a friend who had been watching my little Doberman, Amber, Voltan's little sister, who said that she must have eaten something or was poisoned. She had died.

Feeling that things happen in threes—my leg getting broken for the second time, my dad dying, and my dog dying—I wondered what else was going to get thrown at me in this time of loss. If not for my faith I would have had nothing to sustain me. Faith is what gets us through. The faith that my mother instilled in me was impenetrable. My mantra had become, "My faith will make me well!"

I returned to the healing waters of the hot springs. More Acuscope and Myopulse treatments, back into the tub, more pulling on the leg and soon I was actually running. I would swim a mile every day and ride my bike around the lake every other day. The running created the most discomfort, but I refused to succumb to the pain and it gradually diminished. Treating myself several times a day for almost a year, I was slowly but surely rebuilding myself.

"In His image, in His image," I repeated over and over in my mind while I trained, honoring the Creator by honoring my body. With my mother's faith inside me again, I knew my body would once again provide me with the life I desired. Unfortunately, Dar's would not.

CHAPTER FOURTEEN

If You Can Force Your Heart And Nerve And Sinew
To Serve Your Turn Long After The Are Gone

I got a call from Dar after he had heard that I was in a rough place. He offered his condolences regarding my father's death. He realized the things that I had tried to protect him from were now happening, but he loved his wife and was still trying to work things out. "She is the mother of my new little boy," he continued, "and he is just incredible."

After a long talk that night, I felt that our friendship was on the way to repair. He told me he was off to do a film in Page, Arizona, called *Million Dollar Mystery*. He would rather be at home with his wife and new baby, but he had some great stunts to do for this film. One would be on a motorcycle, where he was going to hit the guardrail head first, fly over the handlebars, and land on an airbag 75 feet below. It sounded great, and I knew that Dar would nail it.

The Fatal Flaw

Three days later, on November 21, 1986, while half-listening to the news, I heard a report that the world's greatest stuntman was killed in Arizona. Tragically, it was true. We lost Dar to a stunt gone wrong.

We later found out from George Fischer, the stunt coordinator, that Dar had gotten a call from his wife that clearly upset him on the day of his big stunt. However, he did not want to talk about it, and he told George that it was no big deal as he continued to prepare for the big guardrail hit. George said that he was concerned when Dar headed for the guardrail at full blast. He hit it dead on, did a front handspring off the front handlebars, and landed perfectly in the airbag below. Dar had pulled it off perfectly and once again walked away without a scratch.

Unfortunately, that was not the end of the story. George continued to tell me the events of the day, which included another call from his wife not long after he had completed the big stunt. Dar left his trailer visually upset, slamming the door just as he ran into George. George asked him if he was okay, and Dar said that he was fine. His next scene was a simple chase scene sequence. He would be following the big van with the bad guys in it. They were going to release a bunch of volleyballs and his job was to dodge the volleyballs. One of the balls got stuck up underneath Dar's front wheels, which slammed him to the ground so hard that he probably had a concussion, but he refused any medical attention and went to his trailer. He only had one more scene that day and it really was not considered a stunt. What happened in that trailer while he rested his pounding head, we may never know. What we do know is that 30 minutes later when he was called to the set he was visibly upset. His normal demeanor of the happy jokester was gone, replaced by an intense focus to get the last shot in the can. George told me that he had called down to base camp and made sure that the medical crew was still in place even though the stunts were done for the day. The production manager assured him that the medical team was still there and he would hold them. We later found out this was a bold face lie. They had been released after the last stunts were performed to save the production company a miserly $500.

George called for the bike riders for the final run by the cameras. They would be chasing the same van down a dirt road and would go past the cameras as they rounded the turn at 85 mph. All went as planned as the bike riders raced past the cameras; they went around the turn and all slid toward the outside of the turn. Dar was furthest out so he just stood up on his pegs as he left the road. According to George, it looked as if Dar was going to do the same stunt he did earlier, although this time there was no railing or an airbag below. Dar left the side of the road standing on his pegs. Just below, unseen by the cameras, a yucca plant lay directly in Dar's path. Dar was impaled on that yucca plant, lacerating his liver.

George called for the medical team and found that they had been dismissed hours earlier. He radioed for the police officers and for anyone that knew CPR. Dar was bleeding badly. They radioed for a helicopter but all were in use in other areas of the state. They loaded Dar into the back of a police car. He was in and out of consciousness as they headed to rendezvous with the ambulance service or the helicopters, whichever got there first. Dar did not receive any medical attention for one hour and fifty-eight minutes. He bled to death. The world's greatest stuntman, son, husband, father of three boys, my best friend and mentor was dead.

We fought the movie company for a wrongful death suit. We lost. We raised money for a foundation in Dar's name that would be for his children and other children of stuntmen that had been killed. Stuntmen from around the world came to Dar's memorial and brought their priceless footage to donate to the production that Gary Benz created to benefit the families of stuntmen that had been killed. More than $100,000 was raised, but unfortunately the money disappeared. The only person besides Gary who had access to the account was Dar's wife. To this day, I still feel a twinge in my gut when I think that if I had not introduced Dar to his last wife maybe he would still be here with us today. There was no stunt that Dar could not perform and pull off with the utmost safety. He was absolutely brilliant. God bless you Dar.

1986 was a year to remember for tragedy. I broke my leg twice, my father died, my dog died, and my best friend was killed. But also in that year my body miraculously recovered from an injury when everyone said that it was impossible. I was sure of one thing: God was watching over me every step of the way. So were my mother, my father, and their team of guardian angels. God had a bigger plan for me, and as Jesus Christ did his forty days and forty nights, I, too, had to walk through the wall of fire.

Yea though I walk through the valley of the shadow of death, I shall fear no evil. Thy rod and thy staff they comfort me.

My spirit felt born again. I firmly believed that I was becoming one of God's white light warriors. I assigned myself the task to stay clear of the devil's deceit and false promises and to bring light to those without. (the definition of darkness being "without light").

Tithing

The meaning of my life had become very clear, to give back and help others heal themselves. Learning to listen to the voice within and supply my body the fuel it needed made all the difference. Some lessons would still have to be learned the hard way but my path was clear. I had found the reason to a troubling question to many: why are we here? The answer for me was to heal the place and bring peace to it. To create Heaven here on earth is our mission. Dream big, and that is my dream. Heaven here on earth is ours; all we have to do is choose it!

One sunny afternoon I joined Dennis and our new friend Johnny G (the innovator for the cardio vascular exercise commonly known as "spinning") for a ride around the lake. He was a South African long-distance bicycle racer training in the high altitude of Big Bear for a grueling race from San Francisco to New Jersey.

The winding lake road has several blind spots, and just as we came down a small hill Johnny G and Dennis made a quick left turn around one of these blind spots. I glanced back, didn't see anything, and began the turn as well.

A split second later came screeching tires, and the next thing I knew I was riding the hood of a green Volvo. My bicycle had been knocked out from under me and had tumbled down an embankment. By the time the car came to a halt I was clinging to the bumper for dear life, executing a stunt I was not going to get paid for. Dennis and Johnny had heard the braking car and looked in time to see me disappear under the car, thinking I was surely injured or even dead. My stunt training had paid off. By holding onto the front of the car, I survived with only a few scratches on my butt and a bent rear wheel.

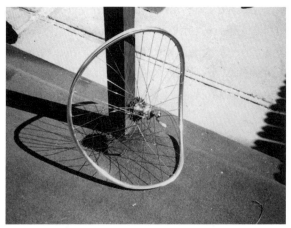

Letting the bike take the blow this time

There were no obstacles, not even a Volvo, that could keep me from my training, and I was growing stronger and stronger. Dennis got me up early one morning and handed me some paperwork.

"What is this?"

"Your entry form for the California State Triathlon Championships," he said. A lump forming in my throat, I thought back on all the dark clouds of fear. I remembered the doctor's prognosis: "You will never walk again without a severe limp. You will be crippled for life." Could I really do this? Was I really proving the doctors wrong or was I just fooling myself? Hell, I had just survived getting hit by a car, my father dying, my dog dying, breaking my leg twice, and my best friend and mentor killed in a freak accident.

My First Triathlon

I finished in the middle of the pack in my first triathlon one year from the date of my injury and called the doctor in Honolulu who had bolted my leg back together again to tell him of my accomplishment. He said what I was doing was the stupidest thing anyone could be doing on a leg as badly injured as mine. He actually called me the stupidest human being he had ever met and said that he was sure I would be arthritically crippled within the year.

Now I really wanted to prove how well I had recovered. I continued to race in the next two California Championship series triathlons, again finishing in the middle of the pack. Triathlons became my new passion, and I tried to compete in one every month, each time proving to the doubters that it was possible to come back stronger than ever.

While running into old friends at some of the events, it was hilarious to hear the wild stories floating around Hawaii about my injury and disappearance. I had been beaten up by the mob in one, and a pissed off boyfriend had knocked the crap out of me in another. I explained that I was indeed injured in a non-stunt related accident, and always added that the cause of the injury did start with the same three letters as stunt, but the other letters were "pid," as in a stupid-related accident. I could not deny that alcohol was just a stupid way to get hurt.

My prayers had been answered, and I was left in awe of the power of my two healing instruments. I decided to make electro therapy my way of tithing to repay this gift. We could show others suffering from debilitating pain that there was hope. No matter whom I went on to treat, the skeptics and the believers alike, they all got well. How could something this good be available and so few know about it?

I threw myself into my therapy sessions with every ounce of my effort. I have never worked that long and that hard than I did in those days of discovery, but the hours and days flew by, patient after patient, recovery after recovery. These were days of constant revelation, finding my true power and the power within us all, and the lessons were just beginning.

My first question was whether I could teach others to get the same results that I was seeing. I knew from the first horse I treated that this was no fifteen-minute modality, although that was the line they were using in marketing the devices to doctors. You could only bill fifteen minutes on one insurance code of E-stem the way they were doing it. With Dr. Chaney's wife at the helm in the billing department we got creative, including using codes for myofascial release, biofeedback, multiple areas of treatment, and neuro muscular re-education.

The checks began coming in and our receivables soared to over $20,000. We had to bill under Dr. Chaney's license and once the Chaneys were paid they would write us a check. So far everything was going great. It was a win-win for everyone.

The Acuscope consists of a computer inside a rectangular casing. A variety of probes can attach to the computer with slender cables. Their job is to pick up the micro-amperage current existing within our body's cells between two probes and then send back out to the body an adjusted current according to what the normal, healthy body current ought to be. It is a sensitive feedback loop from the body to the machine and back to the body. A thin layer of special gel is applied to the skin under the probes to facilitate the pick-up and delivery across the cellular membrane. What make the system even more elegant are the many different possibilities for correcting areas that need healing.

Like the many different routes in a city from one location to another, the more systems of communication the practitioner knows about the more messages he or she can develop to tell the body to heal. For example, I could put the probes on two sides of a gaping wound and the wound would begin to close faster than without the treatment. I could also add knowledge of acupuncture to the treatment. Acupuncture is based on the existence of fourteen major channels of communication that interact with each other in reliably consistent ways. Along the channels, like amplifiers along an electrical grid, are acupuncture points. I had learned to hurry the healing message not only by placing the probes near the area of discomfort, but also by figuring out which channels were involved and placing probes on important points along those channels. There are also micro-systems within the ear and on the hands and feet that healers from generations past have identified.

To work on horses or other animals, or to work on the feet of humans, there were flat metal plates instead of probes, giving a general healing reading of that zone of the body and a more diffuse healing message in response.

I had two different machines, the Electro Acuscope for neurological repair and the Myopulse, designed specifically for connective tissue repair: muscles, tendons, ligaments, and bone.

I received the basics of treatment when I bought the machine, but my instructor primarily used a very few handheld probes. Rarely did I see use of the other specialty probes designed for the ear, the teeth, the lymph system, and the reflexology points located on the hands and feet.

I trained one of Dr. Chaney's massage therapists to conduct the actual protocols that I was slowly developing. I learned far more from my work on myself and the horses than I ever learned from the training staff where I purchased the machines. I had been treating myself for two hours, three times a day and even slept with a machine to get the results that I did. I would fall asleep with the plates on my knee then wake up and put the Acuscope on charge, put more gel on the plates, switch the wires into the Myopulse, and let it run on a continuous setting until I woke up again.

The protocols that I was developing made sense to me. My first training was based on how I personally treated every client. I would always ask, "Where do you hurt?" and have them put their finger on it. I'd put a drop of electrolyte gel there and treat around the area of pain, going through the frequencies that we humans resonate at in hertz: delta (0-3.5 Hz), theta (3.5-7.0 Hz), alpha (7.0-13 Hz), and beta (13-40 Hz and above). I read the dial to see if the feedback told me the body was pulsing micro-amperage current properly through the cells of the area of discomfort. Next I would use the Myopulse the same way, and at the end of this methodical process I would have cleared the body of dissonant currents at all the frequencies that humans and animals resonate and then I'd finish off with the Y-shaped probe and a relaxing massaging motion.

If the pain did not diminish I would use another frequency, and if still there were no results I'd switch back to the Acuscope. Voila! The pain would drop dramatically every time.

I explained to Nancy, the first student I trained, that once you have laid a foundation with specific points, ask the patient to move the joint around or to bend over if it is back pain. If the pain is gone, you're done with the treatment. If not, bring out the Y-probe and massage the area using an acute frequency, normally starting at 40 Hz, then have the patient move again. "Your first two days will be direct to the area of most pain, and the third day will treat systemically using probes designed for ears, teeth, hands, feet, or spine," I instructed Nancy.

The machines included special ear clips and a headband that held sources of micro-amperage current at specific points around the skull. They were great to let the patient experience their most relaxed and de-stressed states of mind (in alpha and theta brain waves). "Time permitting," I counseled, "do this to everyone and the results will be spectacular." My trainee began to treat exactly the way I taught her and she too got excellent results.

Now I was paying someone at a fraction of the cost in my time and money to do what I had been doing, and I could spend more time training. I knew now that I could be duplicated, which meant my earnings could dramatically increase. I did not have to see the general public, just the VIP patients who came especially to see me. Life was good.

The Chaneys' Defection

Dennis and I would train every morning, pushing each other to work harder and faster on our road bikes. We had recently met an ex-Olympian, David Brinton, who was a Velodrome racer in the 1986 Olympics. He was going to be competing at a bike race two hours west of Big Bear Lake in Dominguez Hills. David had experienced our treatments and said that if we took a booth at the race he would spread the word to the other racers about our miracle machines and our incredible altitude-training center in Big Bear. We took David's advice and got a booth. We literally took our show on the road with anticipation of generating business and at the same

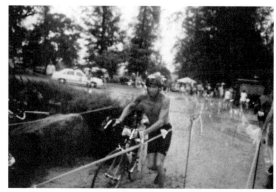

One mile swim, fifty miles on the bike, and a 10 mile run – I was back

time interesting investors in building a world-class altitude-training center on our hot springs property. The day was incredible and a lot of interest was generated. Dennis spent the day working on drawings of an Olympic caliber pool, high diving platforms, and a world-class fitness club.

After a long, hot day in Dominguez Hills we headed back to the hot springs. As we pulled in something looked very different. Dr. Chaney's Winnebago was missing. The good news was that the instruments were safely in my bedroom where I left them. But the Chaneys and over $20,000 of our money in receivables were gone!

Dennis went in chase of them. It seems they were concerned about the harmonic convergence and headed for Sedona Arizona in case it was the end of the world. When Dennis finally caught up to them, thirteen people were living in a one-bedroom apartment waiting to be beamed up.

We never saw or heard from them again.

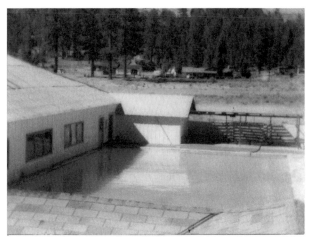

The out door pool at Eagle Valley Mineral Hot Springs,
Big Bear California, 1987

The Gift Of Divine Presence

Whether you saw it as doomsday or a new beginning, the day of the harmonic convergence would change my life forever. August 17, 1987, was built up as a special day. Predictions of prophecy, hope, and fear were all attached to the day's astral phenomena. With the planets aligning in a way they had not for thousands of years, one could only wonder what it would bring. (The Period in History known as the harmonic convergence was defined by Jose Arguelles as "the point at which the counter-spin of history finally comes to a momentary halt and the still imperceptible spin of post history commences." It was the fulfillment of the prophecy of Quetzalcoatl known as the "Thirteen Heavens" and the "Nine Hells." The prophecy stated that following the Ninth Hell, humanity would know and experience an unprecedented new age of peace. The hell cycle ended on August 16, 1987, and would be followed by 25 years, ending on December 21, 2012, thus beginning as biblically predicted the 1,000 years of peace on earth.)

I awakened just before dawn and immediately felt a strange sensation; every imaginable emotion seemed to be emanating simultaneously within me. After heeding the strong desire to look at the stars, I emerged from my trailer to find everything quite normal and calm in the predawn shades of blue and gray. But the feeling inside was growing stronger and more powerful. With my senses heightened in stone-cold sobriety, I walked out into the frozen grass of our neighbor's pasture where 25 horses made their home and could only believe that I was experiencing the sensational presence of the divine.

I cast out my arms, gazed up into the heavens, and silently communicated, "Come to me." I closed my eyes and repeated the incantation: "Come to me." When I opened my eyes I found all the horses in the pasture approaching, gathering around me. The mares, their colts, and even the stallion, which never came near anyone except the mares, moved closer and closer until they completely surrounded me. This story may be hard to believe, it was hard even for me to believe, but it happened. It was a moment in my life, in time, that I have never forgotten, such a feeling of connection and communion with all entities of life. Then, just as suddenly as it had come, the feeling left me, and the old hum of fear crept inside of me, propelling me to scatter the overpowering presence of the horses and yell, "Go on, get out of here!" They all fled instantly, bucking and kicking off into the early morning dawn.

I went into the pool house, now filled with a cloud of mist so dense that you couldn't even see across the width of the pool. Seated with my legs in the water, I prayed and thanked God for this moment of clarity and expressed my complete gratitude for the miracle of my healing. A reply came not from my head but from my solar plexus as I felt a comforting warmth wash over me like I had never experienced before.

A voice, an indescribable resonance, spoke, "I AM WITH YOU!" I guess so, I thought, thinking that the gathering of the horses was surely bigger than me.

"You are healed!" the voice continued. "You will surf, you will snow ski, and you will even fly your hang glider again, but now you work for me. You must give back to others what your experience has taught you, how to heal."

That morning changed my life. Everything my mother had told me became tangible in my life now and it was clear that I had a purpose. I was simply inhabiting this body to do something special. To change the face of medicine, as we know it today from the invasive and poisoning practices of surgery and drugs to a non-invasive and naturally synergistic approach allowing the body to heal itself.

Everything in my life had been leading to this mission. Prepared as a child, watching my mother and her suffering, offering only forgiveness in return, I too would be patient with forgiveness and tolerance, but would ceaselessly search for ways to introduce this new direction with love and compassion.

Before championing such a radical departure from the norm of modern medical practice, we had to search for every flaw. Just as we had walked the entire scaffolding of the Astrodome's roof with Dar, searching for the slight flaw that could bring down the entire stunt, we would look for a crack in this vision, in this miracle machine. After over 24 years of searching, I have never found the flaw. It just isn't there.

A Poor Combination: Romance and Business

David Backstrom called me a day or two later and said that he had an investor who would like to back us in a medical center in Hawaii. David had already contacted Barry Nutter, a chiropractor friend on Oahu, and he was all for it. David asked me if I was interested in running the chronic pain division with my instruments.

From the way David sounded, his investor was someone that he was dating. I immediately was worried. Mixing pleasure with business can be deadly. He assured me they were only friends. She would provide $35,000 in seed money and we could start immediately, but I would be the one going over and setting everything up since I had the connections on Oahu. His investor said that she would provide $100,000 to assure marketing money and to insure that we would not be under-capitalized.

I informed Dennis that it was time for me to go. The Chaney defection felt like closure to my year of healing and I was ready to return to Hawaii and the business I loved. Now I would be returning with another gift that would soon subsidize me in ways that I never expected. David was offering me an opportunity that was really too good to be true.

I headed back to Hawaii to get things set up with Dr. Nutter, and everything seemed to be going well. We included Barry in all of our plans and introduced him to our potential investor. We had found a location that would work for all of us and began negotiating the deal.

I immediately sensed that the investor was madly in love with David but unfortunately David did not feel the same way. She continued to quiz me about David and I could only answer that I was unsure about his feelings for her.

David flew in and tried to smooth things over but when answering the direct questions that were asked him regarding his feelings for her, he was honest and told her the truth. She stormed out, and along with her went the $65,000 in investment money needed to secure the location and the deal. Shortly thereafter, the money ran out and we were on our own once again.

Barry took over where we left off, found an investor, and asked us to join him, only this time we would be working for him and not vice versa. I began seeing patients in his office and it was not long before the news media got hold of the miracles going on in a chiropractic office. A few weeks later we were featured on the evening news with a story about our treatments on the world surfing champion, Sunny Garcia, and a stuntman, John Thorp, and his dramatic recovery.

We made Dr. Nutter the hero when the news showed up. I gave him a basic script to follow since he knew little or nothing about how I had gotten Sunny pain free. I had to coach him on the treatment that was being featured in his office during the news interview by whispering in his ear the science behind it or in laymen's terms how the cell holds a charge. He did well for a doctor who had never performed a treatment in his life except in front of the news cameras.

The clinic was an instant success and the word of mouth publicity from extremely happy and pain-free patients generated a waiting list of patients who wanted to experience the miracle machine and the results that their friends had been experiencing.

Once again I began training another assistant, Susan Summerall, to back me up. I repeated the same general protocols I did with Nancy. Susan did it exactly the way I showed her and she too had a new career. It was a win-win for everyone. I received a rental on the instruments from Barry's office and a percentage of each treatment.

CHAPTER FIFTEEN

And So Hold On When There Is Nothing In You Except The Will, Which Says To Them: Hold On!

Return To Magnum

I went back to training for triathlons and letting everyone know that I was back, pain-free, my leg and knee healed, and ready to do what I loved, the stunt business.

It was not long before the phone started ringing again. After hearing the truth behind my disappearance, the doors to my stunt career began to open once again. The stunt coordinator for *Magnum P.I.* at the time was Tom Lupo. We had always gotten along and I had never let him down in any stunt. As soon as he started explaining how he had an actor my height and weight having real trouble with a fight scene with the star of the show, Tom Sellek, my heart started to pound.

"So you're ready to come back to work?" he asked

"You bet!" I proudly replied.

"Well, get your ass over here. I'll see you tomorrow."

When a stunt performer is seriously injured, he must demonstrate that he is not a liability to the film company. Breaking into the industry is hard enough, and plugging back into it can be even harder. But now I was given a chance to return to the work I loved.

The voice, the message from within on the morning of the harmonic convergence in the pasture, had said I would ski, surf, and hang glide all over again. As far as I was concerned, I was fulfilling my new destiny. My invitation to return to the show came out of the blue and I felt obliged to honor the offer.

The first day back on set felt like a return home. The act went off without a hitch as far as the production was concerned. Tom accidentally hit me square in the mouth, apologizing profusely, but I was getting paid to take a hit here and there and was happy to walk back to my trailer without complaint.

The jobs continued to come my way after my successful return to *Magnum P.I.*, and I was thrilled to be invited back into the elite fraternity of stuntmen. However, the words delivered to me that morning inside the pool house kept coming back to me, reminding me that my true comeback was not yet complete: "You will surf, you will snow ski, and you will even fly your hang glider again." It was time for me to fulfill those prophetic words, to finish the breakthrough after the breakdown.

I felt a new challenge come over me, a challenge to not only continue to heal myself, but the newfound ability to help facilitate others to heal themselves as well.

I had witnessed amazing recoveries, including my own. I saw this challenge as the biggest stunt ever, to heal myself completely and show others that they too could heal themselves. This would be the challenge of my life.

I decided to give my orthopedic

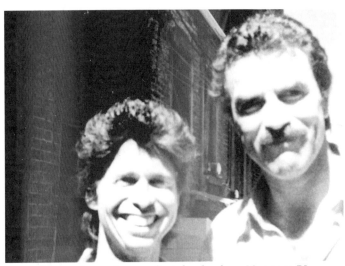

Tom and me after my first day back on Magnum PI

surgeon a call to let him know that I was back in town and that his predictions were wrong. I did not get a knee replacement as recommended, yet I had just run three triathlons on a leg he said would never bend. With a disbelieving chuckle he replied, "Well that confirms you must be the stupidest human being I have ever met! To run on a leg that is majority bone on bone was just plane stupid. You will probably be arthritically crippled soon."

I dismissed his opinion once again and climbed on my bicycle for a ride to the beach.

On my ride to the beach I could only think about basic science and that every cell in the body replaces itself with a new cell every seven years. I would have to wait seven years to prove my prognosis to be correct. I was out to show the medical community and those doubting doctors with their prescription pads and surgeries that there was a new way of healing the body by adding the perfect electrical current, and it was not invasive and it was not with drugs but it was done electrically. My body was healing itself completely naturally, and I was facilitating it by giving it the right food, fuel, exercising, detoxifying, and something that was relatively unknown, the body electric.

A Few Pins And Screws

I took off on a bike ride from my house to Sandy Beach then over the top of Koko Head Crater. As I glowed about my recovery my knee suddenly locked and my bike immediately flipped, landing me hard on my face. Thankful for my helmet, I could not figure out what I hit. My ego was crushed when I finally realized that the reason for my fall was that my knee had locked in a ninety-degree angle and I could not move it! I was crushed. The doctor must be right.

I got myself to my feet and since I had locking pedals I locked my left foot into the pedal, kept my right knee out of the way, and rode home using one leg. When I got home I carefully maneuvered myself to a stop and then in slow motion fell to the ground. I hopped into my house on one leg. As I sat by the phone ready to make the call, in defeat, to my doctor, I noticed a red protrusion from just below my patella. That is strange, I thought. It must be a bone part coming loose and I am in for more surgery. Since my options were limited on how I was going to drive myself to the doctor or find someone to help me, I decided to push on the protrusion. When I did it went back into place and my knee moved freely once again. I couldn't believe it. I had just gone from being a totally defeated, stupidest human being on the planet to the self-healed genius.

I still had to call the orthopedic surgeon. Because it was Saturday I figured I would get an answering machine. I was amazed to hear his voice on the other end of the phone. I told him what had happened and he told me to come on in. He met me at the door of his office with a scalpel in his teeth and a pair of pliers and a screwdriver in his hands. I was thankful this carpenter- orthopedic surgeon had a sense of humor. He asked me to walk for him and then marched me into the X-ray room, laid me down, and took a few pictures.

When the photos were developed, he looked and looked and said, "This is incredible. You barely have any cartilage there and you are basically bone on bone but your joint actually looks polished. One of the pins that I put in holding your tibia plateau in place was the culprit. You have healed so well that the pins are working their way out." He made a slight incision, removed the two pins (the third seemed to be firmly in place), put one stitch in my knee, and said, "This is just amazing. You see what exercise will do."

The surgeon did not want to hear anything about the Acuscope and Myopulse. "John," he insisted, "you recovered because it was your mind over matter and you are one strong-willed man." I told him he was one great carpenter and that he did not trust his own work, and, more importantly, the gift of the body and its amazing ability to heal itself. I walked out of his office on cloud nine and back on course for the Tin Man Triathlon, a half-mile swim, twenty-eight miles on the bike, and a ten kilometer run.

Once again, I finished in the middle of the pack. Just to finish was the victory for me. I set my goals higher, and the next race that I competed in was the Kauai Loves You Triathlon, which was a one-mile swim, fifty miles on the bike, and a ten mile run, basically half of an Iron Man.

The day of the race was pouring down rain and the surf at Hanalei Bay was over ten feet with a strong current. The one mile swim turned into a two and a half mile swim for most since the current swept everyone out to sea and only the strongest swimmers continued on. Over 60 competitors had to be rescued and could not finish the race. I was one of the 100 that made it through the pouring rain, the multiple bicycle crashes, and the final ribbon at the end of the ten mile run. If this was mind over matter it did not matter. I was back at the top of my game. To be honest, I had never been in this kind of condition in my life except as that kid called "Guts" playing football in middle school and high school, and pain-free too boot.

Through word of mouth I soon had all types of holistic practitioners showing up at my stunt trailer or my home asking if I would help them with their pain. I had them sign a release that I was not practicing any medicine but was just doing demonstrations since I did receive a commission from my sales, and everyone walked out with the same amazed look on their face. Some were pain-free for the first time after suffering for years.

I knew my body was in shape. I was in good enough condition to run, cycle, and swim, but could I return to the adrenalin-rush sports like big wave riding, skiing, and even flying? My mind still had a few obstacles to overcome before I hit the surf. Although the surgeon had created a workable leg from the jigsaw puzzle presented to him, my foot had been attached crooked, making my leg look more like a hockey stick. Not wanting to look like "a grime" (a beginner), an even bigger fear I had was that I would not be able to get to my feet quick enough before the wave pounded me. Yet I had to trust those words I had heard that early morning before the sun rose. "You will surf again." I knew I had to give it a go. With a lump in my throat the size of a golf ball, I listened to the news. I heard what I'd been waiting for. The first big south swell had hit.

To Surf Again

Upon hearing that the surf was up, I pulled into the parking lot at Fort Derussy right in front of Threes, Oahu's perfect south shore break, and was slightly relieved to find a full parking lot. My fears still lingered: "What if I can't get up? What if I have a bad wipeout and re-injure my leg?" Just as I was tempted to seize this available excuse not to surf, a beautiful little Hawaiian girl approached my car to say she was leaving and offered me her spot. My escape revoked by the generosity of a smiling angel, I knew, without a doubt, that it was time to face my destiny.

I sent up little silent prayers and took a few deep breaths while removing my board from the top of my car. Watching the break, I walked slowly to the beach, and then began waxing my board thoroughly, very thoroughly. "Quit stalling," I whispered to myself.

I came to the end of the jetties just as two other Haoles paddled back in and noticed one was bleeding over his right eye and the other held his board's snapped off fins in his hand. "Hey bro," they yelled, "don't even think about going out there. The water is full of Mokes and it must be kill Haole day." The hostile local Hawaiians had delivered a clear message in the form of a few knocks to the head and some busted fins. "You won't get a wave out there today," they continued to warn me.

Without a reply, I timed my dive into a coming wave, determined to change the vibe. I began my paddle out, baptized anew by the cleansing turquoise waters of the Pacific.

A little weak in the arms from not surfing for so long, I took my time getting out to the perfect six to eight foot right-hand peelers. Out in the line-up I discovered the crew that the two terrorized surfers had warned me about. The Hawaiian junior surf team was in the water, and these kids were hot. However, my fears of the stiff competition for waves that they would pose was assuaged when I saw the leader of their pack, their coach and my good friend, Ben Aipa.

Ben had shaped my boards and had been a solid surfing buddy for years. "Bruddah John," he greeted me while paddling over, "where you been?" I gave him a brief description of my injury and recovery. "Yo Bruddah, that is one mean looking break," he said, astonished at the sight of my leg. "How can you stand on it?"

"It may look bad, but it works."

"So what, you think you can surf on it?"

"That is what I'm here to find out."

"Well, the waves are perfect," he said, nodding in support of my test. "And don't worry about the little farts. I got them under control."

I positioned myself on the outside and lined myself up with the same old coconut tree on shore, preparing for action.

Always with someone looking to drop-in on me, I waited patiently and watched several waves pass through. Soon everyone had caught a wave, leaving me all alone on the outside as a giant set emerged upon the horizon. It was now or never, and I turned my board around. Everyone stuck on the inside was yelling and screaming now about the huge approaching set. Ben was yelling, "Go Bruddah, go," and paddled over to block the little crew from jumping in late, giving a Haole like me the prize wave of the day.

The ocean began to suck and pull, and the doubts flashed across my mind: "What if I wipe out? What if I blow my takeoff? Maybe the leg won't work. They will laugh at Ben if I look like a kook." Then that inner voice demanded, "Quiet." Calmly stroking into the rolling wave, I let its immense power quickly grasp me. Feeling a bit unstable while pushing to my feet, the large drop was definitely shaky, but as soon as I planted my fins and made the bottom turn, the wave lined up perfectly before me. The beaming smile on Ben's face as he paddled over the top lip in front was the last sight before the wave curled over, slotting me right into a perfect tube so far back in the hollow revolving chamber that it really didn't seem possible to make it out. Still hidden deep inside the aquamarine barrel, I leaned into the blue wall and accelerated, my board working deftly under the control of my feet and legs. Hope rose as I drew closer and closer to the light, but I was very aware of the threatening lip looking likely to knock me to the jagged reef below. This tube went on for a lifetime, definitely the longest tube ride for this old surfer. A dream ride.

The roar of the collapsing wave grew louder until the exploding spit shot me out into the warm Hawaiian sunshine. This ride had been the entertainment for all the guys paddling out, and they generously encouraged me with their cheers to execute a sharp cut back and then pull into the tube once again to finish off the epic wave.

As I paddled back out, Ben caught a big roller and gave me the Shaka sign while I hooted his wave. Feeling set free upon the ocean's churning waters, I joined the celebration as we all proceeded to catch wave after wave that day. The sinking sun on the blue horizon topped off the three-hour session, and I thanked God for holding me up. I had indeed surfed again.

Yawning with satisfied exhaustion, I sat on my board peacefully anticipating the imminent green flash when one of the little Hawaiian rippers paddled over to me and started chuckling.

"Hey brah, you even smile when you yawn," he said.

"It is just one of those days," I returned and had to laugh with him, realizing for the first time that there had been a shit-eating grin on my face for hours.

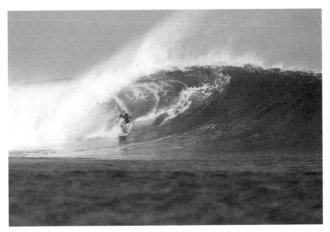

At 56, still finding tubes in Indonesia

To Fly Again

I awoke to a cool breeze the following morning from the northern wind. It always brings a big smile to all the wind riders of Hawaii, whether sailors or windsurfers, but the north wind is most special to the hang glider pilot.

Carried by the momentum of the successful return to the surf, I called my buddy Duff King and asked what his day looked like. With a sudden urge to fly a hang glider, I asked if he wanted to accompany me. Duff was the kind of guy who lived to be in the air, a pilot for Hawaiian Air and a phenomenally talented hang glider pilot. He was cautious and precise, and I could not think of a better friend to help me return to the air

Duff expressed immediate concerns, questioning if my leg could handle the landing. "Hell, if I can surf, I can surely fly," I said, trying to sound convincing even to myself. But deep down I was apprehensive, knowing as well as Duff that the takeoff would be easy, but it is hard to run doing forty if you miscalculate your landing. Flying is easy. It is the landings that can kill you. Even if I survived, I couldn't afford another injury. On the other hand, I was determined to.

We met at Makapuu and the conditions could not have been more perfect. My anxiety was evident in my preparations; the glider set up took almost half the normal time. With Duff's help, I carried my glider to the edge and I hooked myself in. Down on my knees now, I again offered my prayer up for the Father, Son, and Holy Ghost. Upon my amen the words returned: "You will even fly your hang glider."

Duff lifted the nose of my glider into the wind and without a second of hesitation I launched as I had done hundreds of times before, an act as natural as breathing. The lift was intense, strong, but as smooth as glass. An unconscious scream, "Ahyoooou!" burst from my lips; I was flying. I soared down to the green wall, then headed off to the Pali and could not stop thanking the divine hand for supporting my flight. Whales jumped below, emerging joyously to share in my celebration of life and the moment off the point at Makapuu.

The dream state eventually faded away as the sun began to set, a cool reminder that I had to land soon. The landing being my true test, the doubts flooded back: "Could my leg handle a running landing? What if I blew

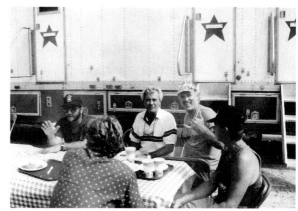

James Darren (Moon Doggie) , Duff King and John Thorp on the set of "Raven"

my landing?" Then my voice inside brought a fierce rebuttal, "Stop. Trust yourself."

I came in over the trees and lined up for my descent to Waimanalo Beach Park, now scattered about with families enjoying the beautiful tropical sunset. Spotting a deserted section of the beach, I guided my craft down. "Just like riding a bike," I assured myself as I turned for my final approach. With the cool wind in my face, the land rapidly drawing near, I reached out with my feet and they gently found the soft sand, a perfect landing to end another perfect day.

Returning immediately to my knees, I stayed down in gratitude and prayer and then opened my eyes to find that little children had surrounded me. A little Hawaiian girl with wondrously round eyes like a deer came up to me with a big piece of watermelon. "Hey Bruddah, you like some watermelon?" she asked, as I unhooked myself and accepted her gift. She then asked me if she could fly too. Echoing the wisdom of my mother, I told her there was nothing she couldn't do if she really wanted to.

There must have been 20 kids surrounding me and we all watched with smiles as Duff came flying in with a perfect landing as well. He walked over to me and my clan of dreamers.

"Hey Juan," he yelled. "You're back." I had been blessed with a second chance to fly, to soar with the beautiful innocence of a child.

To Ski Again

Several times a year the dormant volcano of Mauna Kea, one of five volcanoes which together form the island of Hawaii, presents a majestic snow-capped summit, living up to the Hawaiian translation of its name: white mountain. Rising almost 14,000 feet from sea level, the highest point in the state, Mauna Kea is actually part of the largest mountain range on the planet if measured from the ocean floor. It seemed only fitting that the completion of my tripartite prophecy of recovery might come on such a grand peak, so singularly difficult to access and ski, as it is without lifts and services.

One of my buddies, Sam Nottage, the same buddy who helped me teach Dar to fly, had a friend who worked at the internationally renowned observatory atop Mauna Kea, and he gave us a day-by-day report of the conditions. Any cold and wet spells from November to March could mean limited but perfect snow pack lining the slopes of the cinder cones. After an especially wet winter week, we could see the white cloaking Mauna Kea, and we waited for word from Sam's contact of when we would be allowed back up on top. Finally calling us back, he told us that the snowplow would clear the road tomorrow and we could follow it up, leaving us all alone to partake in the perfect unadulterated powder. I caught the next plane out of Oahu and was on the big island by sunset.

"There is a swell running and we can get in about an hour of surf before sunset," Sam said excitedly in greeting as he picked me up from the airport. We had a fantastic sunset session, dear friends on a deserted beach ending another charmed day. Content to wait on the beach for the others to catch their final waves in the now-fleeting light, I couldn't help but steal glances down at my disfigured leg. My foot went to the north instead of the south, definitely crooked. The fear crept in once again: "Would I be able to hold my leg straight enough to ski? Would I make a fool of myself and fall flat on my face?"

But just as before, my anxious questioning was immediately ruled out by the powerful words originating from deep inside: "You'll surf, you'll snow ski, and you will even fly your hang glider, but now you work for me." I had given myself over to this destined path twice already and my faith had held me up; I had no reason to doubt it would be any different atop the volcano.

We were up before the sun and quickly loaded the heavy-duty jeep we would take to the top. Sam's wife did not ski so she was going to drive the jeep, which would act as our ski lift. We filled up two extra five-gallon gas cans to ensure us plenty of runs. After a three-hour drive to the top, creeping along behind the snowplow, we arrived at the surface of the moon, the cinder cones protruding white and extraterrestrial. Immersed in the clouds, towering above the Pacific, I was set to fulfill the final and perhaps most strenuous challenge upon my leg, to snow ski deep powder.

Fitting into my old ski boots was alarmingly painful, but after a session of deep stretching the pain eventually subsided. We hiked to the summit behind the observatory, locked into our ski bindings, and let out a simultaneous, "Let's do it."

The snow was heavenly powder, knee deep and light as a feather, and my leg felt strong and agile as I pushed from side to side. It was beyond comparison. We skied pristine slopes, dodging jagged lava rocks peaking through the white blanket until ending our first run by the side of the road where Sam's wife was already waiting with the jeep. "Just like riding a bike," I thought, and jumped into the jeep as excited as a young boy, ready to do it again.

We made run after run until we barely had enough gas to get home. Riding home, I looked again at my twisted leg with new appreciation. My leg worked fine in the snow, and the final stage of the prophecy had been realized.

With a few hours of daylight remaining when we got home, we decided to take advantage of the still pumping swell. I had always desired to surf and snow ski in the same day. Another perfect sunset, another perfect surf session, and another dream manifested; all shared with smiles and dear friends.

My life was back in full glow. At each stage of recovery, my faith had delivered gifts far exceeding my expectations. Worried that I may never walk or even stand again, I never could have imagined that I would soon be surfing and skiing in a single day in Hawaii. I can only use one word to describe my state at this point, bliss. As my wife, Lisa, would say, the "bliss I plan."

A Fall Guy's Revenge

I was surprised one morning by a phone call from none other than the Six Million Dollar Man. I could recognize that Kentucky accent anywhere. "Hey John, I am coming over to meet with your old buddy Glen Larsen regarding a show based on a stuntman," Lee Majors reported. "Glen has put into motion a new television series, *The Fall Guy*, and he's asked me to co-produce, star, and even wants me singing the opening theme song. He's hosting a party at his Hawaii Kai estate and I want you to go with me."

I reminded Lee how Glen had sold me out on *Magnum P.I.* and used me as his "fall guy." I was still not feeling too good about him, although I had been cordial when I'd run into him since then.

"Don't sweat it John, that's just the nature of the beast," Lee said. "You've got to forget about that Glen Larson and Don Bellisario fiasco. Glen told me he thinks the world of you and that there would be a place for you in the show. I'll be in town next week and we will have some fun," he promised.

The following week I was with Lee at Nick's when we ran into Glen and J.C., engaged in a slight embrace as we approached. I had always gotten along really well with J.C. and held no grudge against her, but for Glen, sadly I could not say the same. Glen greeted us warmly and asked if I was doing all right. I assured him that I was doing just fine.

"You're not still mad at me are you John?" Glen asked.

"No, it's no problem," I lied.

He asked us to join them and began talking about *The Fall Guy*.

"See John, I told you I was going to do a series on stuntmen and there is definitely a spot for you."

I was leery of his promises at this point. J.C. was sitting very close to Glen and I could not help but notice her hand in his lap. With a slightly guilty smile, she leaned over and told me how incredible it always was to watch me fly and asked if I would take her for a ride sometime. I told her that I had just rigged up a parachute behind my boat and would be happy to take her paragliding. She asked if I could take her up the next day if I was coming over with Lee. Glen said that sounded great and they looked forward to seeing both Lee and I tomorrow.

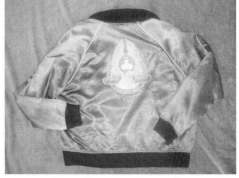

The jacket Lee gave me from "The Fall Guy" series

I pulled up in front of Glen's house with the boat, the parachute, and a couple of friends to demonstrate the safety of paragliding. J.C. ran right out and could not wait to go for a ride. She said that Glen would just love to see her parachute behind the boat. We chatted a little, and then she whispered to me that Glen was getting a divorce and that they were an item. What else could I do but congratulate her as I prepared her harness and instructed her on how to maneuver the parachute.

The wind was perfect as the parachute filled smoothly and lifted J.C. off the beach like a butterfly. I took her around the bay and landed her gently on the sand. Several of the writers came out and were brave enough to go for a ride as well. Then J.C. said that Glen just had to go for a ride, and I thought if he does, boy would I ever give him a ride, the f------ traitor. She was persistent and eventually came running out of the house with Glen in tow.

"Glen wants to go for a ride," she beamed.

He looked me square in the eyes and asked if this was safe. I said of course it was but I must have been doing a poor job at concealing my sly smile.

"Now John, you really are not still mad at me are you?" he asked.

"No, not at all!" I lied once again.

Now Lee came walking over, knowing full well about the bad feelings I was still holding for Glen. Lee started raising concerns about Glen's weight as a possible problem, but I could tell he was just looking for an out for Glen. He took me over to the side and said, "John, now don't hurt him." I guaranteed him that Glen was in good hands, but he could sense what was coming. It did not matter how much power or money he possessed, I was going to teach Glen a lesson.

I adjusted the harness around Glen's midsection and gave him the basic instructions. "When I say run, you run," I told him, and he gave me a look of "Oh shit, what have I gotten myself into?" My two helpers adjusted Glen and held him in position for the wind to fill the chute. I yelled run and off we went, a perfect takeoff.

As soon as we were clear of the reef, I initiated my plan. If you turned the ignition key off and on, the boat made a loud backfire explosion, so I did just that and as the boat lost power Glen began coming down. Just as his feet hit the water, I gave it enough power to dunk him into the ocean briefly before immediately pulling him skyward again. I repeated this several times, dunking him and then dragging him forward and then back into the air. I could see Glen glaring at me, but I just shrugged my shoulders and pointed to the motor; gee, I'm sorry, boat problems.

I eventually landed him in the shallow water unharmed except for a bruised ego. Everyone knew that I had gotten my payback. Honestly, I really did not care if I ever worked with him again. I did not trust Glen as far I could throw him or drag him. He had given me a real education on the ways of the movie business and it had not left a very good taste in my mouth, reminding me of that Hollywood stench that I had been introduced to by Redd Foxx. Within days, the word was all over the *Magnum P.I.* set that John had dragged Glen Larson around the bay out in Hawaii Kai. Maybe I was not such a bad guy after all.

The Fall Guy eventually went on to be a big hit, running for five successful seasons, but before it got off the ground Lee and Glen got into a pissing match over who was producing the show, resulting, funny enough, in a jacket war. Glen was handing out jackets with Glen Larson Productions on the back and Lee was tossing around Lee Majors Productions jackets of his own. Not surprisingly, I have kept Lee's jacket, which has a big red heart on the inside inscribed, "With Love from Lee Majors." I got one of good old Glen's jackets too, but there was no "With Love" on the inside lapel. I have worked with a lot of let's just say confident and self-assured men in many fields, but the egos in the movie business are unsurpassed. As I pulled my boat away from Glen Larson's estate that day I reconciled with the reality of a cold and fickle industry.

One show that actually lasted more than a couple of seasons was *Jake and the Fatman*. The show started in Honolulu after the end of *Magnum P.I.* and shot over a hundred episodes.

I got to play the part of a cowboy drug-dealing killer in the pilot episode. I had a pretty substantial roll as the hit man trying to kill Jake, played by Joe Penny. Joe's stunt double, Todd Keller, and I would be working together for the first time. Todd got a little nervous when I told him that he was going to be my airbag for the stunt, which required me to jump off the top of an eighteen-wheeler and land right on top of him. Todd was a good stuntman and we pulled off the stunt without a scratch. Todd had been working with Joe for years and was one of the only guys I had ever met that came with stunt school training.

We always felt sorry for the kids who paid thousands of dollars to go to a stunt school and then are never hired on a television show or feature film. This is something that the owner of the stunt school will never tell them. When their training is complete and their wallets are empty, they spend years hanging around the honey wagons they see parked along the roadside knowing that a movie or television production is being filmed at that location. They wait patiently for the stunt coordinator to come by so they can introduce themselves and hand off their resume, nothing more than a sad exercise in futility. You had to be related to someone or know someone and even then it was almost impossible to be hired. Even experienced stunt performers with television and movie credits would line up and kiss the ass of any stunt coordinator who could get them hired.

Dar was one professional who never begged for a job. He was one of the star performers and honored members of Stuntman's Association, but he was also very interested in joining Stunts Unlimited. Unfortunately, Dar had done a television special entitled The World's Greatest Stuntman, and in the

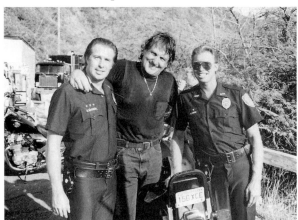

Todd Keller, Dick Ziker, and me on the set of "Jake and the Fatman"

world of the biggest egos the vote, which had to be unanimous, was against letting him in despite even Dick Ziker's lobbying for his acceptance. The truth is, however, he was so good he did not need an association. His talent was all he needed.

The stunt business had also come to me. Being at the right place at the right time resulted in on-the-job training for most of the stunts outside of my expertise, and then a relationship of mutual respect with Dar took me to the next level.

As tough as it is to get there, once you are on set it is a fantastic time. I always had a good time working on this show and getting to know everybody. William Conrad, the "Fatman," was always full of stories.

One story he shared was about how he was the voice of Marshal Matt Dillon on the radio show *Gunsmoke* way back in the late forties. When television boomed in the fifties, the producers of the show were ready to bring it to the screen. Since the radio audience was familiar with Williams's voice, the producers gave him the opportunity to read for the part.

William showed up for the interview and was introduced to a tall handsome actor by the name of James Arness, who had also just auditioned for the television version of his character. William sat down in the same chair that James Arness had just gotten up from and was handed the familiar script from the radio show of which he was the star. He barely needed to glance at the script since he was Marshall Dillon every night for the millions of radio listeners. He began reading the lines with the deep resounding voice of Matt Dillon. When he finished the scene, he knew he had nailed it! He looked up into the producers' smiling faces. All they could say was, "William, without a doubt, you are the voice of *Gunsmoke*." William just smiled and as he got up to shake their hands. The chair got up with him, stuck firmly to his large backside. He may have had the voice of Matt Dillon but he sure did not have the body. At that moment, he knew that his career as Marshall Matt Dillon had come to an end. Six-foot-six surfer James Arness would be the new Matt Dillion. *Gunsmoke* went on to become one of the longest running television series in the history of television.

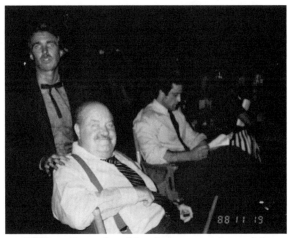

William Conrad and I enjoying ourselves while Joe Penny reads his script

William Conrad, best known for his starring role on the TV series *Cannon*, was a seasoned star and team player and a joy to be around on the set. He flowed with the many punches that were thrown in this business and knew that the only thing to do was roll with them. Conrad felt blessed to spend his time in Hawaii and even more so that his show decided to make its home there.

Joe Penny on the other hand hated Hawaii. Apparently, it was just too hot for him. Joe was difficult to work with and never seemed very happy. It might have been due to his hair falling out and having hair plugs surgically implanted. The make-up department had to spray black hair dye on his scalp to hide the plugs. The tropical heat made Joe sweat and sweat, and due to the hair dye, black streaks would run down his face, making him look like a woman with her mascara running. This obviously had a negative effect on his general mood.

Believe me, if he was a good guy on the set, I probably would not have even noticed or remembered such embarrassing details about my time with him. Being well-liked and respected on the set goes a long way toward a successful career.

"Serendestiny"

To use the words of my friend Mark Victor Hansen, "serendestiny" would find me on my next film. I would work with George Fischer, the last stunt coordinator who worked with Dar. It was a film entitled *Fists of Steel* with Carlos Palomino and Alexis Arguello, two world champion boxers.

George loved Dar and he assured me that he had covered all the bases. He felt terrible that not only did we lose the lawsuit with the movie company but also about the missing money scandal hanging over everybody's head, especially heavy for Gary Benz.

Just before I performed one of my biggest stunts of the film, a producer yelled, "This one is for Dar, John," as I was doing a back flip off the second floor of the ocean liner while still firing shots at Carlos Palomino as I headed for the ocean surface. The stunt was serenely familiar to Dar's early defining backwards plunge while he continued to fire his gun at Burt Reynolds although mine was from a much lower altitude.

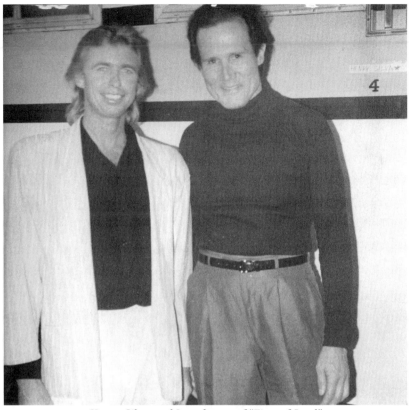

Henry Silva and I on the set of "Fists of Steel"

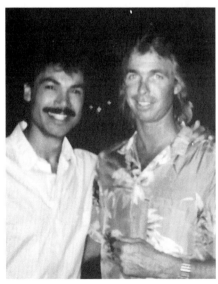

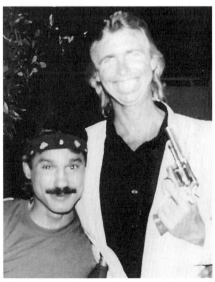

Carlos Palamino "World Champion Boxer" and I on the set of "Fists of Steel"

Alexis Areguello World Boxing Champion and I on the set of "Fists of Steel"

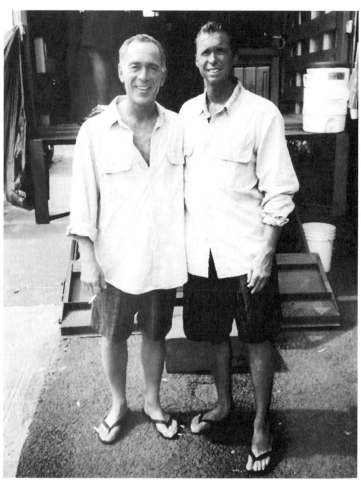

Doubling for Bruce Weitz co-star of "Hill Street Blues"
and I on the set of the "Birds in Paradise"

CHAPTER SIXTEEN

If You Can Talk With Crowds And Keep Your Virtue

On one of the final episodes of *Magnum P.I.,* I was working with the horse wrangler who had been flown in from Los Angeles. He was demonstrating how he trained horses to perform stunts without getting them injured. The use of trip wires and other old school ways that were used in the Western movies in the '60s and '70s had long since been outlawed due to so many horse injuries. Here was another calculated risk taker who loved horses and made sure that both horse and rider came out of the stunt unharmed. I was fascinated with this horseman's attitude and spent every minute with him to learn his specialty act. He would dig out a pit where the horse would fall, then fill up the whole with foam rubber chunks and cover the last foot with earth and leaves, making it look just like the surrounding area. Then he showed me how he could do a flying lead change at the same time turning the horse's head in the opposite direction; the horse had no choice but to go down. Once the horse went down with the rider, who was also a highly skilled horseman, he would hold the horse down, making it look like both horse and rider had been killed. Only when the director yelled "cut" would the rider roll off, the horse get to his feet, and the handler lead him up the dirt ramp and out of the hole. This was demonstrated to me several times and then he looked at me and asked, "Want to give it a go?"

Loving horses and considering myself a good horseman in my own right I said, "Sure!" with that slight apprehension of working with an animal once again, only this time it was with a highly intelligent one and not a billy-goat. I climbed on and took off on a trot, then into a cantor, and circled the horse around until Wrangler Tom signaled me forward. As I slowly cantered forward he yelled, "Now!" I used my opposite leg to get him to change leads and the reigns to pull his head around in the opposite direction; the horse went down right on the spot, landing soft as could be on the foam pads beneath. Needless to say, I was impressed. I would have a new talent to add to my stunt bag of tricks.

Everything that is great has its time, and *Magnum P.I.* was coming to an end. At the rap party everyone was sad that this great show was coming to an end. The surprise at the party was an announcement that Tom had agreed to one last season for the benefit of all the other actors. Everyone was delighted, especially me since my redemption was complete and I had resumed a spot as a utility stunt performer. The last season flew by, with even a hang gliding episode thrown in.

A year later we held the final, final rap party and the show came to an end. At that party I met Jim Reynolds, a self-made multi-millionaire in the commercial real estate business in Honolulu, who would soon become one of my best friends and mentors. I knew his wife, Stephanie, an accomplished actress and model who had appeared on several commercials, television shows, and, naturally, *Magnum P.I.*

The Sport Of Kings

Stephanie introduced us and was surprised that we had not already known each other because we had many mutual friends. Jim was an avid horseman and one of Honolulu's top polo players. We immediately had a wonderful mutual respect and a friendship was born. I was explaining that I had recently learned the horse fall stunt and he quizzed me; if I knew how

to fall off I must be able to ride fairly well. He asked me if I had ever thought of playing polo, but I explained that it was not in my budget. He said that he was the owner (patron) of one of the best polo teams in Hawaii that consisted of Ronnie Tongg, his sons, Ryan and Rustin, Kimo Huddleston,

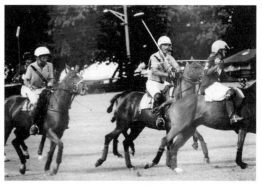

Playing polo on Kauai. Players from l to r: John Thorp, Bill George and Gordon Smith

and Kawika Manoa. I was surprised and honored when he asked if I would like to join the team. He had horses for me to ride and an instructor who would give me private coaching. It was an offer I could not refuse.

The first time I hit the ball was under the tutorial of Tommy Campos, who just happened to be Don Ho's ex bodyguard. (Remember his bed? Well, so did Tommy!) That didn't slow me down. I was addicted. Tommy saw the gleam in my eye and my ability to ride but would never let on that he recognized that I was a horseman. The first horse he put me on was Mona, a well-trained thoroughbred beauty. I cantered around the field with the mallet in my hand and pulled up in front of Tommy, expecting some slight recognition that I could ride. All Tommy could say was, "You ride like a monkey fucking a coconut." I was shattered.

Tommy asked me if I really wanted to play polo, and I said absolutely! "Well," he said, "if you show up here every day we should be able to get you playing." Tommy would spend hours with me until my hands were bleeding and my butt had sores that were very slow in healing. There was rarely a kind word from Tommy, just constant verbal abuse. I grew to love this old Hawaiian man and understood his abusive style was the way he showed he loved you.

Soon I was treating all of Jimmy's horses with the Acuscope and Myopulse with the same incredible results. Tommy was naturally my biggest skeptic, but after seeing lame horses heal very quickly he asked me if it would help his low back. "Without a doubt," I said, "just look at my knee."

"You're just disfigured and crazy," he responded, but in his heart of hearts he knew that I had something that was miraculous in what it could do.

Tommy had a big van and he would lie in the back with his pants pulled down so I could treat his low back. I knew that he was hurting, and since he had given so much of his time teaching me the sport of kings I really wanted to help him get out of pain. I knew that I could do it but his van had very little circulation and Tommy found enormous joy in farting out loud while I worked on him, then he would laugh like a banshee.

It wasn't long before I reached my limit. I told him, "Make a choice: You can stay in pain or you can stop farting while I am treating you!"

Tommy would love to tell that story over and over again as my success in the medical world came to the attention of the news media, governors, and ex- governors.

It wasn't long before I was driving with Jim to the polo matches on the north shore at Mokuleia in his one-of-a-kind, black convertible Ferrari Testarosa and scoring my first goals for team Reynolds. Once

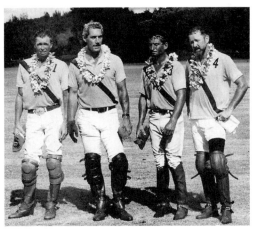

After a hard fought Polo Match our Los Lobos Polo Team from L to R: John Thorp, Bill George, Greg Davis and Bob Miller

again I was divinely blessed to be amongst the elite as I made my way up through the ranks in the polo world and the hook was firmly set. Jim Reynolds left the polo world, but I would continue paying my fees by doing aerial stunts in my hang glider, dropping money and prizes from above and then making a spectacular but very dangerous landing onto the polo field. The Honolulu Polo Club would use my daredevil aerial stunts to attract viewers to the field. Once landed, I would have my horse brought over to me, put my boots on, and play polo. Always a showman, what an entrance!

Dar's Constant Presence

Even in death, Dar continued to inspire me forward in the stunt world. The next film would be *Trench Coat in Paradise* staring Dirk Benedict (my old football-watching buddy from the night of Glen Larson's betrayal), Bruce Dern, Catherine Oxenberg, and Michele Phillips. Larry Rapaport, the production manager, contacted me and we talked about me taking the co-stunt coordinator position along with George Fischer, since he was still in town. I had never met George before Dar's death and now I found myself working with him on my last two shows.

If George would co-coordinate with me, the network felt confident in giving me a shot, as this would be my first stunt coordinator spot on a full CBS movie of the week. Larry gave me the good news that I would be the co-coordinator along with George. Little did I know that I was being hired to be fired.

I was to learn later that I was only selected to create a spot for the director's boyfriend, who was unavailable for the first few days of the shoot. Her plan was to bring in a local stuntman and make it look like they were helping me break into the second unit directing and stunt coordinating position. However, if my work didn't look perfect she would find an excuse to bring her boyfriend in for a little paid vacation in Hawaii. He was standing by to take my job as soon as they found the smallest cause to get rid of me. It was a plain and simple set-up.

The first night on the set I was setting up for a fight scene with Dirk Benedict. I would be doubling for the bad guy in a fight with Dirk, and then I was going to be attacked by a large parrot. I had a perfect stunt double for Dirk, but the director insisted that he do the fight scene himself. Dirk was really nervous about getting hurt and clearly did not want to do the scene. The director wanted the set dark, with the only light coming from a small table lamp. I knew that with the lights so low no one would be able to see the fight scene, and I debated with the director over the lighting. I also directly questioned her decision to use Dirk in the scene despite his obvious fear. I went through the choreography of the fight scene with Dirk and showed him exactly how I planned to keep him injury-free, but he was still baffled by the necessity of his presence in the take. "Why does she need me in this shot if the lights are going to be so low?" Dirk asked me, but I was just as confused as he was.

I told Larry about the discrepancies over the shot and he agreed that he did not understand her lighting technique for an action-based fight scene, but he too had to go along with what she wanted; after all, she was the director. I knew the shot was going to look bad, but having no choice I went ahead with her ideas and got Dirk through the fight scene without a scratch.

Triumph And Disaster, My Constant Companions

Sure enough, the following day I got the call from Larry that the dailies looked horrible and they were bringing in another stuntman from the mainland to finish coordinating. Once again, I was shattered. It went from the happiest day of my life to one of the lowest moments of my life, all in 48 hours. Nothing seemed to have changed in this backstabbing industry.

Two days later I had dinner with Larry and he explained how I was set up. A few days later, the director's boyfriend showed up to take over my place. I got a call from him when he arrived and to my amazement, he happened to have done a lot of work with Dar in the past and remembered meeting me at Dar's house. He offered me a utility stunt position and then apologized profusely for taking my job. He confirmed what Larry told me, I was hired to be fired!

The good news was that Larry Rapaport stood up for me and I did receive an official credit as the stunt coordinator for the film. Using that credit and Larry as my reference, I went on to get a stunt coordinating position on a television series entitled *Byrds in Paradise*, another CBS television series based in Hawaii. It starred Timothy Busfield as a single parent running a high school in Hawaii. Unfortunately, the series only ran for one season and it was not picked up for the following year.

The entertainment business can give you some of the biggest highs in life and it can also provide you with some of the biggest lows. My personal recommendation is to stay away from it unless you have nerves of steel and can deal with rejection and the rampant egos racing about recklessly, crushing lives without a second thought.

If Neither Foes Nor Loving Friends Can Hurt You

A month after getting seriously burned for the second time in the industry, I got a call from none other than good old Glen Larson, who was back in town producing a show starring and co-produced by Cheryl Ladd. The executive producer credit belonged to J.C., Glen's previous assistant who had successfully made the transition from secretary to new wife. Glen came through as he said he would all those years earlier, offering me the stunt coordinating position for this new Hawaii series, *One West Waikiki*.

Of course with Glen it was never predictable work and before one big stunt Glenn called me at the last minute and said, "John, I am really sorry, but we have already booked the helicopter for another scene. You will have to do the best you can by shooting from the road."

Luckily, I had an ace up my sleeve and planned to introduce my flying cameras, which would utilize ultra light aircrafts. We were able to mount cameras on the ultra lights as well as being able to carry the cameraman. At first glance, the cameraman thought it looked a little too dangerous, but after a few minutes in the air he relaxed and was soon having the time of his life. The filming went perfectly, and when Glen saw the dailies, he asked in amazement, "How did you ever get that shot?" Not only did we get the shot, we also brought down the production costs by thousands of dollars.

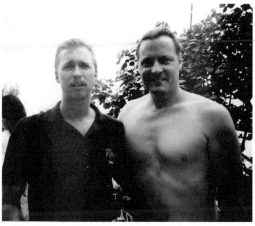

Doug Barr, co-star of the TV series "The Fall Guy" and me on the set of One West Waikiki

One scene called for a hang glider to be seen through the driver's window as a glider swooped down on the car. Flying along the roadside could only be done on a perfect wind day. The weather cooperated and we got the shot, although I did have to use Glen's son, Chris, as a traffic controller. Glenn had failed to notify the Honolulu police department that we would need a few officers to regulate the traffic. Once again there was a ploy to save some dollars in manpower and the legal permits to tie up traffic at the Makapuu lookout, where we would be filming. Over the years I had learned to roll with the punches and be very creative. Chris might have to dodge a few cars, but the bottom line was that everyone was happy when you got the shot.

In another episode, they had hired a group of male strippers called Manpower. J.C. and Cheryl Ladd had found them in Australia and decided to fly in these pretty boys to play the good guys in a murder mystery. They had some training in martial arts, as that was part of their strip review, but stunt fighting and actual fighting are very different. These macho men strippers had never seen how a fight scene for the screen was actually choreographed.

I explained to these rookies that you never hit anyone and that it was all about the angle of the camera. Stuntmen train for years to do a bar

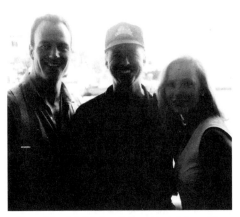

Cheryl Ladd, Richard Burgi and I on the set of "One West Waikiki"

room fight scene, one of the most difficult scenes to shoot. I was given just a few hours to train these male strippers to pull off a professional looking fight scene that normally would have required all well-trained stuntmen. It was evident after a few hours these guys from down under were not going to be able to do this without a few punches actually being landed.

I told my stunt team to pad themselves up real good, and we let these guys actually make contact with us. Otherwise we would never get the shot. The first roundhouse kick delivered by the male stripper caught yours truly in the mouth and my front tooth was folded back like an electronic bowling pin. I looked at the cameraman and asked, "I hope you got that shot." With a grimace he agreed and offered me a handkerchief to wipe the blood from my mouth.

It still came down to the same idea: sacrifice your body to glorify your soul. Everyone loves you if you get the shot, but I had to learn to define myself on a different scale than the approval of the industry. I learned to hold the integrity of my life up against lives of men like my father, Nick Nicholas, Dar Robinson, Buzzy Trent, and Jim Reynolds.

My passions began to change as I watched people's lives change when they came to me in chronic pain. I would always say, "Take a look at the sign outside my trailer. It says Stuntman, not Doctor. I will be glad to help you if you are willing to do your part, which is to eat a healthy diet and have a good solid exercise program." It was not long before the word was "Go see John," whether in the stunt trailer, horse stall, or even in the back of Tommy Campo's stinking van. No matter where the location, the results were the same. Their pain went away and stayed away.

Gods Plan, "But Now You Work For Me!"

In 1990 I enrolled at the Institute of Oriental Medicine under the direction of Dr. Lucy Lee, O.M.D. and Dr. Cyrus Loo, O.M.D. I felt that if I could learn to place needles in the precise acupuncture points along channels and meridians I would amplify my results using the Acuscope and Myopulse by incorporating the points without using needles. I would replace the needles with two non-invasive probes that do not penetrate the skin but send a message to the computers. The computers in these two machines decipher the information they receive and then send a corrective signal back to the area of injury at one hundred times per second. Cybernetic space age technology combines with Chinese medicine. This combination of the oldest form of medicine and this new form using artificial intelligence designed for the human electrical pathways was the basis for my future protocols.

It wasn't long before I got a call from the vice president of Castle Medical Center asking if I would be interested in a position at the hospital. It turned out that one of his top nurses had come to me, her position unbeknownst to me, and had a dramatic recovery from the debilitating headaches she had been suffering with for years.

Dr. John Monge was a truly great human being. He told me that he was a very competitive marathon runner in the 50 and above bracket but he was unable to run due to a hamstring injury. He asked me if I could help him. I assured him I could. What he asked me next surprised the hell out if me. If you can fix me, would you take a position at the hospital?

At first I was leery and hesitant about coming down to a hospital. As far as I was concerned, hospitals served you junk food and were hosts for disease. I nicknamed them roach motels and sarcastically would add, "You check in but you don't check out!"

Dr. Monge told me he would pay me approximately $500 a day and if things went the way he anticipated with all the dramatic results he had heard about he would allow me to expand the program to their three centers: one at the main hospital, one at their world renowned Work Well Rehabilitation Center, and another at their outpatient center in the Kailua professional center. I countered with, "But I am not a doctor, I am not licensed in anything." He assured me it was not a concern, as I would be covered under the hospital's license.

"And by the way," he added, "you were concerned with what we fuel our patients with. As part of the Seventh Day Adventist Church, Castle Hospital is a Loma Linda Division Hospital, a nonprofit, and we serve our patients a vegetarian diet. They do not eat junk food here." Things were sounding good. They were fueling their patients correctly. I would be working with the top physical therapists, so the patients would be given the proper exercise program and I could electrify and detoxify them. My acronym of F-E-E-D (Fuel, Exercise, Electrify, and Detoxify) was going to be placed in mainstream medicine. Now all I had to do was perform.

With still a few doubts in my mind I once again explained that I was a stuntman and that was my life. I was not going to give that up for a nine-to-five job. He assured me that if I would share my technology with them he would be glad to work with my schedule and I could do both.

Dr. Monge was determined to run again. He said, "Come and treat me for a week. It will be worth your while, and if you are successful with me we will talk about a future with the hospital. Wouldn't you like to prove to the world what you believe in? Don't you want to prove that in healing yourself was the truth and you didn't just use mind over matter but real medicine with real results?" He pushed the right buttons and the following Monday I showed up at Castle Hospital's Work Well Rehabilitation Center. And as they say, the rest is history.

I began seeing their chronic pain patients and Dr. Monge. Sure enough, he was able to run again. He is still dancing today.

A month later there was a full-page spread on the front page of the Loma Linda Castle Medical Center newspaper that read, "Stuntman brings technology that saved his life and his career." I already had a full schedule and now a waiting list weeks deep. Dr. Monge asked if I had someone else trained, so I brought in Susan to help me out and paid her more money than she had ever made in her life. Now I was able to compare the results with the clinical protocols I had developed. With almost a hundred patients a week I was able to find things that no one else had ever been able to prove before. I found astonishing ways to find the root and cause of their problems. Pain was just a symptom. Often the painful area was really not the problem but was just a referred pain. I enjoyed playing Sherlock Holmes: What was the cause? What had triggered this event? How could I bring the patient back into homeostasis and allow that person's body to heal itself just like mine had, and now hundreds of others?

Naturally, all the hospital's doctors were skeptical. "Which of my patients do you want to see?" some of the orthopedic surgeons would ask.

"Your malpractice cases, naturally!" I volleyed back. "Don't send me your easy ones. Send the ones that are suing you and the hospital." That shut them up, and it was a great way to start.

Once Again Looking For The Flaw

One of the first patients was brought into my little treatment room. The doctor explained to me that he felt she had a spondylosyndesis and her sternocleidomastoid was totally in spasm. I had no idea what a spondylosyndesis was nor where the sternocleidomastoid was located. When the doctor left the room I asked the patient where she hurt. She pointed to her neck and I began there. I also treated down her spine and under her scapula. I asked her to move her head and she almost started crying while she guardedly started to turn her neck, then move it up and down. She looked at me with tears in her eyes and asked, "What did you do?"

"I just removed some blockage and resistance in the area and brought the tissue to rest and the muscle out of spasm. I will still need to see you for the next three days." She thanked me profusely and left. That night I went and bought a *Taber's Cyclopedic Medical Dictionary* and looked up the big words the doctor used to describe her condition.

Spondylosyndesis, I learned, is a binding together possibly caused by a surgical formation of an ankylosis between the vertebrae.

Spondylosis is a degenerative arthritis of the cervical or lumbar vertebrae which puts pressure on the nerves.

The sternocleidomastoid is one of two muscles arising from the sternum and inner part of the clavicle.

I had my first three large confusing medical terms down.

The following day when the patient returned, she was thrilled. She had slept better than she had in years. Her neck was still 90% pain-free and she was demonstrating full range of motion. I had her put her neck into a position where she could still feel the slight residual pain, treated there, and had her move her neck. She was pain-free once again. The doctor stopped by to see how she was doing, and she immediately blurted out, "This is a miracle. Why did you not give me this treatment sooner?" He had a shocked look on his face and began to stammer.

"As you can see, doctor, her sternocleidomastoid is no longer in spasm and your diagnosis of her condition as spondylosyndesis or a spondylosis may be incorrect. As you can see, in two treatments she is totally pain-free and has full range of motion without discomfort." He had the strangest look on his face when he asked, "So what is your medical background; I thought you were a stuntman?"

"My background, Doctor, is first I do no harm, and second I have healed myself. The treatments I do you do not consider medicine; I call it common sense medicine. As I said before, feel free to send me any patients that you are unsuccessful with using standard Western medicine and I will show you what common sense medicine can do."

Later that day he stopped me in the hall and asked what I could do for his tennis elbow. "Stop by tomorrow and let me show you what I can do." I treated his epicondyle problem (love the big words these days) and in one session his pain was reduced by 90%. Three days later I watched him walking up and down the hall bending his arm in all kinds of contortions and in no pain no matter what he did.

Between working on television shows and my time at the hospital my life was abundant. My stunt business and Dar had always told me to search for the flaw; the flaw, no matter how small, could kill you. But no matter how hard I tried to prove this technology wrong it just never seemed to fail.

To say my life was good at this time was an understatement. I had a wonderful and beautiful woman in my life that I had met at a polo match, Cyndi Chambers. We later became engaged. I had trained many staff members at Castle Medical Center to become technicians. Castle had purchased three more medical centers on Maui, and I staffed each with technicians. I had overseen over 10,000 treatments, including personally, and my technicians were under the umbrella of a major medical center. The results were unheard of. Our success rate was suspicious, to say the least. But no matter how hard they tried to disprove what we knew to be the truth they couldn't do it. How could my team be the only ones getting these incredible results all of the time? Was it just because I silently prayed over everyone? Everyone that I trained was a Christian. Maybe that was it!

CHAPTER SEVENTEEN

Or Walk With Kings—Nor Lose The Common Touch

On an eerily lit day in Burbank, California, my father took my young hand and led me out into the front yard of my childhood home. Our neighbors already lined the street, excitedly chattering, and my father knelt and talked of the coming performance of the sun and moon. He explained for the first time to me how the sun, earth, and moon cast shadows and created what we saw as the different shapes of the moon each night. After handing me a piece of exposed film, he told me we were about to do something that I had always been forbidden to do: stare at the sun. The earth, moon, and sun were coming into alignment, and we gathered with our neighbors to witness the earth falling into the shadow of the moon, my first solar eclipse.

He continued to explain that the exposed film would protect my eyes from any damage by the very powerful sun but warned me still not to look directly at the eclipse. I felt the magic of this mystical event that demanded our attention but could also bring us harm if we were not careful. I stood in awe, sharing an event that captivated young and old, as the universe revealed its immensity, its perfect design and balance.

7/11/91: The Total Eclipse Of The Sun

I had not thought of this day until receiving a call at the beginning of the summer of 1991 from my good friend John Allen, whose stoically calm, prosecuting attorney demeanor was oddly replaced by an almost childlike excitement. The source of his joyous wonderment was a total eclipse of the sun that was coming on July 11 and that could only be captured in its totality from limited locations in Hawaii, Mexico, and Central America.

John was desperate to witness the event from the decidedly prime viewing location, the big island of Hawaii, but could not find a single available hotel room or a flight. His call to me was a last ditch effort to at least secure himself a place to stay on Oahu, where the eclipse could be viewed in an impressive 98% of its totality.

He was welcome at my home in Oahu, but John, not content to settle with 98%, laid out his plan, his attempt to persuade me to go with him to the big island. Money was no object. He would hire a helicopter, private plane, or boat to take us to the perfect spot. Another total eclipse would not occur in Hawaii for another 150 years, and he stressed that it was now or never for the two of us.

The eclipse was spreading a contagious excitement, and I must admit I was beginning to feel its enticing power tugging at my soul. The excitement continued to grow inside until erupting into an overwhelming desire to be a part of this stellar event.

Already apprehensive about neurotically racing around the islands in search of the perfect spot, I also couldn't stop thinking about the possible weather problems. Can you imagine how disappointing it would be for those who had traveled all the way to Hawaii to find the entire spectacle occluded behind rain and clouds?

John continued his attempt to convince me to go with him. He would cover all the expenses, a tempting offer that would have to be refused. He was welcome stay with me if all else failed, but I was going to be experiencing this mystical event from my hang glider.

High On The Moon

This was the final stage of my recovery, the universe coming to find me. It had been over five years since I had gotten involved with the Electro-Acuscope and Myopulse, and the power of my own recovery had created a momentum that propelled me to aid in the recoveries of thousands of patients. I was caught up in an increasingly challenging and demanding practice at Oahu's Castle Medical Center, but the eclipse caught my attention and gave me a moment of repose to evaluate this new path. Why had this come to me? Had I been preparing for this since my childhood?

The eclipse would be my chance to unify all experiences with faith, my personal testament to the communal power that inspired me to live, heal, and now soar.

Swept up by the momentum and power of the coming phenomenon, I explained honestly to John why I could not accept his generous offer and that I would be in the air viewing the celestial event while flying my hang glider. The ominous shadow was once again coming to my front yard, only this time my front yard was the wind currents over the cliffs of Oahu. It felt only natural that I venture out into the hands of the divine natural order to face the coming darkness and pass into the new light, a defining opportunity never to come again in my lifetime.

I repeated to John that I would do everything in my power to get him to the Big Island, but after that we would each have to find our own unique experiences of the eclipse.

"I always knew you were a little bit crazy," John replied. "I knew it ever since that night you flew your glider off into the full moon."

I had forgotten about that night, but now it all made perfect sense.—my attraction to the mysticism of the moon and the desire to reach out for it, fly into its magnetic pull.

I was still working at Nick's then and John and a group of my friends surprised me with a visit to the restaurant. They were in a festive mood, many commenting on the eerie feeling in the air that night. I had decided earlier in the day that I was going to make a flight off Makapuu at exactly midnight to celebrate the full moon, and I briefed them on my plans. They didn't think I was serious at first, but at 10:30 they found out just how serious I was when I walked up to their table and asked, "Are you boys ready to really get high? Let's go flying."

A cautionary and admonishing questioning peppered our ride up to the cliff: "Are you nuts? How many people have been killed up there already?" I was getting a little nervous but was undeterred. From what I had already experienced, I knew I was about to share something with them that could get them higher than anything they could ingest into their systems. Even though they would not personally be flying, the energy of a midnight takeoff into a full moon night was enough to give everyone present a buzz never experienced before, something they would not soon forget.

Accompanying John was a very special and respected group of friends, including Barry Hilton, Charlie Galento, Duff King, and their girlfriends. Duff had agreed to launch me, and I felt my energy level rising to a pre-adrenal rush as we approached the top. I could feel the full moon drawing me into its power, asking me to join with it, embrace it, and become one with it. Nothing was going to stop me from doing just that.

Gliding in and out of clouds as we waited on the top, at times the moon left us all in total darkness. I did my best not to show my healthy apprehension, and it was the desire to share this experience with my friends that pushed me forward.

The takeoff was straight vertical as I climbed upward to touch the silver clouds that awaited me, filling my body with adrenaline and inspiring a primal scream, "AHH YOOU!"   I enjoyed a smooth and flawless flight, dancing in the bright sky before my good friends, until the unexpected crept in as I came down for a landing. On my final approach to the landing zone, a huge cloud covered the moon, leaving me and everyone else in total darkness at the very worst time.

In the darkness, we are left with only ourselves, left without direction from anywhere but within. I yearned for the direction of light, and suddenly it was there. Duff, below in his car, shined his bright lights on what I thought was the landing area, but little did I know that he had parked his car well to the right of where I was clear to come down. He was actually parked in the middle of the road, which I didn't realize until I was only feet away from the pavement. I didn't see the erect stop sign until it was too late.

I tried to bank right, but was too low and clipped the stop sign with the tip of my left wing, which spun me around into a 360-degree turn. Somehow, I proceeded to land on my feet and walked away with only a slightly bruised ego. Duff didn't realize that I couldn't tell from the air where he was located, and neither of us expected the immense dark cloud to cover the moon just as I began my final approach.

To this day, well over 30 years later, whenever I see anyone from that group they inevitably mention that special night. It was truly a powerful night for all involved, and I knew that the eclipse could provide the same type of experience, only intensely magnified by the unparalleled rarity of the stellar experience. It was now or never for this vehicle I was using to travel through life, my body, to join with one of life's truly mystical events, the total eclipse of the sun.

Totality

"Nothing there is beyond hope, nothing that can be sworn impossible, nothing wonderful, since Zeus, father of the Olympians, made night from mid-day, hiding the light of the shining Sun, and sore fear came upon men." Archilochus (c.710 - 676 BC)

John Allen arrived as planned and was successful in obtaining a flight to Maui. I was committed through and through to have my own experience.

The week prior to the eclipse was, as predicted, stormy and cloudy with the wind and rain howling day after day. Spending the majority of my time studying the weather patterns, I was deeply focused, consumed with my preparations. Cyndi reminded me that I had hardly said anything to her all week.

It was one thing to fall in love with a stuntman, but it was another to try to live with one. She clearly had a hard time understanding why I would do these things that could get me killed, why I would jeopardize everything for this one stunt. It was hard for her to believe that I truly loved her when I put my life on the line time and time again.

"John, why do you have to do this?" she would ask. "We have everything going perfectly. If you love me you won't do this." It was true; things had never been better. I was financially secure for the first time in a long while, my body was beyond recovered, and my medical technology was thriving and continuing to astound the doctors at Castle Medical Center. I had only one answer to her question of why this flight was necessary. I tried to reassure Cyndi that if everything was not perfect, I would back off and not do it. "I've never seen you back off yet!" she quietly said. I took her into my arms and said, "I'm still here aren't I sweetie? Don't worry, I won't let you down."

The edge keeps me clean and honest, living every day to the fullest, and this is the only way I can live. Cyndi was slowly realizing that she would never be able to change me. The one thing that was changing was our relationship, which would be put to the test in the next couple days.

The day before the eclipse was perfect. The sun was shining and the wind was out of the northeast. It seemed the universe was going to cooperate with us after all. However, it was indeed too good to be true. The clouds rolled back in that evening on the back of more snarling winds, and any hope of a restful night of sleep was gone. I was up checking the skies every hour. Any glimpse of the stars and my heart jumped, only to be dampened by another large cumulous collection.

At four o'clock, before the first rays of dawn, the phone rang. It was Duff asking how it looked. The conditions were switching so rapidly the final decision would come down to the moment of takeoff.

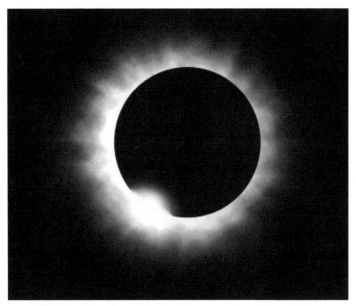

John Thorp is the only person to ever fly a hang glider into and during the total eclipse of the sun.

CHAPTER EIGHTEEN

If Neither Foes Nor Loving Friends Can Hurt You

I got off the phone with Duff and immediately called my film crew, which consisted of Bill and Gay George, to let them know it was a go. They were up for the task. Bill had even rented the long lens we needed, and if the weather would cooperate, we were set to capture the moment on film. Duff showed up 30 minutes later with his hang glider on the roof of his car, and I had already loaded everything on my car the night before, so as soon as Bill and Gay showed up the adventure was on.

Since there was really nothing left for her to say, Cyndi was very quiet all morning, but we held each other's hand and felt the love we shared as we passed through the gate and began a very nervous ride to the top of Makapuu. We were amazed to find more than 50 spectators gathered at the summit, all awaiting the spectacle.

A Lonely Arrival At The Edge

The grey clouds and cold wind strikingly ominous that dark morning, the conditions looked poor. I tried to remain optimistic, but first light confirmed our worries. As the weather only worsened, it looked like a flight was going to be impossible. Having seen the weather switch on the drop of a hat from this launch spot, I suggested to Duff that we go ahead and set up anyway. Just a slight window was all we would need to get airborne. Under a tense silence, we walked down to our cars, removed our gliders, and carried them to the top.

My dream challenge was indeed taking on mythical proportions. Duff continued to walk up to the launch platform to check our wind conditions in hope of an improvement, each time without luck. If anything, things were looking worse. Remaining faithful, I continued to set up my glider but could feel Duff growing more impatient by the minute. He was leery of the conditions but also did not want to miss seeing the eclipse, and we could see that Diamond Head looked clear, standing out as the only potential viewing option. He took one last look at the conditions and yelled down at me, "It looks like shit; there is no way I'm flying in this."

He knew better than to try to talk me out of it. He had never been successful in the past and knew he would not be successful today. What I didn't expect was that he would refuse to launch me. "I'm not going to be a part of your death," he said. "But if you are really set on flying, see those two guys over there? They are both hang glider pilots. Maybe they will launch you."

The only way he could see the eclipse was if he left immediately, which left launching me out of the question. Without a word of protest, I watched him throw his glider on top of his car and then speed down the mountain toward Diamond Head. My ace in the hole gone, I was on my own, which somehow seemed fitting for this personal test. I couldn't condemn Duff's decision not to fly; he had his reasons and I had mine.

I recognized one of the pilots but had never seen the other before. I was not overly excited about putting my life into the hands of someone I barely knew, especially in these conditions, but I was going to do everything humanly possible to fly. I introduced myself to the unknown pilot and asked him if he would launch me. He readily agreed.

The familiar pilot was Andy Andrews, a good pilot I had seen fly several times before, and for a while it looked like he might attempt the flight himself. He too eventually decided that the wind and clouds were not something worth dealing with. The other pilot was already in position on the launch platform and was giving me a blow-by-blow report of the shifting conditions.

Like just another takeoff, we went through a last minute check of my glider and found everything looking airworthy. Andy, holding the nose of my glider while I checked my harness, asked what kind of parachute I had. I didn't have a parachute. I explained that I had never flown with one because throwing a chute at Makapuu would blow you back into the cliff and bounce you all the way down the face. Andy offered to sell me one, but I scoffed it off and even joked about my clever ruse of stuffing towels in my chute pocket to appease the club rule that called for chutes on all flights.

Once again seeking the guidance of intuition, I got down on my knees. I asked all my guardian angels to watch over me and had a distinct feeling that my old friend and mentor, Dar Robinson, now joined the ranks along with my faithful mother and more recently my father as well. I whispered, "Hey Dar, give me a hand on this one."

Andy helped me carry the glider over to the platform, where he handed the nose to the other pilot, who was tied in and set to launch me. Overcome with a strong inclination that he was more nervous than I was, I asked Andy if he would launch me instead. It was a little uncomfortable dispelling the other pilot, but I had long learned to trust instincts over comfort. He understood and gladly passed the chore over to Andy, who was surprisingly calm.

Once again, I was standing out over the edge, watching my past, present, and future float, twist, and merge in the sharp, unruly winds. The weather was not cooperating, the wind blowing parallel to the ridge and the clouds completely engulfing us time and time again. Looking down the ridge, I saw that the clouds stretched all the way to the ground. Not a good sign, in fact, the worst.

A Leap Of Divine Faith

We waited and waited on the edge as I continued to ask Andy what the wind felt like. "Like shit," he would return, unable to keep from laughing out loud at the absurd conditions. The wind would quickly gust up to 30 mph and then just as suddenly completely stop. Although everything on the surface was saying not to fly, something inside assured me that I could do it, motivated me to stand out on that stormy cliff calling for wind reports with the time of the eclipse rapidly approaching.

Then, in a matter of seconds, the small window I was looking for opened before us. Andy said he could feel a little wind at his back, and I knew the moment was here. It was now or never. With my nod of affirmation, he

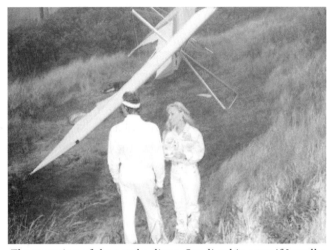

The morning of the total eclipse, Cyndi asking me if I really thought it was all worth it

lifted the nose of the glider into the wind, taking me past the point of no return. I committed and went for it, feeling my body turn to spirit at the precise moment my feet lifted off the ground, and I stepped out into endless space.

Instantly dropping 30 feet, plunging toward the jagged rocks jutting out below the launch platform, I struggled desperately through severe turbulence to get my feet into the harness, which had been yanked harshly into my crotch during the difficult takeoff. Horrified gasps escaped from the crowd as I barely missed crashing into the cliff before finally situating myself correctly into the harness. Now in a determined fight to gain altitude, I remained within mere feet of the ridge. Inch by inch, I slowly continued to rise, overcome with relief once I felt myself climbing, right into the

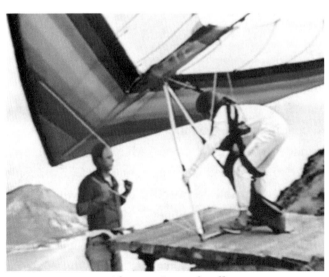

A long wait at takeoff

engulfing cloud cover. Visibility less than an arm's length away, there was only the feeling of rising to trust until my glider suddenly broke free from the consuming and blinding gray into a brilliant blue sky. I was just in time.

There, in all its mystical glory, was the eclipse just starting on its fleeting path toward totality. I radioed to Bill to see if they were seeing the majesty that I was now facing, but he reported nothing but clouds. Initially disappointed that I had not mounted a camera on my glider to capture this view, the serene energy of the celestial event quickly halted any anxiety.

I felt drawn to the presence of the rolling lunar shadow dimming our life-giving star. I looked back toward the cliff and found it still buried in clouds and radioed to Bill to pray for a break. I prayed to myself that those I loved below could share in this powerful moment.

A Light At The End Of The Tunnel

"There is a God," Cyndi could not help but scream, accompanying the roar of the spectators below and signaling to me that our prayers had indeed been answered. An unknowable hand pulled a drawstring to part the curtain of clouds, and the stunning celestial performance left all in awe as they too wondered at the first glimpses of the eclipse, now nearing 90% of totality.

However, just as quickly as the spectacle had been revealed, all was suddenly hidden; once again, my glider disappeared into the clouds. Patient and accepting, I waited, somehow positive that the cover wouldn't last, and less than a minute later I emerged to fly

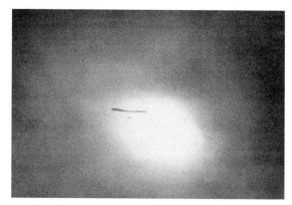

Heading for the light at the end of the tunnel

unobstructed directly into the eclipse. The extinguished sun hung before me, choked off by the black disk of the moon at totality. Facing the darkness, I felt open to embrace the new light already seeping out around the edges, the radiant glow of the solar corona seemingly displaying the beginning of all light.

"I just knew there was a God! I just knew it," Cyndi was captured expounding on the film recording at the moment of totality. The spectacle came and went, fleeting and ephemeral, but the midday re-dawning of the sun connected us all, with everyone and everything in that moment.

Surely lifted up for this renewing experience, I would need the same divine hand to get me down. The turbulent and cloudy conditions battering and blinding me at every corner, I was doing everything possible just to stay in the air, locked in an intense fight for control.

Whatever window had been opened was now dramatically slammed shut, and I knew it was time to get home. Bill, thrilled that he had at least ten minutes of great footage, radioed that the filming was a success. They were heading down to the area I had designated for my landing, and I took the opportunity to radio to Cyndi that I loved her and that I would see her on the beach. Continuing to battle with the ever-changing wind conditions, it would be very difficult to stay aloft until they were in position to film my landing.

Unbeknownst to all of us, half the island had driven out to Makapuu and Sandy Beach in search of the best view of the eclipse, creating Oahu's traffic jam of all traffic jams. It was bumper to bumper from Hawaii Kai to Kailua. After two grueling hours in the air, the struggle to stay up was becoming more and more difficult by the minute. Just when you think the hard part is over, something even more unexpected happens.

A thick, low-level wall of clouds rolled in and completely engulfed me. Having gone in and out of the clouds all day, it didn't really concern me at

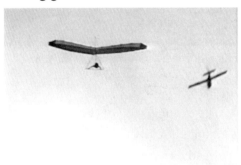

first, thinking I would simply break out at any minute. It didn't, and it got worse when it began to rain, my hands now so slippery I could barely hang on to the control bar. I was completely grayed out, flying blind.

Blinded by the dense cloud cover, I had no idea how close I actually came to a midair collision

Then, in the distance, I could hear something coming closer and closer. A helicopter, I first thought, but I was soon able to make out the distinct drone of a small airplane flying in Makapuu's restricted airspace. That was all I needed, to share this maze of cloud cover with a renegade plane flying in zero visibility. A genuine cocktail for disaster.

The worst danger, however, was still the cliff. At one point, I actually thought I could see green directly under me, but I told myself that I was imagining it, or at least I hoped I was. I knew that I was below ridge level when the thick clouds rolled in and believed that I was probably headed out to sea. For over 15 minutes, I could not see a thing, consistently greeted by only white blankness at every turn.

During my airplane pilot training we were taught to trust our instruments when we were caught in the clouds, since attempting to fly by the seat of your pants in clouds could bring on the often fatal condition of vertigo, leaving you unable to tell if you are up, down, or sideways. I did not have the privilege of instruments today and was left with no choice but to trust my own instincts. Reminding myself to remain calm, I flew the glider simply to the best of my ability, hoping and praying that at any second I would not slam into the cliff I could no longer see.

I radioed continually to Bill that I was grayed out and lost in the clouds but received only garbled replies and eventually only the lonely sound of empty static. I attempted to radio once more, desperate to know how far down the clouds went and encountered the most radical turbulence yet. My glider was tossed completely out of control. Fighting to regain command, I was left shaken and confused at what could be causing such violent turbulence.

Finally getting a slight break in the clouds, I could not believe my eyes. Houses and a marina, where the hell was I? Incredibly, my glider had been blown over the backside of the cliff and was caught in a downdraft, a hang glider pilot's worst nightmare come true. Once again, the glider pitched upward radically and then tumbled, this time placing me upside down in my sail, an impossible situation to rectify. To make matters worse, a web of high-tension wires stretched out before me everywhere. "I really am going to die," I muttered.

"I'm in trouble," I radioed frantically to Bill, still on my back in the inverted glider but talking all the while plummeting to the sure death awaiting me below. Calling and calling with no response, I had to accept the fact that I was alone in this nightmare, left with only my fight and my faith.

Then, when all seemed hopeless, the glider was miraculously propelled out of the inverted stall, somehow righting itself. Thankful to be flying again but still facing the imposing wires below, an image of tomorrow's newspaper headlines flashed before me: "Man Killed in Hang Glider." But I promptly chastened that fear and made up my mind not to be fodder for the evening news. Feeling Dar's presence conjured up his promise before he jumped from the sky-high CN Tower: "If the wire breaks, you will find sand in my eyes because I will be fighting with my eyes wide open all the way to the ground." Deciding to do the same, I committed myself to the greatest fight of my life.

With the wires boxing me in, I knew I couldn't get over the set immediately in front of me, so I headed for a ridge parallel to the wires in hope of finding some lift. The glider barely cleared the charged strands while I still battled the most violent turbulence I ever encountered in my life. Miraculously, the glider had not broken up after being so ruthlessly tossed about. Everything was unfolding in slow motion while I prayed that my reactions were in fast-forward. Not so proud of my pack full of towels now, I longed for the parachute that Andy had offered me before the launch.

No one had ever flown in this area and lived to talk about it. Jagged lava rocks lined most of the terrain below, offering a sure and gruesome death if I went down here. The thought crossed my mind to try a water landing at the marina, but at the speed I was flying, I'd probably be knocked out on impact and drowning wasn't a pleasant thought either. If I were meant to find an opening, I would find it.

Then I saw it. A slight clearing bordered by a patch of vegetation lay ahead at the end of the marina, and I figured the high bushes and trees just might provide enough of a cushion for a crash landing. If I could make it there, that is, as a large set of wires still blocked my approach. Another miracle gave me just enough lift to get over this last high-wire hurdle, and

I turned my glider for the final approach, heading straight for the clearing at literally breakneck speed.

I hit the bushes at approximately 50 mph. Like an intrepid adventurer of a Hollywood blockbuster, I burst through the jungle, cracking and crashing through the branches and bushes. The glider finally came to an abrupt stop embedded in a tree. I unhooked myself from the glider and dropped about five feet down, my body returned to the earth to complete the final miracle. I had survived.

The glider looked undamaged and I was equally unharmed. I crawled about two hundred yards through the bush until I found the slight clearing I had seen from above, where I found a road. I stood on the side of the road until a car came into sight and stopped before me. They offered their assistance and explained how they had feared I was going to crash into their backyard as they watched my volatile decent. They added that the sound of me hitting the jungle was horrendous, leaving them astounded that anyone could have lived through such an impact.

They volunteered to help me find the rest of my crew, and we set off, patiently battling the traffic until we could get into radio contact. It had been well over two hours since our last garbled radio communication. The last thing they heard was my broken message, "I'm in trouble." When they couldn't find me anywhere along the beach, they knew something had happened. Cyndi was beside herself with worry; the worst thoughts crossed their minds as the radio returned only haunting static. No response meant no John. Radio communication was impossible from the other side of the cliff, but once we got around the corner by Makapuu, I was finally able to reach them. Calling out that I was alive and well, I could hear the relief and joy in the shouting voices on the other end.

I lived to see the footage after all and lived to fly again, but Cyndi was clearly running out of patience with me. Realizing how close I had come to dying gave her more than an uneasy feeling. She told me she would always love me but that she had to let me go; I had scared her for the last time. It hurt deeply to hear those words, but I understood. She was not the first loved one to tell me this and she probably would not be the last. Loving someone unconditionally is a difficult task and I accepted the sacrifice in the pursuit of my path.

Thankfully not the way I had feared while upside down in my rapidly plunging glider, I was featured on the news that night. There on the screen was the beautiful image of my glider flying directly into the total eclipse, capturing and sharing my silent prayer and celebratory gesture of life.

A sobering news segment followed and detailed a tragedy that did occur during totality. A skydiver, in an attempt to film the eclipse, was killed when his parachute prematurely deployed and pulled him through the struts of the plane, sending him falling to his death. He had made over 3,000 jumps, a master skydiver.

It could just as easily have been me; my own story could have ended in tragedy. To this day, I cannot think of a rational explanation for how I got over the cliff.

Ordained as the White Light Warrior I pledged to be at my mother's funeral, a force much stronger than me decided it was not time for me to die, and I knew the gift I had received could only be repaid by continuing to give, to work, and to heal.

I have been asked if I will ever fly during an eclipse again. The answer is, "If it comes looking for me." Destiny is not achieved. Destiny finds us when we are open and willing, when we are faithful, when we are fearless.

The Business Of Medicine

It was now totally clear to me that God was not finished with me yet. I had a lot more living to do, and my mission was clear to me now. I would share with the world the gift of how the body heals itself electrically.

We slowly trained ourselves out of a position with Castle Hospital. They had purchased several sets of instruments. Their staff was now trained thoroughly and their results reflected it.

I began placing my trained technicians, soon to have a new title as Electro Toxicologists, in other medical offices. This is where I became acutely aware of the business of medicine.

Castle Medical Center was a non-profit hospital. It was run like a champion professional sports team. Everyone got paid, but the "business of medicine" was replaced with their motto, "this is a patient-focused health care facility," a term I would use in all of my future clinics.

Due to the notoriety and the publicity generated at Castle and the news article that went out to over 300,000 people, I was considered a big fish in a little pond in Honolulu. Hawaii may be a state, but in reality it is a small town and the word spreads fast. Many surgeries were eliminated by our treatments, so I thought that the insurance companies and medical professionals would recognize what I was doing as a very good thing.

I found it very interesting that private doctors who brought us onboard did so mainly for the bragging right that they had the same amazingly successful therapy as Castle. Soon I would be rudely awakened again and again to the continued reality of the business of medicine.

Oh to hear a doctor say, well we had that patient preapproved for surgery and now the patient is saying that they do not need it. One doctor casually said to me, "I am a surgeon and I like doing surgery. Besides, I get paid a lot of money for doing it." I volleyed back, "You may be a great surgeon but didn't you take an oath that said, 'First do no harm?'" That didn't go over well. Taking a scalpel and cutting into a person who may have avoided the knife is just plan wrong. On the other hand, it may not be the great surgeon but the anesthesia that kills them.

What was also becoming very clear to me was the attitude that the patient did not matter, only their insurance reimbursement did. The better the insurance, the easier to get an approval on a surgery that a patient may not need. As long as they were covered, who cared? "I can make you better than new," some doctors would say.

Another sickening reality: the sicker the patient, the more money they were worth. This profession that I was trying to do the right thing in was not agreeing with my plan. My plan was a financial disaster to the world of allopathic medicine.

In many of these so-called medical centers, the doctor, chiropractor, and even the physical therapists were in bed with the attorneys who were sending them their patients.

The attorney would instruct the patient to go to a particular clinic that he or she was in alignment with, knowing that the tort laws in Hawaii restricted an attorney from getting involved in a lawsuit unless there were over $20,000 in medical expenses. The industry insiders were not too happy with me when the patient got well and was discharged with a bill averaging $2,500 to $4,500, not $25,000 to $45,000.

I had proven that I could get their patients well for a fraction of the cost and they did not have to go through surgery and weeks and weeks of rehabilitation. Another doctor actually told me to stop showing off and getting people well so quickly. "This is a business my dear boy," he said, "I will just stop sending you my patients until we have them over tort and then you can show off and get them well. If you keep getting them well so quickly the attorney will stop sending me patients."

That was it! I was done! I would open my own clinic and make them all look bad.

Now all I had to do was raise the money to open a mini medical center. I told a few friends what I was planning, wrote a business plan, and then miracles began to happen.

Three people from different areas of the world told me that I needed to meet a gentleman by the name of Bernie Dohrmann. They said his expertise was putting together the money people with the idea people. He held a business seminar six times a year by the name of IBI (Income Builders International). Bernie would be coming to town and he would be holding private and group meetings with potential students.

I was very skeptical of such a deal. I was not a seminar type of person. I was a stuntman. No rules kind of guy. The final straw was when David Backstrom, my getaway driver from the Orange County hospital, called me from Maui and said that he had just sat in on a meeting with Bernie and he had mentioned to Bernie that I wanted to open a clinic. Bernie was planning on being on Oahu the following day, and if I would like to meet with him he would meet me for dinner. Once again serene destiny was upon me.

The following night I met Bernie Dohrmann. He looked the part, gold Rolex watch, flashy suit, and Italian shoes. He has got to be hot in that three-piece suit, I thought. I introduced myself and we shook hands over his meat loaf, mashed potatoes, and a large diet Coke. I gave him a quick run down on my history at Castle Medical Center and the clinic I planned to open. I showed him the article from Castle Medical Center and handed him my business plan.

He took one look at my business plan and said, "You have what it takes. My next seminar will be full of medical doctors that would love to get involved with what you have." He was running a special. Normally it would be $5,000 to attend but the special would be a two for one deal. If I signed tonight he would pair me up with another student, making my total for the class $2,500. The closer: "Do you have a credit card?" he asked.

He looked me dead in the eyes and said, "I guarantee you will raise the money you need to do your medical center." I handed him my gold American Express. He was slick, but he said everything that I needed to hear and added a few bonus points by saying that his seminar would be directed to the wellness and alternative medicine fields and it would be perfect for me, especially with the business plan that I had written.

He padded my ego further with, "John the world really needs to know what you are doing. Since you are signing up tonight and since I am late for a meeting, I will have a one-on-one session with you tomorrow. Meet me at the hotel at 11:00 am and I will personally prepare you for the seminar." He had set the hook and he wasn't going to let this fish off the line.

I showed up at the hotel a half hour early and found a line out the door to Bernie's meeting room. I was impressed that he was that sought after. I felt really good about the decision that I had made as I took my seat in the waiting room.

I had scheduled some VIP patients to be seen at my house at 1:00 pm. I sat there reading and re-reading my business plan as I patiently waited my turn. I watched 11:00 am come and go; 11:30 passed with not as much as a word from anyone. At 12:00 I was starting to get angry. At 12:30 I was done. He had my money. He promised me a full hour private meeting and not one person even came out to tell me he was running late. I had a sinking feeling in my stomach when I headed into the room ready for a fight.

"EXCUSE ME!" I said in a loud voice. I had an appointment at 11:00 and it is now 12:30. Is this the way you treat the people who have already paid you for your seminar? I have people in pain that are showing up at my house for treatment, and I am not going to let them down like you have me. I'll be back later to get my money after I see my clients, and you better have it ready for me." With that, I stormed out and headed for the elevator.

Bernie was in hot pursuit. He apologized profusely, saying that he was so sorry but he had not been told that I was waiting and his schedule was not in his control. "You sure were in control last night when you told me to be here at 11:00 am. I have people waiting for me and I respect their schedules." He repeated how sorry he was about the scheduling. He assured me there would be plenty of people there that would be willing to invest. With a sincere look in his eye he said, "John, please, you just have to be there."

He handed me the welcome packet he had for those who'd signed up. "Here," he said, "take this. I will make time for you, I promise." "Well, you have my credit card," I hissed. "Don't worry, I will be there. Because if you are full of it, I will be there to handle you the way we do in the stunt business, and it is not pretty."

As you can tell I still had some anger issues to deal with, but I had become very passionate about the medicine that I had now worked with for almost 8 years. Happily, everything Bernie promised came true. I made life-long friends at that seminar who also became patients, like Mark Victor Hansen, Jack Canfield, Wally Mento, Captain Steve Hogan, and Rand Brenner.

My First Clinic: The Balanced Body Center

Within 90 days my clinic was funded and the Balanced Body Center in Kahala came to life.

The training program that I developed at Castle Medical Center worked so well that I applied for a vocational program for a student that had been a past patient. The state approved to pay for his training if I would agree to give Scott Wakefield a job after he completed the course

Scott became my head technician, and his wife, Trisha, left her job as the office manager for an orthopedic surgeon at Castle and became my office manager. Brian Davis was my physical therapist, and Dennis McKenna's daughter from a previous marriage became a massage therapist and Acuscope technician.

We were featured on three local news channels, and that packed my little 650 square foot clinic. We generated a great cash flow. Also, with Trisha's knowledge in medical billing, she had the skills needed to bill insurance companies.

Our treatments using the Electro Acuscope and Myopulse were being reimbursed by workers' compensation at $135 per hour treatment. Our average workers' compensation patient was getting well in half the time it would have taken standard Western medicine. We prided ourselves in the fact that we were improving health care quality while lowering health care costs.

The Balanced Body Center was running comfortably in the black and was generating profit. The best thing was that the clinic ran without me. I did not need to be there on a day-to-day basis. Naturally, when the ex- governor

George Arihoshi needed his sore shoulder treated and requested me to treat him personally, I gladly did. George had held two terms as governor of the state of Hawaii, and after I got his shoulder back to normal his wife also became a patient.

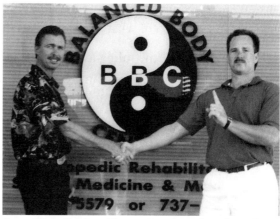

Scott Wakefield and I, opening day of my first clinic, the Balanced Body Center

I had personally made a point to the former

governor about how quickly we were getting patients back to work. Once again my ego was getting the best of me, making everyone else wrong. I explained to him that our average workers' compensation benefit, per patient, was between $2,500 and $4,500 for complete resolution of an injury. The average of most other patients seen by conventional therapies was between $15,000 and $40,000 for partial resolution of the injury. Remember, the law in Hawaii stated that an attorney could not sue for personal injury damages unless the medical charges were over $20,000.

Governor Ben Cayatano had recently taken office and noticed the same things that troubled me. There was no motivation to get people well quickly. Everyone was in on the take. I saw guys out in the water surfing, but limping into their doctor's appointment. They were healthy enough to surf but not enough to go back to work. Who was paying for all of this abuse of the worker's compensation? We were. That was why our workers' compensation insurance was so high. This was all about to change drastically.

No Good Deed Goes Unpunished

One of the first things Governor Cayatano did was lower all the workers' compensation benefits. Our reimbursement for the use of the Electro Acuscope and Myopulse went from over $135 per hour to $24 per hour, overnight. We suffered, even though we were the good guys who had personally brought attention to the cronyism between the doctor and the attorney and had proven that our common sense medicine was getting people well for 10% of what other medical offices were charging.

On July 2, 1995, the ruling took effect and several clinics closed within months due to lack of reimbursement. The Balanced Body Center had established a large cash clientele who understood that we had no relationship with their insurance company and we expected to be paid by the patient for services rendered. The patient was given a super bill with the billing codes to submit to their insurance company for reimbursement. We would survive this dramatic reduction in compensation. For one thing, the news media was always ready for a new story with another celebrity and another amazing recovery. When you have medicine like this you let the media do the talking for you.

A Confrontation With A Grand Master

I can't say enough about my good friend and new mentor Bernie Dohrmann, the business networking seminars that funded my first clinic, and the fact that he tirelessly gives everyone the opportunity to use new tools in the world of the free enterprise system. He has been gracious to feature me at several of his events because he, too, has been my patient. The following last two stories are directly linked to Bernie and IBI (now known as CEO SPACE).

I was being featured at a networking business seminar at IBI in 1994. At this seminar was a female Korean kung fu master dressed in full flowing gowns and a host of followers dressed in the same manner. She gave a spectacular demonstration, letting someone shoot arrows at her while she blocked them with the swift flick of her arms. Very impressive, I thought. She was called a Grand Master, although I have seen too many circus shows and dog and pony shows to be fooled by all this hoopla. Everyone has their thing, but when she began parading around a woman that was diagnosed with cancer and telling everyone that she had cured her of her cancer with her magical powers that is when I decided that if she got into my face the show would end here one way or another.

Sure enough, she walked up to me with all of her followers in tow and said to me, "I know you are a healer and have healed many, but I too am a great healer and have also healed thousands. You and I should talk."

"You have got me all wrong," I commented, "I am no healer, nor are you."

Her group got silent. No one called out the Grand Master. I continued, "How dare you drag around this poor woman and tell everyone that you have healed her. Even Jesus Christ said he never healed anyone. When confronted on this issue he would say, 'Do you wish to be well? The blind could see and the lame could walk but not by my powers but by the powers of God. I have not healed you; your faith has made you well.'" With a voice coming from deep inside (my friends would say "in that John Thorp tone of voice"), I reprimanded her. "You are not God," I told her, "and if this woman truly is healed from her cancer her faith has made her well, not you and all your hocus-pocus."

"How dare you speak to me like this!" she said as I watched her body begin to shake all over. I felt the power of my Lord and Savior Jesus right by my side as I said once again, "I am no healer but I am a facilitator in helping people heal themselves. I help awaken the Jesus Christ that dwells inside each and every one of us." At any minute I figured this little woman was going to kick me right in my private parts, but at this point I was so full of the power of the Holy Ghost that I was divinely guided and protected. We stood there staring into each other's eyes until she turned and walked away grumbling and mumbling incantations and shaking like a leaf.

It didn't take long for word to get back to Bernie Dohrmann, the organizer of the event, that his buddy the wild and crazy stuntman turned doctor had gone up against the Grand Master in a showdown of wills and survived. Most importantly my private parts were still intact.

Bernie immediately called me up to his room in the presidential suite to have a good laugh about what he had heard, but he wanted to get it from the horse's mouth. I sheepishly began explaining that something just came over me and I was channeling from above. The words just flew out of my mouth as I slayed her darkness. "Are you nuts?" Bernie countered, "That lady could have killed you," he said laughing out loud. "Only you could have done something like that."

Unfortunately the woman who was being paraded around died a few months later, proving my point about the great Grand Master.

CHAPTER NINETEEN

If All Men Count With You But None Too Much

It was at this time that an actor friend of mine who had recently starred with Lee Majors on a short-run series entitled *Raven* assured me that he had the needed funds to reproduce the Balanced Body Center in California. I would have to check with my investors to see if they were willing to take a chance to move the clinic to California. I had a gut feeling that this move was just not right. But I had witnessed what a big fish in a little pond could do and we had proven we could be successful. Once again, another challenge. How would a guppy do in the ocean of mainstream Western medicine in a state the size of California?

My actor friend had contacted an old friend of his who dealt in commercial real estate. He had found a medical office building that had recently been sold to a new group of investors. The Westwood Medical Plaza building was over 50% vacant and he was negotiating a deal for us to move in. Things were moving very fast. As far as I was concerned, too fast.

He continued to assure me that he had the needed funds to pull this whole thing off, but when it came down to signing the papers his credit was not the best and I would have to be the sole name on the lease. I had been flying back and forth from Hawaii trying to keep the Balanced Body Center going. I had recently got back together with Cyndi, so between my personal life and the dramatic change in front of me I was slowly slipping back to my old friend, the occasional shot of tequila.

My friend assured me that even though he had a problem with a bank that had caused his credit to be challenged he knew enough people to raise the $500,000 it would take to move my whole staff out to California and to fund a major medical center. I knew what it took to start the Balanced Body Center, and that was a small 650 square foot clinic. This clinic would be almost four times that size and the rent was $5,000 per month. I was nervous to say the least, as so far I had been financing all the preliminaries on my credit cards.

I flew back to Hawaii and called a meeting with my investors. I asked if they were ready to roll the dice and told them that other investors would be getting involved as well. The newspapers in Hawaii were full of the problems with the new healthcare reimbursements in Hawaii, and our group was well aware that the Balanced Body Center was no longer doing as well as it had in the previous year. Scott and Trisha felt we could do it. They believed that my friend, the rising star, could raise the money.

They were mesmerized with his star status and felt that if he didn't personally have the money he must know plenty of other movie stars who had money to invest. I knew the other side of the coin. I had seen so many actors who had their fifteen minutes of fame, and some of them had hours of fame, but they were still broke and living on their star status. I ran a restaurant, and when the check came the so-called movie stars never reached for it.

To Risk It All, Once Again

I finally agreed to make the move and contacted one of the best attorneys I knew who lived in California. His name was Steve Knapp. I had met him through Dennis McKenna. Steve represented Dennis is his heyday and had kept him legally out of trouble. Steve would be my corporate attorney and oversee everything. Steve was not only good but also great. He negotiated a deal with the Westwood Medical Center that would include tenant improvement of over $80,000.

I asked if I could bring in my own construction crew to do the improvements and if I brought the remodel in for under the $80,000 if I could put the balance toward my lease payments. The office manager agreed to that. Steve found some small print that said the building had the right to move me if I was given 90 days notice. Then, I would have to move my suite to somewhere else comparable in the building. He struck that part of the lease and wrote in that the management of the building could not move me into another suite until my 5 year lease expired.

Steven explained to the building management that since Thorp Institute was a start-up medical corporation and an alternative one at that it would make our medical center look unstable if we were moved from suite to suite at their discretion. The building manager went along with our request and formalized our lease with the stipulation that we could not be moved under any circumstances for a period of 5 years. Her job was to get tenants into the building, which we later found was up for sale again.

I hired Barrett Mahon, the son of Barry Mahon, who you will remember was Errol Flynn's personal manager. Barrett's construction crew came in and demolished the existing suite and built me a state of the art beautiful 2,500 square foot clinic with six treatment rooms and five plush medical offices for the doctors and myself. They did such a great job that the building used my office suite to advertise what future tenant offices could look like. With the money I saved by having Barrett do the remodel, I ended up with a balance of a year rent free.

My actor buddy was still trying to raise money, but after several months everything was still being put on my credit cards. He did borrow $40,000 from his sister and brother-in-law and contributed another $10,000 from his own savings. He was one big zero short, raising $50,000 not the promised $500,000. The stress of funding this major medical center and paying everyone's salaries and moving expenses on my credit cards was killing me. Stress is the cause of 80% of all death illnesses, and my stress level was over the top, contributing to an increase in alcohol intake as well.

I know that my actor friend in his heart of hearts really felt he could raise the money. I am very grateful to him for his friendship and his belief in my mission. He went out on a limb to borrow the money from his family, and I know he tried his best. It was just not enough.

Steve Knapp began drawing up a private placement memorandum in order to raise the money within the limits of the law. Not only was I responsible to pay everything with little or nothing coming in, I was also responsible for training everyone to be technicians in the office. The 18 hour-a-day marathons in getting this all together was driving me to drink more and more, and my relationship with Cyndi was also being strained.

The one good thing was that Barry Hilton was spending most of his time in Mexico at his house in Cabo San Lucas and he allowed me to rent a room at his house once again in Malibu for Cyndi and me.   Barry was seldom there so the whole house was ours to use, which included tennis courts, a riding arena, swimming pool, and Jacuzzi. We looked good but financially I was in debt and maxed out on most of my credit cards.

I did have several great meetings with the medical community, and Dr. Mark Darrow, MD, JD agreed to hang his shingle in the office. He introduced me to Dr. Anne Meyer, MD, the head of the pain division at Cedars Sinai, and it wasn't long before Cedar Sinai became so convinced of the viability of this treatment that they sent, via prescriptions to Thorp Institute, the following patients: post heart transplant, post liver transplant, carpal tunnel, reflex sympathetic dystrophy, fibromyalgia, tendonitis, ulnar nerve compression, nerve entrapment, TMJ, C7 radiculopathy, ulnarneuritis, thigh hemorrhage, tendon transfer (wrist pain), and a host of others. These were all problems on which Western medicine was having little or no effect.

I had also reconnected with Dr. Cynthia Watson, MD, an integrative medicine specialist in Santa Monica, and she was referring patients as well. Some of the movers and shakers of the movie industry showed up for treatments, and the media followed. We were featured on a tabloid news show called Strange Universe that was broadcast coast to coast. We were holding our own financially but since my name was on the front door many patients only wanted to be seen by me.

I was being pushed to my limit. I was not meant to be inside 18 hours a day. I was an outdoors guy who kept his sanity by surfing and flying my hang glider. I had little or no release other than alcohol from the nightmares I was dealing with. The devil was at my doorstep and I knew it!

I had hired a billing specialist to deal with the insurance companies. The outright lies they would tell us regarding reimbursements that never came sent me into screaming rages at them over the phone. I had no idea of the intricacies of insurance reimbursements even if we had gotten the required pre-approvals. Pre-approvals would mean nothing to them when it came to paying, as they refused on many cases. I got the real meaning of "the check is in the mail." It was total bull!

My lunches with other physicians began to include cocktails to help everyone deal with stress, and soon some other old habits began to come to the surface to recover from the cocktails. I was paying everyone else's mortgages and rent payments and was the last one to get paid. My staff was at each other's throats. My actor friend would come in and out as he pleased and his ability to get along with the staff and the patients was limited. My gut feelings from the beginning proved to be on the mark. I should have trusted myself. I looked very successful, I was the owner of a prestigious medical center, but underneath it all I was in a living hell. I understood the reality that there is no money in getting people well. There is only money in keeping them sick.

I received a letter in the mail that stated that we had 90 days to move to another suite. A fertility clinic loved our remodeled office so much that they had contacted the management group with an offer stating that if they could immediately move into our suite they would rent the entire seventh floor. Our year of free rent was coming to an end and the lease payments would soon begin to the tune of $5,000 per month. I called my attorney, Steve Knapp, and he said, "Don't sweat it John. They cannot make you move, and if they do you can probably negotiate more free rent."

We were offered a bigger suite for the same price on the eighth floor. I was successful in negotiating another year of free rent. The only problem with the suite on the upper floor was that it was right next to the elevator. The elevator made a lot of noise and my meditative treatments needed quiet. The building management assured me that they would fix the noisy elevator. We redesigned a new suite with the same construction team as before. This just prolonged my agony for another year. Fortunately the building was unsuccessful in correcting the noise, so after the year was up and my 5 year lease went into effect I was done with it all. That noisy elevator was my way out. I was close to a nervous breakdown. My fiancé and I were breaking up. I was beat up from the feet up.

I told my actor partner I was done. He argued, "But, we have made it! The clinic is holding its own." I told him "'We have not made shit!"

He was hardly ever there. Trisha, my office manager, couldn't work with him any longer. "What about my investment?" he yelled. That did it! He and his sister had contributed $50,000, a far cry from the $500,000 he said he would raise. I said, "You know what? You can have it all. I am out of here!" Then it was mutiny, when the word got out that I was leaving. All the staff quit. I paid off Scott and Trish what I had owed them and threw in a set of instruments to cover their moving expenses to Washington. My debt to my attorneys was over $60,000 and my credit cards were all maxed out to the tune of $100,000. I was a bankruptcy looking to happen. And it did.

I had watched the things I had given my life for broken and now it was time to stoop and build them up with worn out tools. I found a sweet little house in Santa Barbara with a little treatment room on the first floor. I started surfing every morning, riding my bicycle, swimming, and joined the Santa Barbara Athletic Club. I quit drinking and cleaned up my act. I had my life back. I opened a little office downtown and decided to train others in what I had found to be effective. I began taking everything I had stored in my overworked brain and putting it down on paper. *I put my oxygen mask on and took a deep breath.*

I would see a few patients a day while I wrote down all my clinical protocols. Most importantly, I was taking time for myself. I had reminded myself that I must always put my oxygen mask on first. I began to forgive myself, then others, and began loving myself once again.

I would return to the islands often and spend time with my old friends. I'd go flying with Tommy and surfing and diving with Phil Carr. I began traveling the world and then began writing this book.

My cell phone rang early Sunday morning August 1, 1999. I was on Maui. It was my buddy, Jerry Charlebois. He said he heard that I was on Maui. He had a glider for me, and the wind was perfect up on top of Haleakala.

To Risk It All Once Again

Jerry was in the air the day Duff got killed and had witnessed his crash and his death. It was a very special call to go fly with him, to face another wall of fire in a glider I had never flown and in a harness that I had never used. It turned out to be the same type of glider that Duff was killed in.

When I stepped into endless space Duff was in the air with me. I heard him call my name in Spanish, as he liked to refer to me as "Juan": "Hey Juan, the wind is perfect. It is out of the north, a down range day for sure."

I soared for almost 20 minutes with a lone Mauna E'wa bird that looked strangely like Duff. I have to say, I have made many of those flights to honor passing friends and it has always held true to form; one of the soaring birds comes from off the cliff and makes its rare appearance in such proximity to simply say hello from above. But this flight had an added touch. When I landed in the pasture below I was immediately surrounded by horses, just like the morning of the harmonic convergence in 1987 at Big Bear Lake. I asked the other pilots if the horses were always there. Their reply was that none of them had ever seen the horses there before, and they couldn't believe that they would not leave me alone.

I had walked through the wall of fire that awaited me and came out the other side unscathed. Aloha Duff...

Trusting Yourself When All Men Doubt You

I have shared with you my life, but my mission is to give your life back to you. You, too, can be pain free. You too can heal yourself as I have done. There is no magic pill. It is your self will, trusting in yourself and adding the right fuel, the right exercise, the right electrical input, and the right electrical detoxification. The new world of twenty-first-century medicine will include Electro Toxicology and the global new job opportunity to become an Electro Toxicologist.

The first thing I ask any patient is, "Do you wish to be well?" If they reply yes, then I can help. I can teach them how I was able to heal myself, but it took the following. Fuel: The proper diet, vitamins, minerals, and nutritional products. Exercise: a lot of it. These are things that I cannot do for the patient. It is a fifty-fifty deal. I can't control what they put in their mouths, nor can I make them take a walk around the block. What I can do is electrify them and detoxify them.

Common Sense Medicine

The following is the shocking results of what standard Western medicine is silently doing.

Death by medicine has become the leading cause of death in our country. Over 700,000 people died needlessly last year. What is more shocking is that the total number of deaths caused by conventional medicine is an astounding 783,936 per year.

In the last 10 years death by medicine has killed an astounding 7.8 million people. It is evident that the American medical system is the leading cause of death and injury in the U.S. By contrast, the number of deaths attributed to heart disease was 699,697 while the number of deaths attributed to cancer was 553,251.5.

The estimated 10 year total of 7.8 million deaths caused by conventional medicine is more than all the casualties from all the wars fought by the U.S. throughout its entire history.

There are, however, many things to be thankful for about mainstream medicine. Our intensive care units are some of the best in the world. Our laboratories have the ability to analyze blood, urine, saliva, hair, and stool. You can find out what your body is producing and what it is not producing, and once you have your tests done correctly you can immediately begin giving yourself the nutrients you need by changing your diet and taking appropriate nutritional supplements. In many serious cases of heavy metal poisoning you can receive intravenous drips to remove the heavy metals from your body.

The following guidelines show you how to remove dis-ease from your body and bring your body back into balance.

1. Clean out your intestinal tract with a good colon or intestinal cleaner, a colonic or enema, but make sure you restore the good bacteria when you have finished. If you have taken a lot of antibiotics in your life you have damaged the flora in your gastrointestinal (GI) tract and that flora needs to be repaired. Pro-biotics are available

for this. GI health is one of the most important things you can do for yourself.

2. Get a proper food combining guide. We have a starving nation that is obese due to improper food combining. We have labeled the Standard American Diet "S-A-D." Sorry, you cannot eat a hamburger and a bun or a steak and a potato. The protein and the carbohydrates do not combine well during digestion; they lie in your gut and rot. This creates a lining in your intestinal tract that does not allow you to absorb the nutrients in your food. If you cannot get fuel through a GI tract that is the size of a tennis court when it is laid out, how do you think you are going to get the proper fuel at the cellular level? The good news is that we can to it electrically using computer artificial intelligent assisted Electro Toxicology.

3. Only be tested by a physician who has been certified by the Institute of Functional Medicine. Members of the Institute of Functional Medicine have looked at the world of medicine with new eyes and recognize that they have been duped by the pharmaceutical industry into giving their patients more and more drugs. See www.functionalmedicine.org for more information.

Once your evaluation is complete, go organic. We have poisoned our planet. A recent study indicated that every fresh water stream fish in the U.S. is over the limit in mercury. Eat small, fast open ocean water fish that come from clean water like the outer banks of Hawaii, Tonga, Fiji, and Indonesia. At the very least, wash your plants well. And do not buy meat that is injected with hormones.

4. Do yourself a big favor and buy Dr. Stephen Sinatra's book the *Sinatra Solution* and begin supplementing your body with the nutritional products it is lacking.

5. Then we can run micro-current, perfect current, through your ears, teeth, hands, feet, spine and also do lymph drainage. Using artificial intelligence that only knows homeostasis, we can help clean every pathway electrically. This allows waste products out and nutrients in.

6. All disease is a toxic response, or dis-ease. If you remove the toxicity you remove the response.

CHAPTER TWENTY

If You Can Fill The Unforgiving Minute With Sixty Seconds Of Distance Run

From the break downs here is the break through and the science that substantiates that common sense medicine is here to stay. Remember the last thing that the pharmaceutical industry wants is a painless therapy that gets you well and costs nothing to use but a few cents in electricity. You might think that you do not need drugs!

Introduction To Electro Therapy And Electro Toxicology

Electricity travels via distinct pathways in the body. These pathways include nerves, bones, muscles, and connective tissues. Each cell manifests the property of capacitance, which is the ability to hold an electrical charge (like tiny batteries).

Adenosine-Tri-Phosphate (ATP) is one of the primary molecules responsible for the cells' ability to hold an electrical charge (capacitance). ATP contributes to the active transport mechanism, which is how a cell maintains homeostasis and provides the energy necessary for opening the ion channels' sensitive gates on the cell membrane. This allows nutrients in and waste products out.

ATP is thus responsible for the capacitance level of the cell. It has been demonstrated that areas of the body that manifest pain are often deficient in ATP. We can aid in the electrical cycle by increasing the body's ability to actually produce and store energy in the area of involvement. This is done by charging the tissue in a manner similar to that of a rechargeable battery. The ATP concentration in the areas which are stimulated is increased; hence, the tissue's inherent ability to hold electricity is enhanced. The greater the charge on the cell, the less resistance it has to the flow of electrical energy (internally or externally). Additionally, as the cell charge increases, the cellular function increases.

What does this mean? It means that you have a regenerative cell with an active transport system or sodium pump. This pump is directly responsible for the trans-membrane movement of sodium, potassium, and calcium into the cell and for the movement of metabolic waste out of the cell. A degenerative cell occurs when metabolic waste builds up in toxic concentrations.

How does electrical therapy affect the cell? The work of Dr. Ngok Cheng has shown that ATP concentrations are only affected positively when the applied electrical flow is in the range of from 25uA RMS to less than 5mA. Some pain patients have used electrical devices called TENS machines (Transcutaneous Electrical Nerve Stimulation) to relieve their pain. TENS devices operate in the 20 to 80 milliamp and higher ranges, which deplete the cell's ATP and metabolic processing capabilities.

The amount of current delivered by the Myopulse/Acuscope is measured in microamps rather than milliamps and is within the range found useful by Dr. Cheng. The result is that the cell channels/gates open, allowing nutrients in and waste products out. The lymphatic system and the kidneys can then excrete the waste products, helping to avoid toxic reactions. Toxic reactions can include nausea, headache, sweating, increased pain, dizziness, muscle spasm, bad taste, fainting, and weakness. If the symptoms occur, it is because there is an overload of toxins being released but not flushed out quickly enough by the body's natural mechanisms.

History Of Electro-Therapy

The use of electrical currents in the field of pain management is not new. Torpedo fish were used in antiquity in the Nile region. Patients with gout were required to stand on the fish in the surf and maintain contact until the pain was relieved. In 1971 a porcelain cylinder was found with a copper wire through it in an archeological site dated back to the first century AD. This battery was found in the magician's quarters along with various bowls and artifacts decorated with inscriptions and incantations.

In those days the magician was the physician. He was probably using this battery to remove pain from his patients. Some of the ancient acupuncture needle manipulation techniques can be understood as a way of introducing a mild static charge into the body via the needle.

Transcutaneous Electrical Nerve Stimulation (TENS) came into widespread use in the U.S. in the early 1970s. It was originally developed as a non-invasive method to locate proper sites for implanted electrodes for the relief of intractable chronic pain. When many patients noticed excellent pain relief even before the electrodes were implanted, TENS was born.

Theory Of Pain Relief

Two theories of pain and pain relief dominate the discussion of the use of TENS: The gate theory and theories of the production and function of endogenous opiates, or endorphins.

Melzack & Wall developed the Pain Gate Theory, which suggests that an increased volume of nerve signals from the sensory nerves to the brain will block transmission or recognition by the brain of the slower traveling painful nerve impulses. This blocking "fools" the brain into thinking that the pain is gone. It is thought to occur in the 20-80mA range of stimulation.

The second theory holds that we produce painkillers within our nervous system. Endorphins are our own internally produced painkillers, one type of a class of substances called endogenous opiates. They are generated in response to painful stimuli in nature, and apparently also are produced by certain forms of more intense electro-stimulation. Such intense stimulation usually produces muscle contractions.

Physiological Effects Of Milli-Amperage Microcurrent Devices

Standard millicurrent TENS and EGS (electro-galvanic stimulation) are modalities familiar to most physical medicine professionals. Generally, currents in the range of 20 uA to 120 mA are applied to block neurological transmission of pain signals and stimulate the release of endorphins and other neurotransmitters for the relief of chronic and acute pain. There is very little evidence that a TENS or EGS machine actually heals the cause of the pain, though they can help block the perception of pain and may be useful for that purpose.

Cell Channel Research

In 1991, Drs. Neher and Sakmann (German scientists) were awarded the Nobel Prize in Physiology and Medicine for discoveries in basic cell function. Their research enabled the detection of electrical currents of a trillionth of an ampere in the membrane or surface of the cell. They discovered how tunnel-like structures (ion channels) control the passage in and out of cells of positively or negatively charged particles (ions). Every cell has 20 to 40 types of ion channels that help it communicate and function.

Neher and Sakmann conclusively established the existence of ion channels with the patch clamp technique, which allows detection of incredibly small electrical currents that pass through a single ion channel. The technique records how a single channel molecule alters its shape and in that way controls the flow of current within a time frame of a few millionths of a second.

Neher and Sakmann spent 7 years developing the technique and then spent a decade applying it to describe precisely the structure and function of single ion channels, particularly in the brain. They found that each of the 100 billion cells that make up the brain and CNS (central nervous system) could interact with thousands of others through highly specific connections in a relay system; that, in fact, the channels are not chaotic.

After 5 years they were motivated to understand better how electric currents worked in nerve and muscle cells. Before this, no one knew for sure how the ion channels worked. How many were there? Just a few? Each carrying a large current, or many? Each carrying a small current?

The patch clamp technique has its recording electrode fastened to a microscopic patch of the cell's membrane. The cell membrane is what separates the interior of each cell from its surroundings. Cell membranes help regulate the entry of sugar and other foods that cells need for nourishment and the excretion of waste products. Cells also communicate through channels in the membrane. The channels consist of molecules that allow passage of ions or charged atoms.

The Nobel committee noted that life begins with the activation of ion channels as the sperm merges with the egg in fertilization. All cells have electrical charges within and outside of the cell; the difference is known as the membrane potential. Fertilization changes the potential to prevent other sperm from joining the fertilized egg. All other cells have a characteristic set of ion channels that help them carry out their specific functions.

When Neher and Sakmann applied glass electrodes with microscopic tips to a cell membrane, they were able to electrically isolate a small patch of it and examine individual proteins. The protein served as gates or channels through which only certain ions (particles that are electrically charged) were allowed to pass. They also found that they could remove a patch of membrane and gain access to the interior of the cell. They could study cell physiology in a way no one could before.

At first, neuroscientists used this technique to study the electrical signals from nerve cells that touched off muscle contraction. Then researchers began using the technique to study other cells in the body. They were surprised to find that the electrical activity was also going on in all kinds of cells. Most importantly, the amplitude of current was much smaller than previously thought. The patch clamp conclusively established that applying millionths if not trillionths of an ampere to the cellular membrane activated and opened the electrically sensitive ion channels in the cell membrane, enhancing nutrient intake and waste product departure, thus taking a cell from a degenerative state to a regenerative state in a matter of seconds.

Today

Dr. Anthony Nebrensky developed the Electro Acuscope and Myopulse in 1979. His experience before 1979 was in the development of electrical measuring devices and biofeedback instruments. His background as a physicist led him from missile guidance chip development to using that same technology to scan, search, and seek, like a smart missile, the abnormalities of diseased or injured tissue in the human body at the cellular level. The financial gain in medicine comes from creating a medicine that would create a temporary fix, thus leading the patient to another medicine that would alleviate the symptoms caused by the first medication. The pharmaceutical industry was more interested in people taking drugs than simple cures that cost little or nothing. Medicine is Big Business. Dr Nebrensky said to me, "I retired from this business because no matter how good it was and how much suffering it prevented no one cared." I assured him that there were plenty of people out there who did want to see his healing equipment more widely appreciated. I am one of those individuals, and I feel my troops are assembling. Recently, he received a large contract to build another state-of-the-art healing device. Only this time the world may be ready for it!

CHAPTER TWENTY-ONE

Yours Is The Earth And Everything That's In It And Which Is More You Will Be A Man My Son

The Future

The media has featured us both nationally as well as internationally. The response has been overwhelming. Several national television shows have asked if they could do a feature story regarding my personal experience as well as the thousands of other success stories that have come from the use of the Electro Acuscope and Myopulse. I have turned down these offers until I have a referral network that can handle the demand for this type of treatment. Once I have trained hundreds if not thousands of technicians coast to coast to use the Acuscope and Myopulse and the electro toxicology protocols that have been proven to be effective for over 24 years, I will begin the media blitz. I look forward to marketing a pain management device that has celebrity endorsements, clinical trials, and most importantly a 90% success rate in the reduction of chronic pain.

Epilogue

We would not know light if not for the darkness. Moreover, is it not fair to say that we would not know pleasure if not for pain? We experience pain for a reason, to learn from it and grow past it. With the loss of my mother, I personally experienced an almost unbearable pain at a very early age, and the reality of death has been at my doorstep ever since. Motivated to experience all that life has to offer, I have walked the edge, lost loved ones, and brought my own life within inches of the end.

I believe that these experiences were preparing me to help others deal with their own terrible pain, both physical and emotional. Using the tools of the Acuscope and Myopulse I have taken part in thousands of stories of healing. As founder of Thorp Institute, I have supervised over 40,000 treatments in the past 24 years. The protocols that I have developed are based on clinical findings that have returned over a 90% success rate in the reduction of chronic pain, and I continually ensure that the therapies at Thorp Institute are based on personal experience. I push on with the good news of an alternative path to healing beyond the limits of Western medicine.

The other healing tool, passed on by my mother, I could only appreciate after fully facing the crippling fear of death for myself. I now see that it was through the example of her faith that she passed along what I call a "soulular" wisdom.

Our pure soul does not hold on to the feeling of pain. A soul can only remember its origin, a place of ecstatic love and bliss. Faith sets us free from all pain and allows us to accept the bliss that it is already there. My mother realized her soulular existence through her walk with Jesus Christ, but many paths lead to this divine understanding. Personal faith in the power of a loving soul is bigger than the teacher or the religious vehicle.

In the body, cellular memory holds pain, but we may step beyond the cellular and into the soulular experience if we choose to do so. The spiritual being that we are, the soul will not carry these memories. The body experiences pain and a cell remembers, but the soul cleanses that experience. Our soulular memory remains pure and in bliss. I believe our suffering is over if we accept this new existence.

My personal belief is that we are spiritual beings in these bodies to experience emotion, to love each other, to help bring peace and understanding to this planet, and most importantly to forgive ourselves as well as others. In the school for the soul, graduation day is the day you truly learn forgiveness and unconditional love.

Like the experience of the eclipse, in the moments when I have accepted my place among all people and things I have felt as if I was stepping into endless space and, as the poet says, "slipping the bonds of earth on laughter's silver wings to touch the face of God."

If you seek the connection, you will not be denied. Ask and it shall be delivered. When I had finally evolved and genuinely desired a family of my own, I met my beautiful wife, Lisa Christine Egizii, in May, 2004. We were married in the west Maui Mountains behind the Iao Valley Needle on December 29, 2005.

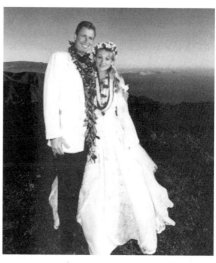

On top of the world with my inspiration -
My beautiful wife
Lisa Christine Thorp

Twenty-two of our friends were flown in by helicopter to this sacred spot where a rare flower grows exclusive to this remote locale. Nowhere else in the world has anyone found this flower. This flower is as unique as my wife, one of a kind.

On April 30, 2007, my wife and I delivered a baby in our bedroom with the help of our midwife, Diane Smith. We were blessed with the greatest miracle possible, our beautiful daughter, Eva Christine Thorp. Then another miracle happened on September 23, 2009. We were blessed with

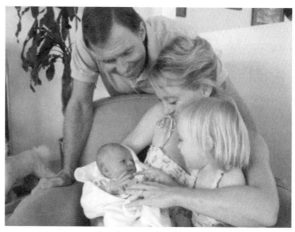

My beautiful family
The most incredible experience of all

another beautiful daughter, Jillian Fay Thorp. I pray for guidance each day to be the best father in the world and that I may pass on to my daughters the same faith and wisdom that was passed on to me.

Almost 10 years ago I wrote a business plan that detailed the building of a medical spa facility in front of one of the best surf breaks in the world, where we could run every diagnostic test possible using blood, hair, saliva, stool, and urine samples. Once we found out what you are lacking, we would immediately add to your diet the needed vitamins and minerals, intravenously if necessary, and at the same time we would be detoxifying your body one single cell at a time using the Electro Acuscope and Myopulse, along with other tools. We would restore your body using oxygen and other gases to kill all the pathogens in your blood.

I figured the perfect site for such a facility would have to be in a remote tropical island and that it would take years of convincing and proposing to make this dream of a five-star, non-toxic hospital for wellness a reality. Little did I know that at the very moment I was dreaming it, a new type of medical facility was being built in one of the most healing locations in the world, as deemed by NASA researchers. Constructed with all non-toxic materials 10 years ago, Sanoviv is a hospital located just south of San Diego at a pristine ecological site in Baja California, Mexico. It is now the model hospital of the 21st Century. Thorp Institute is happy to have a place within this state-of-the-art hospital built by Dr. Myron Wentz, the creator of USANA health products.

It turned out I did not have to build it after all; I just had to show up. Sanoviv has embraced the clinical protocols that I developed at Castle Medical Center, the Balanced Body Center, and Thorp Institute of Integrated Medicine.

I have often been called the doctor's doctor who is not a doctor. I am proud to wear that title, and I will continue to give of myself what I know to be true and what has worked for me and the thousands of others who have sought

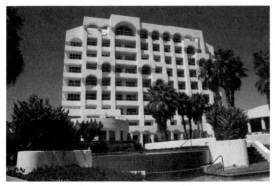

my assistance. Sanoviv is my new playground for healing, the medical spa facility I once only dreamt about. I am ecstatic to contribute my clinical protocols in Electro Toxicology, to bring this new walk of non-drug and non-invasive medicine to

Sanoviv Medical Institute

Sanoviv. I can only offer a sincere welcome to all those in need and interested in riding the medical wave of the 21st century.

I have now started my next book, *From Soulular to Cellular*, where I am building upon my belief that all disease is toxic response. If you remove the toxicity, you remove the response and, subsequently, the DIS-EASE. I must say thank you to another hero of mine who ushered in this new thinking in medical treatment, Dr. Royal Raymond Rife, who was honored in 1934 with a banquet billed as the "End of All Disease." Now thanks to Dr. Wentz and Sanoviv I think we are one step closer to realizing Dr. Rife's bold ambitions. If you can dream it, you can do it, and, if you are lucky, someone just might build it for you.

Dedicated Cast Of Characters
(some were mentioned in the chapters above and a few were not but the ones mentioned below I could not leave out due to the impact they had on my life)

This book was written as a tribute to and for those I love, to the ones that are no longer with us here on earth and to those spiritual beings I am still blessed to be sharing this incredible human experience alongside.

My greatest inspiration will always be my mother and father. I feel their pride, their smiles, and their laughter coming down from above or behind or beside me. Their presence fills me and propels me to do the limitless things that we are all ultimately capable of achieving when upheld by faith. One such challenge has been for me to sit down and write out these guttural feelings that I am so deeply driven to share with the world and, most importantly, with my little girls, one who is sleeping in her big pink bed and the other who is sleeping on her mommy's tummy as I sit here at 4:00 am on a beautiful star-filled night at Mammoth Mountain. There are so many people who have touched my life, and many of their stories are captured in this book. But there are also those who I could only briefly touch upon, and I am taking the opportunity here to add these additional biographies of the dedicated cast of characters of my life.

Barry Mahon, who is no longer with us, joined Britain's Royal Air Force at the age of 17 by lying about his age and was an ace World War II fighter pilot before being shot down over Germany early in the war. The movie *The Great Escape* was based on his adventure under captivity in the enemy prison and chronicled the multiple times he tried to escape. Barry's nickname was "the Cooler King" because he spent more time in solitary confinement, at that time, than any prisoner in the history of modern warfare. He even suffered confinement in a coffin with only a slot at the mouth that slid open so food could be dropped in. Barry, Dennis McKenna, and I were partners in a film company called Production Machine, which pioneered the first computerized accounting system for producing motion pictures. Barry was also Errol Flynn's best friend and personal manager, and they traveled the world together. When my father passed away, Barry took me aside and said, "Anything you may need to talk to your father about, feel free to talk with me. I'm honored to say you're a son to me."

Dick Ziker befriended me immediately and used me whenever he was in Hawaii. He has served as president of Stunts Unlimited (the most prestigious stunt organization in Hollywood) and is one of the best stuntmen to ever be called a stuntman. He is also a great father, having raised a beautiful daughter, Melissa, as a single parent. Dick defied death on a daily basis, but, unfortunately, Melissa was not able to postpone her call. Tragedy struck her at the tender age of 23 when she had a fatal asthma attack and passed away. No parent should experience such pain. The whole stunt world suffered with and for Dick. Dick introduced me to many of his Stunts Unlimited partners, who accepted me due to Dick's recommendations and offered me jobs whenever they came to Hawaii. Dick was always there for me and is someone I will always admire. Thanks Dick.

Bobby Bass (Stunts Unlimited) was one of the most admired and highly respected martial artists in the world. He held black belts in what is now considered mixed martial arts: Karate, Jujitsu, Judo, and Tae Kwon Do. He was a master in all. Bobby also used me every time he came to Hawaii and in many other instances as well. Bobby will also be missed, as he mercifully passed away after suffering a long and debilitating illness, ALS (Lou Gehrig's Disease), in 2003.

Ronnie Rondell, a longtime Stunts Unlimited coordinator, was an incredible stunt patriarch to a family of several sons. Ronnie, like Dick, defied death too many times to count but he too suffered the greatest pain of all, losing his son, Reid, in a helicopter crash on a stunt gone wrong. Ronnie would also use me every time he came to Hawaii and gave me my first opportunity as a stunt driver. He trusted me in a car chase sequence where I doubled for the bad guy, slamming and crashing a Lincoln Continental on a television series called *Hawaiian Heat*. A big thank you to Ronnie Rondell.

John Walbert was one of the first to design and build bamboo and plastic hang gliders in the state of Hawaii. He was also the first to set the record for time aloft in a hang glider, at just over two hours. He flew bamboo and plastics in the very early '70s, and then upgraded when, as one of our team members at Dove Hang Gliders of Hawaii, he started flying Dacron sails and 0/5/8 aircraft aluminum frames. John flew with Harvey Baumgartner, Ray Hook, and I in formation in our blue and white hang gliders, all built out of that little apartment on the Ali Wai Canal in Honolulu, Hawaii. John and his beautiful young female passenger were killed flying tandem while being towed behind a speedboat in Maui.

Jeff Brewer, who went to the Philippines to do stunt work on a film with Chuck Norris, stopped at my house with Dick Ziker and worked like hell to get me on the movie. My best friend and number one helicopter pilot, Tom Hauptman, was originally hired to do all the helicopter work, but since he refused to fly their helicopters and more importantly refused to use the Philippines' gas he was scrapped. The local pilot, Jo Jo, was not doing any stunts in this accident but was merely transporting the actors and stunt people from one set to another when he lost power and crashed, killing everyone on board.

Linda Tracey, who could out-fly most of the guys, was killed doing what she loved, flying hang gliders for a film. When I was towing up out at Morgan's ranch in dedication to Linda Tracey, another Mauna E'wa bird would not leave my wing tip.

Bob Wills, the creator of Wills Wings, one of the best hang gliding companies still manufacturing hang gliders today, was also killed while flying hang gliders. Bob traded records with John Walbert, who could stay in the air longest in a hang glider. John would set a record and then Bob would come over and break it. This went on for years. I remember watching

Bob, hanging from his knees like a trapeze artist in a circus; only he was hanging from his hang glider 1,500 feet in the air. Truly one of the best hang glider pilots ever.

Jim "Wildman" Niece was the first to attempt tow in surfing. I'm not sure if Jim is alive or dead. No one has heard of him since the night before he was to ride outside Kaena Point at 50 feet. I had a lot of fun with Jim, out drinking and out fighting mostly, but it is hard to win a fight when it is five against one, as happened the night before he was to ride Kaena Point.

Tim Rossovich—who could forget Tim Rossovich? Hopefully, he is still here with us. Tim was Tom Selleck's college roommate and played in the NFL. He could also eat a beer glass like it was made of tortilla chips. It must have hurt on the way out because I know his bloody lips didn't feel too good as it was on its way down. Tim and I also became good friends, and I watched him face many challenges. If you are still here Tim, I would love to hear from you.

Randy Craft—You would think that I would have learned my lesson about sailing with Randy, but he got me back out into the Pacific not too much later. He invited me to the Big Island to do a little work on my business plan and to work on sales strategies for Thorp Institute, the company I had created and still run. After a long morning of brainstorming, he said, "Let's get a little exercise and paddle down to Orchid." Orchid is a five-star hotel just down the beach from Pua'ko. Randy has been paddling canoes for 30 years, and he quickly showed me his state-of-the-art designs, which are not only great for paddling but for riding waves as well. He had an extra one of these surf canoes and we decided to go for a paddle break.

We loaded the canoes onto the car and off we went to a little natural harbor a few blocks up from his house in Pua'ko. Randy said the two-mile paddle along the cliffs was a breeze this time of the year. There were a few small waves in the bay, but not enough to prevent us from getting to the open ocean and carrying out this short paddle to the Orchid. I should have known that after our narrow escape years earlier we were tempting the great ocean, which was set on playing rough again this time.

Our plan was to paddle to the resort, have a cocktail on the beach poolside, and have a leisurely paddle home. It all started out as planned, perfectly peaceful. A few small waves headed our way and Randy spun his canoe around and caught them effortlessly. I actually caught a little wave myself and had a fun ride. We headed through the reef and with the visibility stunningly clear we got a spectacular show from the turtles and the beautiful marine life below.

As we rounded the first set of cliffs, the wind started to pick up and the surface became a little choppy, but it was a bright sunny day and it still seemed to be an easy paddle to the resort ahead. I was admiring the volcanic cliffs when I heard a harrowing cry from Randy, "Outside," the call of a big wave approaching.

What was bearing down on us was a potentially killer rogue wave with a 20 foot face. Randy yelled at me to paddle, paddle with all my might as we headed out to sea, racing the breaking face. But as the wave got closer, I knew there was no way I was going to make it over the top. I heard Randy yelling at me to not let go of the canoe. I looked back toward the cliff and then at the huge wave approaching and I thought screw the canoe and dove for the bottom.

I was too late and felt the wave grab me. Then came that terrible feeling of falling off a two-story building as I went over the falls. The weight of the wave pushed me down until it got very dark. I had surf and dive booties on my feet and could feel the pressure of the wave sucking them right off.

It was so black and eerie down there that I knew I had been pushed very deep. When the pressure finally backed off I tried to push off the bottom, but I hit my head on sharp coral, knowing then that I been rolled into a lava tube. I remembered Buzzy Trent saying whenever a wave has gotten hold of you, relax and count. I tried to relax, but my air was running out and I knew that not only was I in a cave but I was also down way too deep, a bad combination.

Then the grip of the wave suddenly released me and sucked me back out. The color of the water turned from black to blue, and I swam for the light and hit the surface. Good news was that I was above water; bad news was that I was less than 15 feet from the jagged cliff side and another bigger wave was heading my way, ready to slam my body into the unforgiving rock. There was no sight of the canoe, so I dove down deep again just as the second wave hit me. The same scenario took me back up and over the falls and rolled me back into that same black hole. I thought of Buzzy, I held my breath and counted, and once again I was released and headed for the surface, only to find another wave on the way. I tried to swim for the wave and get away from the cliff but this final wave caught me again. This time I missed the cave and was able to float to the surface.

I was exhausted and could barely muster the strength to struggle as the backwash continually slammed me up against the cliff and then back away from it in a washing machine-type cycle. Slowly and patiently I made strides away from the cliff. It was at least a mile or so to swim back to the harbor, but after the dark minutes in the cave it was just nice to be alive. The canoe pieces surfaced all around me. The biggest piece left was no more than a foot in diameter.

The fisherman on the top of the cliff could not see me since I was right up against the cliff face, which was slightly inverted. The last they saw of me I was bailing out from the canoe and diving for the bottom. Over 10 minutes had passed without any sign of me.

Randy had also been hit with the first huge wave but had been successful in getting to Orchid Bay by making it to the deep water of the bay, which saved him from the second and third waves. He began paddling back in the direction he had last seen me and was horrified at the site of the canoe in a thousand pieces. He yelled to the fisherman to see if they had seen me, and they gave him a thumbs down. They yelled that they were calling the paramedics, but feared that I had probably drowned. The wind had picked up and now there was a two-foot chop on the water, making it almost impossible for anyone to see a little head bobbing.

Rolling over on to my back and floating freely, I felt everything go into slow motion. The comforting calm washed over me once again as the world slowed down enough to make everything clear. I thought only of survival.

A leisurely paddle for a cocktail at a five-star resort turned into a life or death situation, but I knew it is the easy ones that get you. If not for having spent years surfing big waves, fully understanding the ocean's currents and rips and walking side by side with men like Dar and Buzzy, I would have drowned for sure that day. Most people would have drown, a sad but true fact.

With the horror over, I rested on my back, simply watching the beautiful clouds. I knew I would make it. It might take me a few hours but I would reach the harbor sooner or later. I was broken from my reverie by Randy's voice, yelling, "John!" He had found me and was heading in my direction.

"Holly shit!" he said, "I thought you had drowned. The fisherman on the cliffs said you went down and didn't come up."

I crawled up on the back of his canoe and could only say, "Wow!" We went back to the cliff where the fisherman and paramedic truck were waiting, and overheard them strategizing on where my dead body might wash up. Randy recognized the fisherman and let them know I was all right. "Boy you are one lucky bugger," a Hawaiian man said as we all looked out at the pieces floating on the surface. The only thing in one piece was the paddle, which was floating out to sea. I asked Randy if he wanted to get the canoe and go for the paddle. We both agreed that the ocean had spared enough for one day and she could keep the paddle.

Felipe Pomar and I have been surfing together for over thirty years. I could not leave this most recent challenge off my list. I have been going to a pristine island called Rote in Indonesia for the past four years. My first year there I wanted to film a big swell that hit the island. Felipe had very little if any surf videos of this incredible left. It was easy double, if not triple overhead. The tide has a twelve-foot swing, so in the morning you can walk the mile out on the reef, then a short paddle out through the breakers. It drops off, creating a perfect left that goes for at least a quarter of a mile. Two to three hours later the reef is totally covered and under at least six to eight feet of water. I decided that if I did not film this wave I would have no history of this great spot. I told Felipe the night before that I would take my expensive camera out to film the following day. Felipe assured me that I would have plenty of time to get some good shots then walk back in.

I took a village boy who was Felipe's hired help to help me carry my tripod, lenses, and assortment of things that I would need to get the desired footage. Mike Doyle, another surfing legend, Felipe, my trusted guide, and I walked the reef in anticipation of catching them riding some great waves.

We got some great shots of Felipe, Mike, and even Mike's girlfriend, who also joined us.

The tide started coming in, and coming in fast. So I told Sunny it was time to head in because the tide would be up soon and I did not want to ruin my camera. No matter which direction we headed the water was getting deeper. I kept asking Sunny which direction we should go. He had a wild-eyed look on his face, and I realized that he had no clue what direction to go. As the water got deeper and deeper and his face and eyes continued to become more wild-eyed, he told me that he could not swim. I looked at him in amazement and said, "What do you mean you cannot swim? You are supposed to be my guide!"

I found the highest point of the reef and told Sunny to stay put, but I was not going to leave my camera behind. I walked as far as I could, waving my arms at any boat or surfer to get their attention, hoping that the water would not cover the spot Sunny was perched on. I began swimming for help. That swim turned into a two-hour swim. Mike, Felipe's neighbor, saw Sunny standing there on the reef by himself and took off paddling since he knew that Sunny could not swim. Two hours later I arrived on the beach. I swam the whole way in with one arm in the air holding my camera and doing the frog kick.

It got to that time when you have to look toward the beach and see if you are getting closer or farther away. This could be my last day on planet Earth. Once again it was going to be an easy one that would end my life, and all I was trying to do was film a big day of surf. I was never so glad to see that I was actually closer than farther away. An hour plus later I dragged myself up onto the beach. The people on the beach saw that I was making headway but no one came out to help me. When I reached the beach John Guirney, Felipe's neighbor, just laughed and said what the hell were you doing out there? I explained and told him that Felipe said I could walk in. "Well hell mate, you can't walk in once the tide starts coming in! You're lucky you didn't get sucked out to sea and drown. Ain't no one coming to get you in this neck of the woods, Mate! Hell, I only could see you the last hundred yards or so. With your arm in the air you blended in with the sticks the locals use to grow the seaweed."

Then he told me a story about a guy who took his surf board out there with his mother and all his expensive gear to film the surf, and when he paddled his mother in on the surf board just when they were only a few feet from shore the board tipped over and all his gear went in with his mother. Thousands of dollars of camera gear were destroyed in one quick second. This great surf spot really did not want the rest of the world knowing about it, I guess. That was one long swim!

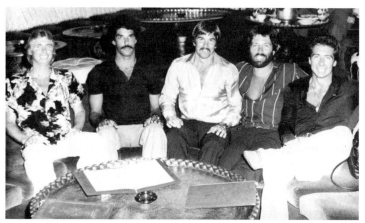

My surfing Buddies in the 70's from L to R John Thorp, Richard Elie (My saviour on the worst acid trip of my life who tragically died as mentioned below) Tom Ramey, Mike Brown, and Felipe Pomar

Rick Elie, my surf buddy featured in the book, caught a bad cold, checked into the hospital, and died of an infection he got while in the hospital.

Rick's tragic death brings me full circle to the purpose of this book. My mission is to improve healthcare quality while lowering healthcare costs, meanwhile creating a global new job opportunity in the field of energy medicine and Electro Toxicology. If the idea of becoming an Electro Toxicologist intrigues you, please contact us at www.thorpinstitute.com or 1(800) ACUSCOPe (228-7267)

Bo Kajer Olsen—The final chapter of Bo Kajer Olsen was, as was usual with him, an incredible journey. I am sure the story tellers will be writing a book about the world famous treasure diver from Capetown. Whether they get the real facts remain to be seen. Before I go on, may I say in my heart of hearts that I have always hoped to find out that every promise Bo had made to me he planned to fulfill and that every story he told me in order to fully enroll me in his plans was also true. The following is the continued heartbreaking tale of Bo Kajer Olsen.

It was about two years after I returned to Hawaii that Bo and I reconnected. My ex-wife, Kim, and Bo had fallen in love and became proud parents of a beautiful little girl, Kassandra. Bo had full custody of his young son, Zechariah, from his second marriage to a young gal who ended up in the care of a mental facility. He was raising Zech on the fish farm he created in Green Valley. Bo had become an expert on fish farming and had received awards from the governor of the state of Hawaii, Ben Cayatano.

Everything seemed to be heading in the right direction for Bo until one day Kim noticed a foggy appearance in Kassandra's eyes. She immediately took Kassandra to a pediatrician and the symptoms were dismissed as insignificant. When the problem did not rectify itself Kim took Kassandra to another doctor and again the condition was dismissed as insignificant. Kassandra was misdiagnosed several times before Kim's fears were justified by a diagnosis that confirmed a rare form of cancer, Retinoblastoma, and the horrible fate that awaited Kassandra. If she was to survive the cancer, her only hope was to have both of her eyes removed. Our hearts were broken that day with the pain of this little spirit and what her life would be like as a blind child. God bless the attorney that represented Kim and Kassandra; they won a million dollar malpractice lawsuit intended to provide a stable way of life for this beautiful child.

Bo confided in me several times about the heartbreak and the stress he was under to try and provide for his daughter, but the only possibility he believed he had to give his daughter and his son the life they deserved was to return to the treasure wrecks he assured me he could find again along the Skeleton Coast of Africa.

My adventuresome spirit was once again aroused. Could I trust him to go after the treasure? Could we survive an adventure that was full of danger not only from the sea but from pirates as well? I was ready to put all my winnings once again and risk them on one turn of pitch and toss.

I could not forget the cannons I saw and the coins that I smuggled out of Africa for him on our earlier adventures. He convinced me that with the right funding and expedition team we could find the treasure that awaited us. He was as confident as I had ever seen him as we talked about buying a boat and returning to the wrecks that only he knew about.

In the midst of this terrible family breakdown there were still many breakthroughs as I watched him succeed in a venture that many had failed in, aquaculture. We laughed as we dragged the ponds with his nets and up to the surface came the most incredible prawns, catfish, and tilapia. I felt like I was with Jesus feeding thousands with the finest food raised in these sacred waters of the Punaluu Stream. The old magic was back, Bo raising perfect food and me helping the sick. It was amazing how our lives had changed.

I was so proud of Bo and his accomplishments. But we dreamed once again about going to recover the treasure on the Skelton Coast. He asked me if I was in. He looked me in the eyes and said, "You know I know where the wrecks are, don't you?" I believed him without hesitation.

A few weeks later, the landlords that held Bo's 40 acre fish ponds redirected the water from the Punaluu Stream back toward the west side of Oahu, where a new development needed the water in order to build what they called the second Waikiki and its first huge new hotel, the Ko O'lina.

Within twenty-four hours Bo's ponds were drying up. He hiked to the source, found the blockage, and with a little dynamite restored the water to the windward side. The local Hawaiian Sovereignty groups hailed him as the savior for their crops and soon rallied behind Bo for the restoration of the water and his fight against his landlords and water rights.

I had introduced Bo to John Allen, mentioned earlier, one of the top litigating attorneys in the country. John was willing to take Bo's case. John loved a fight and water rights and the big guys verses the little guys was a challenge he could not pass up. He won the case, but the settlement was much less than anticipated.

In conducting the case, John's team of investigators had uncovered some incriminating evidence against Bo. If they could find out about this information so could the defense—and this information could destroy the case. Because of this, John settled for approximately $500,000 instead of the

$5,000,000 we had hoped for. However, $500,000 was still a lot more than the $10,000 originally offered by the landlords, and was in my estimation enough money to rebuild the boat we needed to the proper specifications for our treasure hunting along the Skelton Coast of Africa.

We celebrated at John's House in Rancho Santa Fe, California. After John took his expenses and his one third of the net, the rest went to Bo and me. I told Bo that he could keep my portion of the settlement so that we could immediately take the boat, the Antares, to a top dry dock facility, Baja Naval in Ensenada, Mexico. I met Bo there a few weeks after he arrived with the Antares and began filming the rebuilding. That wonderful saying "If you can dream it, you can do it" once again was in the air. Unfortunately, this dream, along with the others Bo and I shared in the past, soon became a nightmare.

Within six weeks the money was gone. Bo called me in a panic that he was out of money. I had given him all the money I had, including all of my savings. The boat and the treasure that waited was my retirement program. Every penny I earned went into the hands of Bo to take care of his and Zech's expenses. At that point I was all in and had absolutely no money left, so I contacted John Allen and asked if he could loan us the

$10,000 to get the boat released and stop the $400 per day fee we were being charged by the Baja Naval boat yard while the boat sat idle. John said no. He refused to lend us a penny because of the discrepancies he and his investigative team had found in Bo's history. As angry as I was with John and now once again uncertain of Bo's ethics, I still promised Bo I would continue to help him.

In desperation Bo contacted his ex-wife, Maureen. He explained to me that he had signed Snake Eyes, the fishing boat he owned in Honolulu, over to her as collateral for the loan she provided. The boat later mysteriously disappeared when I notified Bo that I had a buyer for it so he could repay Maureen. The potential buyer flew to Honolulu to meet me at the location where I had inspected the boat the previous week. To my astonishment, the boat was gone. It had vanished into thin air. No one in the vicinity seemed to know what happened to it, yet it was supposedly being watched over.

When I told Bo that his boat had obviously been stolen, he did not want to pursue it.

Bo always had an answer to my questions, but when he seemed uninterested in the potential sale of the boat, all the trouble I had gone to in finding a buyer, and then the theft of it, I wondered if he had already traded it or sold it to someone else. Why I continued to support Bo when everything was pointed against him I can't explain except to say that I wanted so much to prove John Allen wrong and show him that the information his top team of investigators had on Bo was wrong. I wanted to show him that Bo truly was the Crocodile Dundee character I had bet my life on in Africa.

I confronted Bo regarding the information that John had given me about his past. He said I could believe what I wanted to and he stuck to his story that he was who he said he was.

I arrived at John's office ready to defend Bo once again. John sat me down and invited his investigative team in. They explained to me that Bo was not who he said he was. According to the prosecuting team, there was no record of Bo ever being in the South African Air Force, nor had he ever worked for South African Airways, and his pilot's license had been forged. Needless to say, I was flabbergasted. I felt like I had been kicked in the stomach by a mule. John Allen continued to tell me that the man I had gone to the end of the earth with was going to sail away with our boat and justify it by finding any excuse he could to do so—without me. No matter what John told me I continued to support Bo. I had seen him do brilliant things. How could someone this brilliant be lying, and how could he be lying to me?

I introduced Bo to a group that was working on a treasure wreck in Chile. I set up the first meeting with a friend and patient, Captain Leslie James, and Captain James introduced Bo to the dive team. I felt Bo was in good hands and the trust was building. A few meetings later the deal was supposedly done and the money was supposed to be on the way. Bo and I signed an agreement that stated I would get 50% of all the treasures found in consideration for using my own funds and the investors that I had introduced Bo to through Captain James. I used the last of my savings to fill the boat up with enough fuel to motor 5,000 miles if the wind ran out. We prepared the boat with all the gear including dry suits, new scuba tanks, and all the accessories needed for a treasure dive expedition of this sort.

I had offered a good friend who I considered a little brother to be on the boat as my eyes and ears. He was a surfer and was excited about the opportunity. From the time the boat left San Diego, my friend notified me of the things he overheard—that I was being phased out since I was no longer of value. The new investor group was Bo's new money source, so I was no longer needed.

That all changed when they blew out their sails en route to Puerto Vallarta and the investor's money was no where in sight. I flew into Puerto Vallarta and invested another $2,000 to repair the main sail. Bo was very appreciative and denied all allegations that I had heard from my friend as well as everything that John and his investigative team had found. My dreams of treasure and the redemption of the person I had believed in was what propelled me forward As we set sail to Acapulco I could only feel that all our dreams were coming true. The boat sailed beautifully. I had personally watched and recorded Bo has he brought Antares back to life when she lay gutted in the boat yard at Baja Naval. His brilliance once again could not be discounted. I had witnessed it with my own eyes.

A month prior to setting sail I had been notified that my dear friend, wingman, and roommate for many years, Duff King, had been killed in a hang gliding accident on the cliffs of Molokai. In every hang gliding death that involved a friend of mine I had always experienced a magical encounter, most commonly with an Ewa bird that soared the cliffs of Hawaii. Duffy's death would not be an exception but a confirmation of the spirits that we are.

I took my watch on the Antares, navigating by the stars, while the crew slept below. I felt close to God and could not help but pray for all of those friends who had passed, especially Duffy. To say that the trip was magical was an understatement and the encounter that happened the following day had I not videotaped it would also be hard to believe. But what everyone experienced that morning is something that none of them will ever forget.

The wind had backed off as we crept along in the doldrums under the scorching sun. It was like a scene out of a movie as we floated into a pile of birds diving on the bait fish that shimmered just below the surface. One bird in particular stood out from the others due to his pure white head. He had the head of a bald eagle. This bird dived so close to the boat I actually thought he was going to hit us. Every time he dove he came up with a fish in his mouth, made a loud laughing sound, and flew off. I remarked to Bo that this bird in particular with his bald head reminded me of Duffy since he had become bald in his later years. The bird continued to circle the boat so I yelled out that if it was Duffy then he should land on the boat and prove it to us all. To say we were amazed when the bird did precisely that is an understatement. When I approached the bird he stayed perfectly still as I asked out loud if he was Duffy. The bird answered back with a guttural cry as I moved closer. I climbed up to the tip of the bowsprit and stuck out my arm. The bird jumped onto my arm and sat there as if he had been my pet for life. He even did tricks to entertain the crew. I left the bird sitting on the top of the wheelhouse and went down below to get another camera to record this incredible visit. When I returned, the crew said that as soon as I left the bird flew away. I know you must be thinking that the only reason a bird would land on a boat twenty miles out to sea is if it is injured or very tired. When I returned to the deck I only had to whistle and the bird returned. I repeated the feat once again, all to be captured on video.

For those of you who would like a copy of some of the stunts I have performed, the flight into the eclipse and the phenomenal footage of the encounter with the booby, please feel free to contact me at john@thorpinstitute.com where you can purchase the DVD copy for $14.95. I have always said when your own truth sounds like bullshit to you it is a good thing we have video cameras.

On the way to Acapulco we were boarded several times by the Mexican Navy. They were suspicious of seeing a large boat with what looked like a bunch of surfers aboard. In their minds, we were obviously drug smugglers on our way to Peru to pick up a load of cocaine.

We motored in to a small village to get some supplies and a few beers. As we were setting the anchor we were approached by a boat full of local fisherman asking if we wanted to buy some fish or shrimp. When we declined their offer they countered with, "well how about some mota," the

Mexican term for marijuana. Bo and I thought we would buy just a little, and if we were approached by the Mexican Navy we would simply throw the small amount overboard. The question now was which one of us would go with these shady characters to get a little $10.00 bag of weed. I was the designated one and went ashore with the fisherman and waited on the beach until they brought back the little bag of bud. I returned to the boat and we all shared in the smoking of the herb and had a wonderful dinner at sunset.

The following morning we were approached by another small fishing boat warning us that the Mexican Navy was going to board our boat since they supposedly had photographed me making the $10.00 weed purchase. We threw the remaining pot overboard, pulled up anchor, and headed for Acapulco. Our arrival in Acapulco was uneventful other than that we toasted shots of tequila at a five star restaurant overlooking the governor's bay where the Antares sat peacefully anchored. We spent a week at the Acapulco Yacht Club living it up in the plush environment with hot showers and a great restaurant and pool.

I had accomplished everything I wanted to do and felt the time had come for me to return home to generate some income, since the only way I was supporting myself these days was through sales and trainings for the use of the Electro Acuscope and Myopulse. I had a training scheduled, so I flew out of Acapulco the following day.

Once I arrived home from the trip I began hearing bizarre stories from my trusted friend, Brian. Bo had told him that the Mexican Federales had boarded the boat shortly after I left and showed Bo pictures of me making the $10.00 pot deal. Apparently, they wanted me for questioning. I received several e-mails from Brian letting me know that Bo was trying to discredit my involvement in my co-ownership in the boat, as well as our signed agreement regarding the future treasure wreck operations. He further stated to Brian that I had jeopardized the entire mission and that the Mexican Navy could have confiscated the boat due to my indiscretions.

The e-mails continued from Brian and once again I felt the double mule kick to my stomach as the friend I believed in was truly going to come through as John Allen predicted and sail away with the boat and my dreams.

Still in my heart of hearts I wanted to believe that this was not the Bo I knew for 25 years and had trusted my life with time and time again. I remembered Rudyards verse, "Trust all men but none too much."

Kim asked me to be kind in this final chapter on Bo. She told me how she has forgiven Bo for his lack of support and more importantly his lack of presence in their daughters life. This was his choice not Kim's as he led his family to believe. All of these unresolved issues burned in our stomachs for a final closure to Bo's incredible life.

On July 8, 2010, I received a call from Kim asking if I had heard what had happened to Zech and Bo. She said she knew that I had loved Bo like a brother but that something terrible had happened. On June 29, 2010, the Antares was anchored in Panama in front of Bajo Pipon when five individuals boarded the ship around midnight. They attacked Bo, who was on deck, shooting him and striking an artery in his leg which resulted in his death.

Bo's son, Zechariah, and Zechariah's 6 ½ month pregnant wife, Sujey, were below deck. Zechariah must have heard something and came up to find his father shot and under attack by two individuals. Zech attacked the two individuals, inflicting injury on both of them, and was then shot by one of the other three individuals who he didn't know was on board.

Sujey was also attacked and beaten up about the face. The individuals put an anchor around Zech's shoulders. Sujey heard one of them ask what they were going to do with Zech, and they said they were going to dump him overboard.

She heard one of them ask what they were going to do with the girl and they said to leave her. For some reason one of them said to leave Zech too and it was better that they leave. They took a laptop and some other items, but nothing of real value to justify the extreme action of murder.

Ironically, a week prior to Bo's death he had called Kim and told her that he finally had a group of investors who were going to sponsor him to return to the wrecks in South Africa. He asked Kim to ask Kassandra if she wanted to have him in her life once again. He wanted to make up for all the lost time. Kassandra agreed to speak with her father once again. Bo also told Kim that this would be his way of showing the world and everyone who had invested in him that he truly was who he said he was. He told Kim that he was going to make things right among all those who had believed in him. To this day she loved him dearly, as she sobbed to me over the phone.

As I sit here shocked by the finality of these final few paragraphs I can only feel blessed that my guardian angels have been watching over me as I dodged another bullet. Had my life not changed dramatically in meeting my beautiful wife and becoming a father of two of the most incredible little girls, it could have been me down there once again at the wrong place and the wrong time with a world class story teller. By all means this has been the most difficult part of the book to write. In my heart of hearts I wish this book ended in finding the treasure and Bo becoming the father, partner, and friend he was capable of being. To dream and not make dreams your master—this is one dream that in reality became the final nightmare.

For Kim and me Bo took to the grave any answers he had that could have resolved the issues we hold so deeply in our hearts. He really didn't have a malicious bone in him, although I can't step away from the fact that his first thoughts were always about himself and his needs. His family came second, and maybe that is all he knew. I have always said remember to always put your oxygen mask on first, before you try to help someone else. Bo had put his oxygen mask on me and saved my life. Unfortunately for Bo, his son tried to save him, but Bo's life was done. I forgive you and release you my brother. May God bless your soul Bo Kajer Olsen.

THE END

Aloha Nui Loa,
John Stuart Thorp

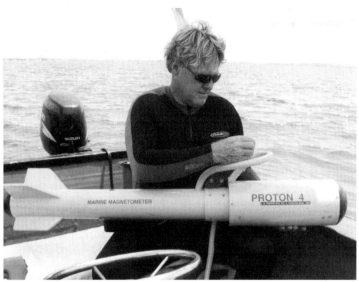

In memory of Bo Kajer Olsen
Born June 1, 1949
Murdered June 29 2010

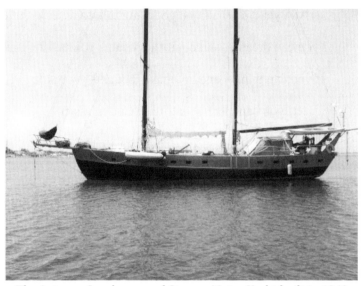

The Antares: Sparkman and Stevens Motor Yacht built in 1949.
A shattered dream. In memory of Bo Kajer Olsen

"IF"

By

RUDYARD KIPLING*

If you can keep your head when all about you

Are losing theirs and blaming it on you;

If you can trust yourself when all men doubt you,

But make allowance for their doubting too,

If you can wait and not be tired by waiting,

Or being lied about, don't deal in lies,

Or, being hated, don't give way to hating,

And yet don't look too good, nor talk to wise;

If you can dream—and not make dreams your master,

If you can think—and not make thoughts your aim;

If you can meet with triumph and disaster

And treat those two impostors just the same,

If you can bear to hear the truth you've spoken

Twisted by knaves to make a trap for fools,

Or watch the things you gave your life to, broken,

And stoop and build'em up with worn out tools,

If you can make one heap of all your winnings

And risk it on one turn of pitch-and-toss,

And lose, and start again at your beginnings

And never breathe a word about your loss,

If you can force your heart and nerve and sinew

To serve your turn long after they are gone,

And so hold on when there is nothing in you

Except the Will, which says to them:

"Hold on",

If you can talk with crowds and keep your virtue,

Or walk with Kings—nor lose the common touch.

If neither foes nor loving friends can hurt you,

If all men count with you, but none too much,

If you can fill the unforgiving minute with sixty-seconds'

worth of distance run—

Yours is the Earth and everything that's in it,

And—which is more—you'll be a man my son

*Written for his son

FDA Disclaimer

The statements made in this book have not been evaluated by the FDA (U.S. Food & Drug Administration). Our instruments are not intended to diagnose, cure, or prevent any disease.

If a condition persists, please contact your physician. The information provided by this book or this company is not a substitute for a face-to-face consultation with your physician, and should not be construed as individual medical advice. The testimonials in this book are individual cases and do not guarantee that you will get the same results.